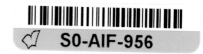

Implementing Differentiated Nursing Practice

Transformation by Design

JoEllen Goertz Koerner, RN, PhD, FAAN
Vice President Patient Services
Sioux Valley Hospital
Sioux Falls, South Dakota

Kathryn Linda Karpiuk, RN, BSN, MNE
Project Coordinator, Nursing
Sioux Valley Hospital
Sioux Falls, South Dakota

AN ASPEN PUBLICATION®
Aspen Publishers, Inc.
Gaithersburg, Maryland
1994

Library of Congress Cataloging-in-Publication Data

Koerner, JoEllen Goertz.
Implementing differentiated nursing practice : transformation by design /
Joellen Goertz Koerner, Kathryn Linda Karpiuk.
p. cm.
Includes bibliographical references and index.
ISBN 0-8342-0569-6
1. Differentiated nursing practice. 2. Differentiated nursing
practice—United States—Case studies. 3. Sioux Valley Hospital
(Sioux Falls, S.D.)—Case studies. I. Karpiuk, Kathryn.
II. Title.
RT89.3.K64 1994
362.1'73—dc 20
93-34421
CIP

Editorial Resources: Lenda Hill

Library of Congress Catalog Card Number: 93-34421
ISBN: 0-8342-0569-6

Printed in the United States of America

1 2 3 4 5

Cover design adapted from logo with permission from the
South Dakota Nurses Association, Sioux Falls.

Table of Contents

Contributors ix

Preface xiii

Acknowledgments xv

Chapter 1   **Context** 1
Rebecca J. Nelson and JoEllen Goertz Koerner

Evolution of Differentiated Practice 2
The External Environment 3
The Internal Environment 5
Differentiated Practice: The Concept 10
Differentiated Roles and Responsibilities 10
Principles of Large Scale Organizational Change 13
Exercise 1–1: Discussion Questions 18
Appendix 1-A: Sioux Valley Hospital Nursing Timeline
    1981–1993 19

Chapter 2   **Culture** 22
Narcy Recker, Kathryn Linda Karpiuk, Elizabeth Hindbjorgen,
*   and JoEllen Goertz Koerner*

Competence 26
Adaptability to Change 28
Decision Making 30
Diversity 31

Communication 33
Risk Taking 37
Summary 38
Formula for Cultural Identification 41
Formula for Change 41
Formula for Professional Growth 42
Appendix 2-A: Integrated Care Committee
    Ground Rules 43

Chapter 3   **Consensus** **46**
Narcy Recker, Kathryn Linda Karpiuk, JoEllen Goertz Koerner,
    and Kaleen B. Santema

What Is Consensus? 46
Building a Group Based on the Consensus Model 47
Roles for a Consensus Group 57
Blocking in Decision Making 60
Pitfalls and Common Problems 61
Exercise 3–1: Group Activity—Reflections 64
Exercise 3–2: Group Activity—Dyadic Risk Taking 64
Exercise 3–3: Group Activity—Most Precious
    Possession 64
Appendix 3-A: Sioux Valley Hospital Staffing/
    Scheduling Committee Group Norms, November 1992–
    November 1993 66

Chapter 4   **Choice** **69**
Kathryn Linda Karpiuk and Chris Nicolai

The Power of Choice 70
Carpe Diem 71
The Gentle Art of Choosing 73
A Lesson from Psyche: A Metaphor 74
Levels of Choice 77
Gender Issues and Choice 78
Pitfalls to Avoid When Making Choices 80
Personal Decision Points 81
Organizational Decision Points 82
Career Decision Points 84
Selection Process 86
Professional Activities 87
Conclusion 89
Exercise 4–1: Individual Exercises 93

Exercise 4–2: Organizational Exercises 93
Appendix 4-A: Sioux Valley Hospital Department of
    Nursing Job Description: Registered Nurse in the
    Associate Role 94
Appendix 4-B: Sioux Valley Hospital Department of
    Nursing Job Description: Registered Nurse in the
    Primary Role 97
Appendix 4-C: Sioux Valley Hospital Department of
    Nursing Job Description: Registered Nurse in the
    Clinical Care Coordinator Role 100
Appendix 4-D: Sioux Valley Hospital Department of
    Nursing Job Description: Director of _____
    Care Services 103
Appendix 4-E: Sioux Valley Hospital Department of
    Nursing Job Description: Clinical Nurse Specialist 105
Appendix 4-F: Role Choice Tool 108
Appendix 4-G: Administrative Standard for Operating
    Procedure for Registered Nurse Incentive Plan for
    Preceptoring 111
Appendix 4-H: Sioux Valley Hospital Department of
    Nursing Job Description Standards: Registered Nurse
    in the Associate Role 114
Appendix 4-I: Sioux Valley Hospital Department of
    Nursing Job Description Standards: Registered Nurse
    in the Primary Role 119
Appendix 4-J: Sioux Valley Hospital Department of
    Nursing Job Description Standards: Registered Nurse
    in the Clinical Care Coordinator Role 124

Chapter 5   **Continuity** **129**
Pamela A. Koepsell, Rhonda Jensen, Joan T. Reisdorfer,
Cindi Slack, Sandy Young, Anthony Weber, Tricia Fjerestad,
S. Jo Gibson, and Nancy J. Paulson

Definition 129
Communication 130
Collaboration 130
Collegiality 131
Accountability 132
Consultation 134
Case Management 134
Integrated Care 135

Benefits of Integrated Care 136
Operationalization of Integrated Care 139
Communication Tools 158
The Future 166
Conclusion 170
Exercise 5–1: Formulas for Implementing
    Integrated Care 172
Exercise 5–2: Steps to Complete a Financial Analysis 172
Appendix 5-A: Sioux Valley Hospital Perception of
    Nursing Care Questionnaire: Physician 174
Appendix 5-B: Perinatal Database 176
Appendix 5-C: Admission Database 180
Appendix 5-D: Sample Integrated Clinical Pathway 182
Appendix 5-E: Sioux Valley Hospital Exceptions to
    Clinical Pathway Codes 185

Chapter 6   Consultation 188
Rebecca Johnson Blue, Linda Birch Bunkers, Carol McGinnis,
*   Lois J. McMahon, and Phyllis Newstrom*

The Process of Knowing 188
Consultation at Work: Case Studies 192
Team Building through Consultation 192
The Art of Showing 198
Consultation and Empowerment 199
The Evolution of Successful Consultation 201
Theory-Based Consultation 204
Overcoming Ambiguity 206
The Transformation of Consultation to Collaboration 209
Exercise 6–1: Consultation Exercises 212

Chapter 7   Community 214
Connie K. Schmidt, Diana Berkland, and Doreen S. Miller

Systems Theory 217
Input 218
Change Theory 224
Output 230
Feedback 232
The Future 233
Conclusion 235
Exercise 7–1: Community Building Exercises 236

Chapter 8   **Corporate** **238**
Cindi Slack, Judith K. Crane, Vicki J. Tigner, and
*   Richard M. Jones*

Corporate Culture 241
Structure 243
Action Council 248
Communication 249
Controlling Health Care Costs 254
Exercise 8–1: Pulse Exercise 264
Appendix 8-A: Sioux Valley Hospital Dakota EDGE
    (Employees Delivering Grassroots Excellence)
    Action Council Bylaws 265
Appendix 8-B: DRG 410: Chemotherapy Administration
    Option 1 272
Appendix 8-C: DRG 410: Chemotherapy Administration
    Option 2 273
Appendix 8-D: DRG 410: Chemotherapy Administration
    Option 3 274
Appendix 8-E: DRG 410: Chemotherapy Administration
    Option 4 275
Appendix 8-F: DRG 410: Chemotherapy Administration
    Option 5 277
Appendix 8-G: DRG 410: Chemotherapy Administration
    Option 6 279
Appendix 8-H: Continuous Fiscal Improvement Report:
    Ongoing Monitoring and Evaluation Monitoring
    Tool 281
Appendix 8-I: Continuous Fiscal Improvement:
    Ongoing Monitoring and Evaluation Standards 283
Appendix 8-J: Aspects of Financial Management 285

Chapter 9   **Compensation** **290**
Eloise Baker, Shari Aman, Roxanne Dietz, and Doreen S. Miller

Systems Theory 291
Creating the Vision 293
Beneficiaries: Patient and Family 294
Beneficiary: The Nurse 296
Beneficiary: The Physician 298
Beneficiary: The Organization 299
Beneficiary: The Regional Community 301
Exercise 9–1: Compensation Evaluation 305

Chapter 10   Celebration **306**
Renee Schulz, Elizabeth Hindbjorgen, Carol McGinnis, E.J. Reid, and Georgia A. Stern

The Need to Celebrate 306
The Power of Celebration 310
Education as Celebration.. 313
Timing 314
Reflections 316
Exercise 10–1: Celebrate.. 319
Exercise 10–2: Celebration Word Search 320

List of Sources **321**

Index **325**

Contributors

Editors

JoEllen Goertz Koerner, RN, PhD, FAAN
Vice President, Patient Services
Sioux Valley Hospital
Administration
Sioux Falls, South Dakota

Kathryn Linda Karpiuk, RN, BSN, MNE
Project Coordinator, Nursing
Sioux Valley Hospital
Nursing Center
Sioux Falls, South Dakota

Contributors

Shari Aman, RN, BSN
Primary Nurse
Sioux Valley Hospital
Medical/Surgical Intensive Care Unit
Sioux Falls, South Dakota

Eloise Baker, RN, BA
Director, Coronary Intensive Care/
   Outpatient Cardiac Recovery
Sioux Valley Hospital
Coronary Intensive Care Services
Sioux Falls, South Dakota

Diana Berkland, RN, BS, MS cand, CCRN
Sioux Valley Hospital
Department of Patient Services
Sioux Falls, South Dakota

Rebecca Johnson Blue, RN, BA, MS
Director, Geriatric Health Institute
Clinical Nurse Specialist
Sioux Valley Hospital
Geriatric Health Institute
Sioux Falls, South Dakota

Linda Birch Bunkers, RN, BSN, MEd
Nursing Administration, Education,
   Research, and Development
Sioux Valley Hospital
Nursing Administration
Sioux Falls, South Dakota

Judith K. Crane, RN, BS, MS
Deputy Public Health Director
City of Sioux Falls
Health Department
Sioux Falls, South Dakota

Roxanne Dietz, RN, BA
Unit Educator
Sioux Valley Hospital
Perinatal/Gynecology Services
Sioux Falls, South Dakota

Tricia Fjerestad, RN, BA
Primary Nurse
Sioux Valley Hospital
Surgical Care Services
Sioux Falls, South Dakota

S. Jo Gibson, RN, MS, CCRN
Clinical Nurse Specialist
Director, Center for Case Management
Sioux Valley Hospital
Center for Case Management
Sioux Falls, South Dakota

Elizabeth Hindbjorgen, RN, BA
Educator, Women's and Children's Health
   Care Services
Sioux Valley Hospital
Nursing Center
Sioux Falls, South Dakota

Rhonda Jensen, RN, BS, MS
Clinical Nurse Specialist—Diabetes
   Program
Sioux Valley Hospital
Department of Patient Services
Sioux Falls, South Dakota

Richard M. Jones, RN, BS, MS
Nursing Administrator, Adult Specialty
   Care Services
Sioux Valley Hospital
Nursing Administration
Sioux Falls, South Dakota

Pamela A. Koepsell, RN, BSN
Clinical Care Coordinator
Primary Nurse
Sioux Valley Hospital
Neonatal Intensive Care Unit
Sioux Falls, South Dakota

**Carol McGinnis, RN, BAN, MS cand,
   CNSN**
Nutrition/Metabolic Nurse Clinician
Sioux Valley Hospital
Nursing Center
Sioux Falls, South Dakota

Lois J. McMahon, RN, BS, MS
Nurse Educator
Clinical Nurse Specialist
Sioux Valley Hospital
Nursing Center
Sioux Falls, South Dakota

Doreen S. Miller, RN, BA, MS
Clinical Nurse Specialist
Sioux Valley Hospital
Geriatric Health Institute
Sioux Falls, South Dakota

Rebecca J. Nelson, RN, MS
Nursing Administrator, Critical Care
   Services
Sioux Valley Hospital
Nursing Administration
Sioux Falls, South Dakota

Phyllis Newstrom, RN, BSN, MN
Director, Education Services
Sioux Valley Hospital
Nursing Center
Sioux Falls, South Dakota

Chris Nicolai, RN, BA, MS
Clinical Nurse Specialist
Sioux Valley Hospital
Department of Patient Services
Sioux Falls, South Dakota

Nancy J. Paulson, RN
Primary Nurse
Sioux Valley Hospital
Perinatal/Gynecology Services
Sioux Falls, South Dakota

Narcy Recker, RN, BA, BSN, MA
Critical Care Orientation Coordinator
Sioux Valley Hospital
Nursing Center—Staff Education
Sioux Falls, South Dakota

E.J. Reid, RN, BSN
Director, Neonatal Intensive Care Unit
Sioux Valley Hospital
Neonatal Intensive Care Unit
Sioux Falls, South Dakota

Joan T. Reisdorfer, RN,C, BA, MS
Director, Medical/Urology/Diabetes Care
  Services
Sioux Valley Hospital
Medical/Urology/Diabetes Care Services
Sioux Falls, South Dakota

Kaleen B. Santema, RN
Nursing Administrator, Women's and
  Children's Health Care Services
Sioux Valley Hospital
Nursing Administration
Sioux Falls, South Dakota

Connie K. Schmidt, RN, BS, MS cand
Critical Care Outreach Coordinator
Sioux Valley Hospital
Nursing Center
Sioux Falls, South Dakota

Renee Schulz, RN, BS, MS
Nurse Educator
Adult Specialty Care Services Coordinator
Sioux Valley Hospital
Nursing Center
Sioux Falls, South Dakota

Cindi Slack, RN, BS, MBA
Administrative Director, Home Health,
  Hospice
Sioux Valley Hospital
Executive Officer, Midwestern Health
  Services
Sioux Falls, South Dakota

Georgia A. Stern, RN
Director, Perinatal and Gynecology
  Services
Sioux Valley Hospital
Perinatal and Gynecology Services
Sioux Falls, South Dakota

Vicki J. Tigner, RN
Director, Neurology and Cardiology Care
  Services
Sioux Valley Hospital
Neurology and Cardiology Care Services
Sioux Falls, South Dakota

Anthony Weber, RN, BSN
Nurse Case Manager
Sioux Valley Hospital
Rehabilitation
Sioux Falls, South Dakota

Sandy Young, RN, MS
Clinical Nurse Specialist, Hospice
Sioux Valley Hospital
Hospice
Sioux Falls, South Dakota

Preface

*It is good to have an end to journey towards; but it
is the journey that matters, in the end.*

URSELA K. LEGUIN

Although each chapter of this book can stand alone, the book is meant to be read
in its entirety. Each chapter builds on the previous chapters, creating a picture of a
nursing care delivery model that has been transformed. There was deliberate intent
to change the care delivery system with the introduction of differentiated practice.
The outcome was unknown, however.

Each chapter incorporates some theoretical information as well as the practical
information we believe readers will find useful. There are exercises at the end of
each chapter to assist nurses to internalize the chapter's concepts. They are intended
to be fun as well as a learning experience. Chapters also have several appendices
with additional practical information.

Chapter 1 describes the environment both internal and external to Sioux Valley
Hospital. The context in which the transformation took place is different from that
of any other health care facility, although there are similarities. Changes can
sometimes be made more easily when the timing is right. The circumstances whence
we came and the present environment are outlined.

Chapter 2 goes into further detail about the internal environment with a discussion about the culture of the nursing department. Each organization and, indeed,
each patient care unit have their own unique culture. The norms and values differ,
just as the norms and values of families differ. These values are threads that run
throughout the rest of the book.

The next two chapters expand on two norms of the Sioux Valley Hospital nursing
department: consensus and choice. How to make decisions by consensus and some

examples of consensus building, including two case studies, are presented. Choice is an integral part of American society and the nursing department's culture. Myth is used to help explain the theory. Choices provided to staff in the differentiated practice delivery system are described.

Chapter 5, "Continuity," is the cornerstone of differentiated practice. Continuity of patient care in today's complex health care environment is realized with differentiated practice. This chapter is the longest because it is the essence of Integrated Care. It has several case studies to enhance the reader's understanding of the differentiated roles.

Chapter 6 is more futuristic, containing a description of the beginnings of consultation and its benefits. Consultation has not been part of the traditional nursing culture and is difficult for most nurses to adopt. Although consultation occurs among all registered nurses, there is particular emphasis in this chapter on the advanced practice role. Because this role is increasingly important at Sioux Valley Hospital, most of the case studies in this chapter are devoted to examples of nurses in the advanced practice role.

The seventh chapter expands on our unique nursing environment with a summary of systems theory and shared governance frameworks. A description of the shared governance structure and communication pattern at Sioux Valley Hospital follows.

Centralized and decentralized corporate affairs are explained in the next chapter. The Ecology of Excellence philosophy, although mentioned throughout the book, is expounded in this chapter.

The rewards and benefits of differentiated practice are delineated in Chapter 9. Although there may be references to the many rewards in other chapters, the authors of this chapter clearly summarize them here.

The last chapter describes the importance of celebration. The reader is presented with numerous ideas of how to celebrate a change in care delivery, or anything else pertaining to the profession. This book is the ultimate celebration for our nursing practice.

There continue to be changes in the model implemented at Sioux Valley Hospital. Nothing ever stays the same for long. But then, health care and the world are forever changing, too.

Enjoy reading this book. It was written with joy.

—JoEllen Goertz Koerner and Kathryn Linda Karpiuk
Editors

Acknowledgments

More than any other book, this one could not have been written without the inspiration and support of many remarkable nursing leaders who showed this practice a new way of being. We would like to express our deep gratitude to these visionary individuals, whose profound contributions reshaped our lives:

- Mary Fuller was the first nurse administrator at Sioux Valley Hospital to move nursing leadership to the executive level at the corporate table.
- Dr Peggy Primm and the Midwest Alliance in Nursing helped us see and value the diversity inherent in associate and baccalaureate nursing education.
- Dr Margaret Newman provided the profession with a theory of health on which we based our practice model.
- Dr Dorothy del Bueno gave us a working definition of competency-based practice along with the political savvy so essential in a professional model of practice.
- Dr Frank Steiner gave us a sense of business acumen along with tools and techniques to develop high-performance teams.
- Dr Tim Porter-O'Grady articulated a vision for shared governance that empowered the nursing practice to embrace its autonomy, initiative, and accountability.

> *If I can see further, it is because I have stood on the shoulders of giants.*
> OLIVER WENDELL HOLMES, SR

Others also contributed to this book in various ways. The following nurses contributed ideas that have been incorporated into the chapters: Teresa Buell, Sheryl Oliver, Mary Selland, and Patty Vaska.

Several secretaries typed various portions of the book. The greatest portion was assumed by Keila Smith. Chapters were also typed by Pat Miller and Kathy Nelson. Lynda Selle produced many of the figures. Dianne Clary, Kathy Nelson, and Crystal Wolfe also assisted with preparation of the figures.

Invaluable assistance with finding library resources was provided by Anna Gieschen, Lenora Bezpaletz, and Deborah Taylor.

Contributions from family members were also greatly appreciated. Dennis Koerner and Dempster S. Christenson were extremely supportive throughout this time-consuming project. Katya and Dempster M. Christenson were also very understanding.

1 Context

*Rebecca J. Nelson and
JoEllen Goertz Koerner*

Drive thy Business, let not that drive thee.
BENJAMIN FRANKLIN

The health care industry is under siege; changing reimbursement patterns present the industry with dwindling human and material resources to provide comprehensive services. Concurrently, patients seeking health care are more acutely ill, expecting more technologic and specialized services that are human and material resource intensive.[1] This scenario is playing out in an environment of outrage at rising prices and lack of access to comprehensive, coordinated services across the continuum of care. The dynamic disequilibrium that is manifest within this chaotic health care scene marks the end of an era.

Economic concerns dominate health care planning and policy decisions as providers seek to become more productive, competitive, and profitable. Professional concerns regarding quality of care and public service often conflict with the profit-motivated business model. Hospitals have duties of citizenship to a larger society and a moral commitment to a broader constituency of publics than stockholders and trustees,[2] creating a moral dilemma for health care providers in choosing among alternative actions.

As corporate representatives of clinical practice, nurse executives are morally obligated to recognize the rights of patients. As employees of health care institutions, they must also uphold the utilitarian and survival goals of the institution. When hospital goals and nursing goals conflict, nurse executives must engage in moral reasoning that is based on professional values and principles that are separate from institutional norms and authority.[3] Nurse executives have a unique opportunity to introduce a professional philosophy into the corporate business model that reflects professional values, capitalizes on professional expertise, and enables the hospital to become more adaptive, productive, and competitive. A professional-based care delivery model emphasizes quality care that serves a diverse public's need. Investment in people through a shared decision-making process leads to long-term economic survival that transcends doing well financially in the short term.

An integrative organizational model, which combines business and professional ethics, professionalizes the hospital corporation. Nursing administration expedites the reframing of its structural dimensions to involve professionals in decision making, to give them greater discretion in their work roles, and to allow more flexibility in the allocation of resources. Broad and empathic decisions are made about the basic mission for the enterprise and its guiding principles for behavior. Human resources are recognized as the corporation's competitive edge, the major source of knowledge, information, and creativity. Nurse executives assist in blending economic and ethical concerns in selecting target populations to serve. Furthermore, research and education along with clinical care are woven into all programs designed for public service.

Effective nurse executives must respond to the restructuring challenge by designing care delivery systems that are bureaucracy smashers. They must create innovative social structures in which persons from different disciplines work together to achieve common goals, replacing the industrial "us versus them" with the concepts of collaboration, partnership, and working together.[4]

According to Porter-O'Grady, "Nursing has long been positioned in dependent employee roles."[5(p286)] Major organizational transformation must occur to draw fully on the creativity, problem-solving capabilities, and special skills of professional nurses. This reform must occur on two levels. The external world of corporate nursing practice must be changed through professionalizing the organization, revising traditional bureaucratic structures and practices, introducing the concept of self-management to humanize the work environment, and providing performance incentives. The internal world of professional nursing must undergo a similar transformation by differentiating the roles and responsibilities of practitioners within the discipline. The focus must be directed toward the enhancement of collegial relationships in which nurses assume different roles but remain professional peers.

> *The history of free (wo)men is never written by*
> *chance—but by choice—their choice.*
>   PRESIDENT DWIGHT D. EISENHOWER

EVOLUTION OF DIFFERENTIATED PRACTICE

A sense of crisis has erupted in the nursing profession. The scope of nursing practice is enlarging as a result of rising patient acuity and fragmentation within the health care industry. Rapid organizational diversification and expansion reflect efforts to adapt to the dynamically changing health care environment. Intensifying physician subspecialization increases costs while decreasing productivity as well as enlarging human resource needs. Furthermore, fragmentation and duplication disrupt information exchange while creating an economic imbalance. Nursing is being called upon to assume broader responsibility in integrating the allocation of human, fiscal, and material resources for improved patient care. As nurses' role in primary care increases, so must their role in clinical care management.

Differentiated practice had its formal origins in World War II, when a shortage of nurses in civilian hospitals led to the creation of assistive roles, namely licensed practical nurses (LPNs) and nursing assistants. Once the war was over and the need for nurses did not abate, these position titles were institutionalized. Throughout the remainder of the 20th century, the education and utilization of these two distinct assistive levels have gradually become more formal and codified. Over the past 10 years, what is new in the dialogue around differentiated practice is the focus on the professional roles of registered nurses (RNs) rather than on the assistive roles.

Historically, RNs with different levels of education have been used interchangeably in most health care settings in one role category: nurse. Nursing practice is not systematically differentiated by education, prior experience, and/or additional contribution to the practice. Without formal recognition or increased compensation, the expert nurse is informally relied upon by patients, physicians, other nurses, and hospital management to a greater degree than the novice.

If nursing is to be viewed as a preferred career choice and if agencies are to retain expert staff, a nursing care delivery model that differentiates scope of job responsibility based on education, experience, and competence must be developed along with differing compensation packages. This will be an evolutionary step in the development of professional nursing that also maximizes cost and quality outcomes for clients and health care organizations.

THE EXTERNAL ENVIRONMENT

The American Nurses' Association began setting the national stage for differentiated practice with their 1965 position statement on entry into practice.[6] It called for two distinct levels of registered nursing based on educational preparation and the resulting competencies acquired. Several years ago the National Commission on Nursing Implementation Project (NCNIP) thoughtfully examined the issue of differentiated practice and created a time frame in which to reach this goal.[7,8]

In 1990 the American Academy of Nursing, in collaboration with the American Nurses' Association and the American Organization of Nurse Executives, convened a conference entitled Differentiating Nursing Practice: Into the Twenty-First Century.[9] This gathering examined the concept of differentiated practice in the current health care crisis. Furthermore, various models of differentiation in the hospital setting and community were explored, and cost and quality outcomes were identified. Finally, the implications of differentiated practice for education and research were also addressed. Shared information provided ideas, new questions, and challenges for nursing to pursue as we plan how the profession will contribute to the public welfare during the next century.

It is important to know the demographics of South Dakota to understand the environment around the nursing practice at Sioux Valley Hospital. Sioux Falls is a city of approximately 100,000 people in a state that has only 686,000 people. It is the largest city in the state and lies in the far southeastern corner, bordering Minnesota and Iowa. The hospital provides tertiary health care to all of South Dakota and the north- and southwestern parts of Iowa and Minnesota respectively. Of the 57 hospitals in the state, there are only 3 larger than 150 beds; 47 hospitals have 30 beds or fewer. The second largest hospital in the state is located in Sioux Falls and is the direct competition of Sioux Valley Hospital (Figure 1–1).

South Dakota is a sparsely populated, rural state with a homogeneous population. Whites represent 91.6% of the entire population; 7.3% of the population are native American, and less than 1% are Asian. Unlike the situation in other large tertiary hospitals, this lack of diversity adds a unique dynamic to the health care system.

On a statewide level, in 1988 a nursing shortage prompted the governor to propose the opening of six LPN schools in response to the lack of qualified nursing personnel. The nursing community had organized the Statewide Project for Nursing and Nursing Education, however, utilizing the differentiated competencies created by the Midwest Alliance in Nursing (MAIN) under the leadership of Dr Peggy Primm.[10] Armed with only a commitment to offer an alternative solution to the LPN

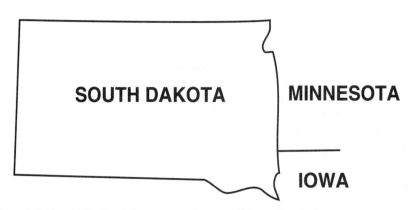

Figure 1–1 Sioux Valley Hospital service area. Courtesy of Sioux Valley Hospital, Sioux Falls, South Dakota.

proposal, the demonstration project tested two roles of RNs in four regional centers. These comprised large and small hospitals, long-term care facilities, and home health agencies.[11] The outcome of that work generated $800,000 from the legislature to open one LPN school and to provide strong funding for associate (ADN) and baccalaureate (BSN) education. Thus the work of restructuring professional nursing began at Sioux Valley Hospital.[12]

THE INTERNAL ENVIRONMENT

In the mid-1980s the nursing service at Sioux Valley was a traditional practice operating in a 511-bed tertiary care hospital. It consisted of three nursing divisions: medical-surgical, critical care, and maternal-child health.

The medical-surgical division consisted of six units housing 256 adult patients. Two of these were 72-bed units; the remaining four were smaller but contained a group of patients requiring more specialized nursing, such as pulmonology, oncology, and neurology patients. More than one third of the 1000-plus nursing staff worked in this division under a clinical nursing director.

The only open heart surgery program in South Dakota began at Sioux Valley Hospital in 1978. This active program of 650 surgeries and 1200 catheterizations per year largely drove the activity of the critical care division. This division consisted of three intensive care units for a total of 39 beds, 48 telemetry beds, the emergency department, and the 80-patient dialysis program. As with each division, a clinical nursing director was responsible for the division and reported to the vice-president of patient services (Figure 1–2).

The maternal-child health division was well known for its sophisticated practice of caring for high-risk maternal, neonatal, and pediatric patients. The only level III neonatal intensive care unit in the state has held up to 50 infants. This maternal-child health nursing practice was a leader in the development of differentiated practice because, during the project year, it was this group that took most of the risk in the role of demonstration units. It was one of the first nursing practices at Sioux Valley Hospital that worked closely with the medical subspecialists and knew the medical model well.

Each unit in the department had a manager called a head nurse. The rest of the unit structure varied somewhat among units but mainly consisted of head nurses, assistant head nurses, clinicians, discharge planners, charge nurses, and staff nurses (Figure 1–3). Twenty-four hours a day, 7 days a week, each division had a nursing supervisor who managed complex bed control issues and patient placement problems. During off shifts and weekends, this supervisor acted as the administrative agent for the hospital system.

The composition of the nursing practice included RNs with ADN, diploma, or BSN educational backgrounds. In January 1990, the LPN role was eliminated.

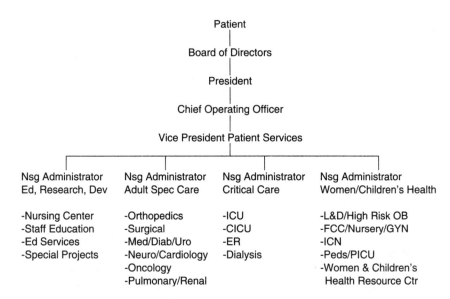

Figure 1–2 Department of Patient Services organizational chart. Courtesy of Sioux Valley Hospital, Sioux Falls, South Dakota.

Assistive staff, such as ward secretaries and nursing assistants, remained. The hospital's diploma school of nursing provided the majority of the nursing workforce until 1986, with nurses holding associate or baccalaureate degrees making up the remainder in equal parts. Master's-prepared nurses, a scarce resource, usually held positions in the school or top management.

Historical precedence was followed by utilizing RNs interchangeably in the one role category known as nurse. The attitude of "a nurse is a nurse is a nurse" describes the culture. The system of assigning patients reflected this belief in that patient loads were awarded by volume and acuity. A nurse provided all the nursing care for the patient during a shift with help from the assistive staff. RNs were required to assume accountability for some of the care provided by LPNs.

In the early 1980s, during a nursing shortage, many creative strategies were implemented to recruit and retain nurses. At that time, there were three major concerns of nursing staff: unavailability of creative schedules; the increasing acuity of patients and workload causing tension among RNs, who were assuming responsibility for LPNs' patients along with their own; and the lack of promotional or learning potential opportunities unless the nurse left active bedside practice. The hospital responded to the first concern for scheduling requests by implementing a 3-day work week program. Unit staff worked three 12-hour shifts a week, with their weekend schedules always including Friday, Saturday, and Sunday on or off (Figure 1–4).

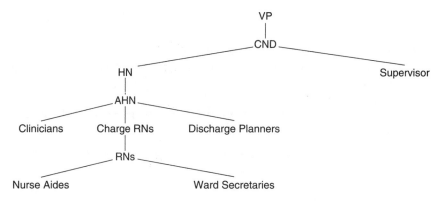

Figure 1–3 Organizational structure before differentiated practice. Courtesy of Sioux Valley Hospital, Sioux Falls, South Dakota.

Significant organizational and clinical efficiencies exist in uniformly operating two shifts a day rather than three. The impact that this program would have on continuity of care was not realized until the increasing demands for comprehensive, coordinated services across the continuum of care were experienced.

The interruption of information flow due to sporadic work shifts caused fragmentation of care and disassociation within the nursing staff. Because they were involved with the hospital only 3 days a week, staff exposure to work life was lessened, and professional socialization became secondary. A blue collar mentality predominated in the culture.

The second important professional issue was associated with the difficulties of utilizing LPNs appropriately in a highly tertiary setting with very sick patients needing significant invasive technologic care. A program of upward mobility and outplacement was established to educate LPNs to RNs. LPNs also had the option to move into technical roles already established in other services, such as cardiovascular services and surgical technician. This was designed to facilitate the elimination of the LPN role in the nursing practice at Sioux Valley Hospital over a 3-year

	Pay Period One													Pay Period Two		
Sun	Mon	Tue	Wed	Thur	Fri	Sat	Sun	Mon	Tue	Wed	Thur	Fri	Sat	Sun	Mon	Tue	Wed
X		D			D	D	D				N	N	X	X	X		D	

Figure 1–4 Sample pay period schedule. Courtesy of Sioux Valley Hospital, Sioux Falls, South Dakota.

period, leaving only one licensed role, the RN. Each person is fully accountable for his or her own practice.

The third issue was addressed with the implementation of differentiated practice. For years, nurses have voiced concern over their inability to enhance their earning potential without going into management or some nonclinical role. At the time of the project, 75 of the 700 full-time equivalent RN positions were paid more than the basic clinical I scale (Figure 1–5). This group comprised management and advanced clinical roles. By differentiating salary consistent with the differentiated roles, the

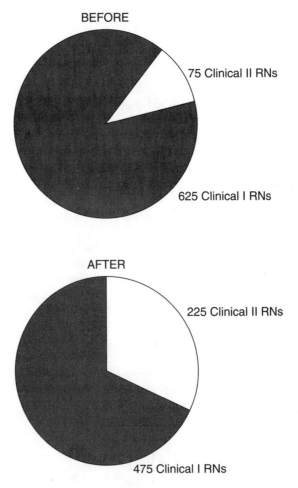

BEFORE

75 Clinical II RNs

625 Clinical I RNs

AFTER

225 Clinical II RNs

475 Clinical I RNs

Figure 1–5 RN pay scale: clinical I and clinical II. RN workforce = 700 full-time equivalents. Courtesy of Sioux Valley Hospital, Sioux Falls, South Dakota.

RN population that is paid more than the clinical I position has been increased by a third. This has increased the full earning potential for active clinical nurses by 16%. It has also changed the organizational chart for the department (Figure 1–6).

The medical staff at Sioux Valley Hospital consisted of more than 300 physicians. The hospital had grown over the last 10 years into a tertiary care medical practice. With the level III nursery, subspecialists in women's and children's medicine joined the staff. As specialization in adult medicine increased, so did specialization among the Sioux Valley Hospital medical staff. Endocrinologists and neurologists are examples of some of the specialties with which the nursing practice worked. In response to the tertiary development of the medical staff, nursing expertise evolved in the highly technologic medical model structure of the hospital. Relationships with physicians were similar to the historical superordinate-subordinate association. Although the hospital had come a long way from the handmaiden era, there still remained many barriers to increased collaboration. Even language was limited to medical terms focusing on diagnosis and treatment rather than including nursing terms that capture human responses to an illness. To begin the project, significant time and energy were needed to educate the nursing practice on nursing diagnosis and the science of nursing. It was through the process of differentiating the roles that articulation of the profession of nursing began, positioning nursing for true collaboration with physicians.

Governance of the nursing practice was executed in the traditional manner. The typical hierarchy and structure existed for management of the unit, the division, and the department. Monthly unit meetings were led by the head nurse, who shared information relating to decisions that had been made. Nursing staff reported problems, including those that were peer-to-peer issues, to the head nurse, expecting resolution. As the roles were differentiated, the skill set acquired by the primary nurses and the associates relating to them became so refined that the staff began

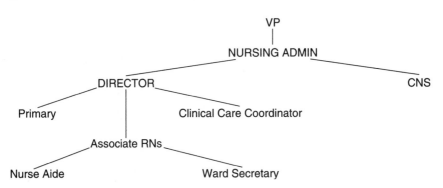

Figure 1–6 Organizational structure after differentiated practice. Courtesy of Sioux Valley Hospital, Sioux Falls, South Dakota.

applying this critical thinking and problem solving in areas other than decisions about their patients. They began to expect to have some influence on issues relating to their practice. This activity required a proactive measure by the administrative team of developing a shared governance structure to guide and facilitate this growth in the staff. Now councils govern the practice, and decisions are based on literature and research (see Chapter 7 for more on shared governance). Other significant events during the past 12 years are listed in Appendix 1-A.

DIFFERENTIATED PRACTICE: THE CONCEPT

Differentiated practice is referred to as a philosophy that focuses on the structuring of roles and functions of nurses according to education, experience, and competence.[7] It establishes that the domain of professional nursing is broad, with multiple roles and responsibilities of various degrees and complexities. It assumes that nurses with different educational preparation, expertise, and background bring different competencies to the workplace.[10] It seeks to ensure that the work of nursing is carried out by the most appropriate nurse in the most appropriate fashion. Comprehensive, cost-effective care is thus provided by the collective discipline of nursing through the integration of those services across the continuum of care into a synergistic whole.[13,14]

Differentiated practice recognizes the contribution of all nursing personnel to patient care delivery as unique and valuable. It creates an integrative web of nursing practitioners across the health care continuum (Figure 1–7). When nurses contribute to patient care delivery by assuming differentiated roles, the aggregate contribution far surpasses that which could be delivered without such differentiation. This model provides the nursing profession with a vehicle to position nurses within the expanding care delivery system in a manner that is beneficial to the health and well-being of patients as well as the health and well-being of the profession and the industry.

Various rationales exist for differentiated practice. First, if properly carried out, it can serve to improve patient care and contribute to patient safety. Second, there is the benefit to be gained from a structure that enables the most effective and efficient utilization of scarce resources. Third, there is the opportunity to provide increased satisfaction for nurses themselves because they are better able to optimize their practice. Finally, differentiated practice provides the opportunity to compensate nurses fairly based on their expertise, contribution, and productivity.

DIFFERENTIATED ROLES AND RESPONSIBILITIES

Nursing practice is based on a body of scientific knowledge (physical and social sciences), knowledge that is derived from experience (leading to expertise) and research (leading to theoretical foundations for knowledge). This base contributes

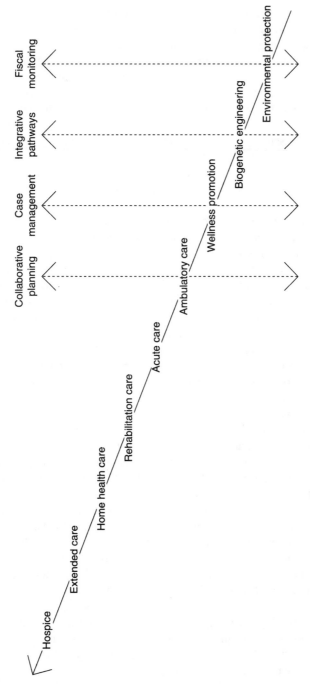

Figure 1–7 Continuum of health care services and integrating factors. Courtesy of Sioux Valley Hospital, Sioux Falls, South Dakota.

to judgment and rationale for modifying actions according to the situation through the nursing process, an essential component of professional practice. Nursing transmits this knowledge through specialized education. There are five levels of basic education for registered nursing (ADN, diploma, baccalaureate, master's, and doctorate); however, all of them prepare for one licensing examination.

The compelling study, Differentiation and Integration of Work Roles and Responsibilities conducted by Lawrence and Lorsch[15], guided the design of new roles and relationships of professional nursing at Sioux Valley Hospital. This Harvard Business School research project identified characteristics of successful organizations and individuals in environments that require differentiation of roles and integration of services. Key differentiating factors go beyond technical tasks to incorporate value variations within the different roles based on time frame, space, personal development, ethical action, interpersonal effectiveness, critical thinking, and commitment to life-long learning. Concepts from this study were combined with the MAIN competencies as well as those developed by the American Nurses' Association to create differentiated roles for professional nursing practice.

The time frame for today's RN (ADN) is based on a vertical focus of activities performed during the shift worked. The integrative function of the expanded RN role (BSN) calls for a horizontal focus from preadmission to postdischarge. This practitioner is concerned with events leading to the specific illness episode that required hospitalization as well as the needs remaining when the client is discharged from the unit of service. A strong focus on discharge planning and accountability for the resolution or referral of all nursing diagnoses represents the expanded activities of this role. The case management role of the advanced practice nurse (MSN) is expressed across the continuum of care for the entire lifespan of the client. Assisting clients with adjusting their lifestyle to a chronic illness or to a peaceful death is the primary function of this comprehensive role.

The scope of interpersonal relationships managed by the different RN categories varies. The ADN, as well as other team members on the service unit, focuses primarily on the client and family. The BSN addresses the client and family as well as members of the total health care team—pharmacy, physical therapy, and other providers—who have input into the total plan of care. The MSN addresses providers across the continuum of care—clinics, long-term care agencies, home health agencies, and acute care centers—that may provide services to clients depending on need on their journey through life with chronic or terminal illness.

Interpersonal effectiveness and capacities of leadership are guided by professional ideology and are strongly influenced by the level of personal development of the individual practitioner. Healthy interpersonal relationships foster conditions that lead to a climate of trust. Open and frank discussions increase efficiency in resolving problems. Conflict must be confronted and brought into the open rather than suppressed through power, control, or avoidance if ethical solutions to complex issues are to be reached.

The ADN resolves problems and issues arising out of the daily activities surrounding client care. The BSN uses more refined skills in confrontation, negotiation, and issue resolution on more complex issues facing a team of health care providers regarding the client. Finally, the MSN must use great political savvy and leadership initiative to negotiate conditions for the client with various health care provider groups across the continuum of care. This role is pivotal for acquiring the necessary resources and services across the continuum of care for chronically ill or dying patients as their condition changes.

Space reflects the concept of structure, which may be defined as a geographic location or a set of policies, procedures, and protocols that govern the practitioner's actions. The ADN works in a geographic environment governed by a set of established policies. This setting also has the full support of a wide range of services and providers. The BSN may work in structured or unstructured settings, which may or may not be governed by a well-defined set of policies. The MSN works in all settings, with geographic boundaries being determined by contextual needs of the client. This professional creates policies and protocols based on the need expressed. A certain degree of skill in problem identification and resolution is needed along with strong clinical competence to move from one area of specialty to another and function effectively. Environments that do not provide the technology and consultation available in an organizational setting demand a high degree of critical thinking and creativity, which can best be maintained through a commitment to life-long learning.

Within a differentiated system, the danger of fragmentation is great because of conflicts regarding the direction to be taken by the organization. Integration refers to the quality of collaboration that exists among departments or individuals to achieve unity of effort in accomplishing the organizational mission. It removes barriers to permit free and equal association among all parts of a whole, encouraging open dialogue among the parts. Three variables necessary for integration to occur are unifying values and vision, creating a structure for shared decision making, and ensuring autonomy of individuals and groups to act based on a common action plan. Integration focused on shared values and vision is essential to unifying the different roles and responsibilities of one professional group into a synergistic whole. A shared governance structure facilitates joint decision making.[16] A professional practice model based on autonomy and accountability completes the framework for an integrative care delivery system positioned to serve the needs of society into the 21st century.

Keep changing. When you're through changing, you're through.
BRUCE BARTON

PRINCIPLES OF LARGE-SCALE ORGANIZATIONAL CHANGE

This book is a composite of the activities and processes that transformed the nursing practice at Sioux Valley Hospital into a professional model relevant to the emerging needs of contemporary society. This was a challenging process for the entire organization, and several themes kept appearing. These themes were to become the guiding principles for the transformative process.[14]

The Context Surrounding Change Is Everything

Change is not smooth and linear but rather a spiraling process, going deeper with each cycle of exposure. An inservice on differentiated practice was given to all nurses involved in the initial project. After several weeks of activity, many questions emerged. As the inservice was repeated, staff could identify issues with which they had struggled along with strategies to deal with them. By the time the staff attended their third inservice, the concept was well in hand. It is only through the lived experience that the essence of a concept is grasped and strengthened through repeated revisiting of the concept. The practice discovered that inservices on the *what* of change with a strong focus on *how to* were not sufficient to motivate staff to the challenge at hand. It was only when the context for the change was painted—the chaotic environment and the social and professional reasons for change—that the staff accepted the challenge laid before them.

As the Essence of a Concept Is Grasped, the Form May Change

Initial understanding of differentiated practice was based on the work of Primm and the Midwest Alliance in Nursing.[10] The ADN and BSN competencies from this work served as the framework for the career options developed by the staff. As work progressed, the literature on research studies about differentiation was reviewed. This led to the Harvard Business School study,[15] which identified that differentiation transcends technical tasks to include differing attitudes and values. Furthermore, the emphasis on the paradoxic connection between differentiation and integration led to the naming of this care delivery system as Integrated Care.

Change Is Messy, Noisy, and Liberating

Redesigning a care delivery model is much like remodeling a house: Double the estimate of time and energy required for completion. Keeping management one step ahead of staff is essential if the project is to succeed. Clear and consistent communication and feedback are imperative in a staff-driven project of this magnitude. Proper support and guidance are essential to directing unleashed energy into productive channels for change.

Differentiating Role Competencies for RNs Mandate Changes in the Socialization and Education of Nurses

As the paradigm for nursing changes, competency expansion does not occur in technical skills but rather in the communication and critical thinking domains of practice. In her transformational theory of health as expanding consciousness, Newman[17] proposes that professional nursing is primarily relational. She envisions emerging professional roles and responsibilities that call for innovation and creativity, empathy and caring, and powerful interpersonal skills to influence and negotiate on behalf of the client and the profession. Nurses practicing in the BSN role at Sioux Valley Hospital were given classes that built on strong critical thinking skills, including business competence, surveillance skills, diagnostic reasoning, and human interaction and negotiation skills along with increased capacity for critical reflection. ADN and BSN schools found that they now had different role models for their students. Thus an innovative research project entitled The Healing Web[18,19] has been implemented to test the clinical education of nursing students in two distinct and complementary nursing roles.

Legal Implications of Advancing Practice Opportunities Must Be Addressed By Experts Who Understand the Work

It has been the experience of some nurses involved with innovation that their activities are misunderstood and restricted by state regulatory boards during a time when adaptation of inpatient treatment modalities to an outpatient setting is essential. If nursing boards are to be effective and supportive of advancing nursing practice, one of two options should be considered. Ideally, all boards should be composed of experts in the field of nursing education and nursing service, so that public safety and nursing innovation to meet changing health care needs would be given mutual consideration. In states that fill those positions by political appointment, a panel of experts must be convened to study the proposed innovation and to make recommendations to the board to maintain a balance between public protection and advancement of nursing practice.

This Is Nursing's Moment and It Must Be Acted Upon Now

We live in a privileged time and place. The advancement of humankind is reflected in transformative movements such as civil rights, feminism, the demise of communism, and the emergence of a global economy. This has given nursing, a predominantly female profession, momentum for healing and growth. The essential ingredient needed for the profession to seize the opportunity is the courage to move forward in unison and harmony. This effort will require us to leave behind our conformity to the old notion of "a nurse is a nurse" and to replace it with a new concept that values and celebrates the diversity that various nursing roles can bring to meeting the total health care needs of society. To do this, we must support and celebrate each other as we evolve toward wholeness, so that we can better assist others in their journey toward the same destination.

Saddle your dreams afore you ride 'em.

MARY WEBB

REFERENCES

1. South Dakota Statewide Project Steering Committee. The South Dakota experience. In: Boston C, ed. *Current Issues and Perspectives on Differentiated Practice.* Chicago, Ill: American Organization of Nurse Executives; 1990:53–67.

2. Benveniste G. *Professionalizing the Organization: Reducing Bureaucracy to Enhance Effectiveness.* San Fransisco, Calif: Jossey-Bass; 1987.

3. O'Leary J. Do nurse administrators' values conflict with the economic trend? *Nurs Admin Q.* 1984; 8(4):1–9.

4. Naisbitt J, Aburdene P. *Reinventing the Corporation.* New York, NY: Warner; 1985.

5. Porter-O'Grady T. Shared governance and new organizational models. *Nurs Econ.* 1987; 5:281–286.

6. American Nurses' Association. *Educational Preparation for Nurse Practitioners and Assistants to Nurses: A Position Paper.* Kansas City, Mo: American Nurses' Association; 1965.

7. National Commission on Nursing Implementation Project. *Nursing Practice Patterns (Differentiated Practice).* Milwaukee, Wis: National Commission on Nursing Implementation Project; 1989.

8. National Commission on Nursing Implementation Project. *Nursing Programs Now and in the Future.* Milwaukee, Wis: National Commission on Nursing Implementation Project; 1986.

9. American Academy of Nursing. *Differentiating Nursing Practice: Into the Twenty-First Century.* Kansas City, Mo: American Academy of Nursing; 1991.

10. Primm PL. Differentiated practice for ADN- and BSN-prepared nurses. *J Prof Nurs.* 1987; 3:218–225.

11. Statewide Project Steering Committee. *Final Report: Statewide Project for Nursing and Nursing Education.* Sioux Falls, SD: South Dakota Board of Nursing; 1988.

12. Koerner JG, Bunkers LB, Nelson B, Santema K. Implementing differentiated practice: the Sioux Valley Hospital experience. *J Nurs Admin.* 1989; 19(2):13–20.

13. Koerner J. Differentiated practice: the evolution of professional nursing. *J Prof Nurs.* 1992; 8:335–341.

14. Koerner J. The relevance of differentiated practice in today's environment. In: Boston C, ed. *Current Issues and Perspectives on Differentiated Practice.* Chicago, Ill: American Organization of Nurse Executives; 1990:35–51.

15. Lawrence P, Lorsch J. *Organization and Environment: Managing Differentiation and Integration.* Boston, Mass: Harvard University Press; 1967.

16. Koerner J. Integrating differentiated practice into shared governance. In: Porter-O'Grady T, ed. *Implementing Shared Governance.* Hanover, Md: Mosby Yearbook; 1992:169–196.

17. Newman M. *Health as Expanding Consciousness.* St Louis, Mo: Mosby; 1986.

18. Bunkers SS. The healing web: a transformative model for nursing. *Nurs Health Care.* 1992; 13:68–75.

19. Larson J. The healing web: a transformative model for nursing; part II. *Nurs Health Care.* 1992; 13:246–252.

EXERCISE 1–1: DISCUSSION QUESTIONS

1. Does education or experience create an expert nurse?
2. Does basic education level reflect the level of practice of professional nurses with multiple years of experience?
3. Do multiple years of experience guarantee that the nurse is expert?
4. Are all nurses practicing in the single role category of RN the same?
5. Does society value diversity with a sense of mutual worth or a sense of hierarchy?
6. Does differentiation of practice create division or synergy in the collective community of nurses?

Appendix 1-A
Sioux Valley Hospital Nursing Timeline:
1981–1993

1981	Mary Fuller began as first vice president for nursing: moved nursing administration to the corporate level
1981	Professional Nurse Practice Committee: first generation of shared governance in the area of quality assurance
1982, January	12-hour shifts started: began as incentive to attract and retain RNs
1983, October	Diagnosis-related groups began: changed health care reimbursement
1984, June	100 LPNs laid off: corporate response to increasing acuity and decreasing length of stay
1984, October	JoEllen Koerner began as vice president of patient services: change in leadership and scope of responsibility
1985, January	Board announced plans to close school: would change nursing recruitment
1985, April	Strategic planning document 1: first effort at strategic planning for the nursing department; completed by nursing administration
1986, May	Sioux Valley Hospital School of Nursing closed: end of 90-year diploma education program
1986, July	Strategic planning document 2: review of Magnet Hospital Study; second strategic plan completed by nursing administration and head nurse group
1986, August	Staffing and Scheduling Committee: shared governance expanded to policy and procedures regarding staffing
1986, Fall	Performance Based Development System: began to use in May 1987; moved to individualized, competency-based assessment, orientation, and staff development
1986, Fall	"Whack on the Side of the Head": interdisciplinary class on creativity and communication for all department heads in patient services

1987, January	Differentiated practice—Peggy Primm: work redesign based on educational competencies of RN graduates
1987, January	Decision to phase out LPNs by January 1, 1990: move to all-professional staff
1987, Spring	Nursing Diagnosis Committee: required decision making; communication process for nursing staff
1987, Spring	Quality assurance: based on research principles
1987, Summer	Summer E nursing program: externship program for third-year nursing students
1987, October	Computer order entry: streamlined paperwork
1988	Acuity system: foundation for costing out nursing charges
1988, April	Ecology of Excellence: business model for clinical staff
1988, June	Nursing Ethics Committee: established to work in collaboration with housewide Ethics Committee
1988, August	Self-scheduling: units design their own scheduling mechanisms
1988, October	Career Pathways Committee: career ladder for professional development and advancement
1989, April	Integrated Care Committee: care delivery system based on differentiated practice
1989	Integrated Clinical Pathways: interdisciplinary care maps
1989, Fall	"Change" course for head nurses: preparation for shared governance leadership competencies
1989, October	Credentialing Committee: process for acquiring privileges to join the nursing practice and to receive annual recredentialing privileges
1990, January	LPN and maternal-child health supervisor positions dissolved: professional and empowered staff
1990, January	"Change" course for supervisors and staff educators: preparation for leadership competencies in shared governance environment
1990, February	Nursing Residency Program: orientation program for new nursing graduates
1990, February	Shared Governance Development Council: decision making for clinical operation assumed by staff representatives at department level
1990, July	Strategic planning document 3: outline for continued development of professional practice for nursing
1991, January	Culture study: foundation for reinforcing culture for shared governance environment

1991, January	Educational incentive for those preceptoring novice employees: reward in form of dollars toward continuing nursing education developed for nurses assisting with the professional development of the nursing practice through preceptoring
1991, Spring	"Change" course for clinical care coordinators and primary nurses: preparation for leadership competencies in shared governance environment
1991, Spring	Unit shared governance councils: decision making for clinical operations moved to unit level, with department level providing guidance and norms
1991, Summer	Housewide supervisor replaced divisional supervisor positions: critical care and medical-surgical nursing supervisors' roles change
1992, January	Peer review process and portfolio: staff assumed authority and accountability for peer evaluation
1992, January	N-Touch computer program beta site: introduction to computerized documentation system
1992, February	Restructuring of critical care and medical-surgical nursing divisions: decentralization of telemetry and expansion of stepdown units between medical-surgical and critical care divisions
1992, March	Integrated Clinical Pathway documentation: incorporated Integrated Clinical Pathways into permanent documentation record
1993, February	End of clinical nursing supervisory positions: responsibility and authority assumed by clinical care coordinators
1993, June	End of pay differential between 8- and 12-hour workday schedule: equal pay scales for all shifts
1993, September	Opened 2 patient-focused care units

Courtesy of Narcy Recker, Sioux Valley Hospital, Sioux Falls, South Dakota.

2

Culture

*Narcy Recker, Kathryn Linda Karpiuk,
Elizabeth Hindbjorgen, and
JoEllen Goertz Koerner*

> *Culture hides much more than it reveals, and
> strangely enough what it hides, it hides most effec-
> tively from its own participants. Years of study have
> convinced me that the real job is not to understand
> foreign culture but to understand our own.*
>
> EDWARD T. HALL

Culture is something that profoundly affects our actions and behaviors and yet is largely hidden from us. Learning about our unique culture gives us a chance to stand back and reevaluate aspects of our working world that we are so used to that we take them for granted.

Understanding the prevalent culture can help individuals and teams operate more effectively. It also helps group members see choices where previously they might have been victims of forces beyond their appreciation. An awareness of culture allows all to question habits, traditions, and ways of doing things that have become ingrained in the lives and working habits of the group. When one begins to identify these hidden forces, freedom for change is possible.

Much discussion and many management books and articles have appeared recently on the topic of corporate culture. Understanding the culture is essential when one is planning for change within an organization. Peters and Waterman[1] identified that the single most distinguishing feature of the excellent organization is the presence of a strong core of values that are both preached and practiced.

When one is considering organizational change, it is critical to take full account of how things are at present and of the needs and values influencing people's behavior. Change strategies must address these issues or the plan will meet with resistance. Fully understanding the characteristics of the current culture is a starting point for change.

Culture is a metaphor and therefore difficult to define. The literature gives many graphic definitions, all of which have relevance to the concept under study. Culture represents a web of understanding that is necessary for people to make sense of and cope with the complexity and confusion of organizational life. The web gives shape to what we do and defines the way in which we do it.[2] Culture reflects the values and expectations that organization members come to share.[3] Baker[4] calls culture the glue that holds the organization together. Culture is the assumed and shared meanings that people assign to their social surroundings.[5] It is the collection of traditions, values, policies, beliefs, and attitudes that constitute a pervasive context for everything we do and think in an organization.[2]

Anthropology transcends these management definitions of culture and integrates these concepts into a world view. Geertz describes culture from an anthropologic perspective: Culture "denotes an historically transmitted pattern of meanings embodied in symbols, a system of inherited conceptions expressed in symbolic forms by means of which men communicate, perpetuate, and develop their knowledge about and attitudes toward life."[6(p3)]

Culture forms and develops over time, representing a living record of authority's past. Present conventions, rituals, and practices reflect the organization's learning and acquired wisdom. These are passed to each new generation of people who join the group.

Symbols carry the meaning that a culture ascribes to them and provide the main access to understanding culture. High-profile symbols include the mission statement, logos, slogans, building and office layout and furnishings, speeches at parties, and retirement rituals. Low-profile symbols are more difficult to define and must be discovered by the new employee. One must learn to decipher what is really being said and how to read between the lines to catch the unwritten, but powerful, rules of "how we do things around here."

Culture is not an individual matter. As people interact, the norms and practices of the organization are lived out, enforced, and reinforced. When cultural meaning is unclear, people discuss events to work out their significance. Culture is about social consensus, seeking accepted common interpretations to help people make sense of their world and operate productively.

Several factors influence organizational culture. Primary tasks, or the organization's main functions, are a large influence. Health care requires a high standard of accuracy and an element of caring that is expected by the public. Thus all who enter are expected to ascribe to and uphold those attributes while working within the organization. Another factor is the size of the organization. The larger the organization, the more formal its culture is likely to be. Large size leads to geographic and communication challenges, which often create or support rivalries. Geographic location is influential as the organization takes on local cultural influences through the employees it hires. Community boundaries and activities also shape the organizational possibilities for development. Senior management has considerable effect on culture through symbolic power. Messages about whose opinions and needs are important can affect the environment and values in a profound way. The culture is not the property of any one group, however; rather, the collective employee pool shapes and maintains corporate culture.

The actual formation of a culture is the response to a complex set of such factors over time. Through our responses, we build a collection of learned needs and beliefs.

To understand better our own culture, the nursing department at Sioux Valley Hospital decided to conduct a study of the patient unit cultures before changing to a shared governance model. The purpose of the study was to help the units identify their norms, values, teamwork, and decision making at the time. By understanding the present culture, the staff could consider making changes to enhance shared governance activities. It was decided to use the focus group process.[7-9]

An ad hoc committee of the Shared Governance Development Council met with a research professor from a local university who had worked with Sioux Valley Hospital nursing staff on other research projects.[10] This committee was convened to discuss the focus group process. The committee, with a few additional members, met again to reach consensus on the questions that would be asked of the focus groups. At a third meeting, the consultant trained the focus group facilitators in leading a group, keeping participants on the topic, and drawing everyone into the group.

The number of groups on each unit depended on the number of staff assigned to the unit. In keeping with the literature, we invited more than 50% of the registered nurses (RNs) from each unit to participate in groups of 6 to 12. Every unit had at least one group; the largest unit had four groups. Head nurses were asked to select a representative sample of their staff for each focus group. On the smallest units, everyone was invited to the one focus group session. The facilitators believed the head nurses would know best the representation requested: nurses with the most seniority, those who were newly hired, informal leaders, and nurses in each of the differentiated practice roles.

When invited to participate, staff were asked to provide information about their norms or usual ways of working together and about differences from and similarities to other units. With this information, we could better understand ourselves and how we operate.

Staff were informed that each of them had a unique perspective that would be important to voice to assess accurately his or her unit's culture. Staff were told that the session would last 1 hour on the date and time established, that the session would be conducted by an interviewer, and that participation was voluntary but would be paid time. If willing to participate, the RN was given a list of the seven broad questions that would be discussed at the focus group sessions (Exhibit 2–1).

Staff nurses were told that the interviews would be taped because of the volume of information that would be covered and that the facilitator would be the only one

Exhibit 2–1 Focus Group Discussion Questions

1. Discuss various types of nurses who practice on this unit.
2. Discuss rules for working together.
3. Discuss rules for organizing and using time.
4. Relate the usual way (ie, norms) of doing things.
5. Discuss rules for telling others what to do.
6. Discuss what the rules are for change.
7. Use three or four words to describe your unit.

Courtesy of Sioux Valley Hospital Shared Governance Development Council Ad Hoc Committee for Culture Study, Sioux Falls, South Dakota.

with access to the information. They were also informed that the facilitators would analyze the information obtained and then meet with the unit to discuss and clarify the results.

Focus group sessions were conducted. Unit participation varied from 40% to 60% of the staff. Careful attention was paid to make sure the facilitators were not from the unit on which they conducted sessions. Each facilitator began by introducing herself, thanking the RNs for participating, and stating the purpose of the meeting. Realizing that many people are uncomfortable when audiotaped, the facilitator assured the participants that she would be the only one who would have access to the information.

After the sessions were completed, the facilitators met to identify terms that would be used to share the trends found on the units. The trends were identified not only by the verbal input but also by the nonverbal behavior that was noted. By having common terms, the unit trends could be compared.

At unit meetings the data were verified with the staff so that changes could be made if needed. Only rare and minimal changes were needed. Trends were reported to the units with supporting statements to clarify the terms used. Comments made by focus group participants without group agreement were not reported.

The trends found were not a surprise. Unit trends were identified; staff agreed with these and stated that their perceptions were now validated. Although part of the same organization, unit cultures differed and sometimes varied widely. See the example in Table 2–1 for focus group results from two in-house, contrasting unit cultures. A deeper understanding of the units as a whole had been gained from this process.

Throughout the department of nursing, the following attributes for staff to be successful and accepted were identified: competence, ability to adapt to change, critical thinking skills used to make decisions, acceptance and use of diversity, and ability to communicate. The acceptability of taking risks to benefit the professional practice and its goals was also mentioned. Each of these items is explained below.

Table 2–1 Two Contrasting Unit Cultures

Unit A	Unit B
Nurse who fits in on this unit	
Flexible	Meticulous
Team worker	Assessment skills
Organized and hard working	Critical thinking skills
Assertive	Communication skills
Rules for working together	
Teamwork	Teamwork
Anticipate others' needs	Anticipate others' needs
Situation dependent	Interdisciplinary
Helping done across roles	
You must be able to ask for help	
Organizing and using time	
Priorities are role and situation dependent	Patient care management
Low priority given to nurses' personal needs	Discharge planning
	Transport services
Usual way of doing things	
Flexible	Creative communication
Feelings about authority	
Hierarchy	Self-governing
"Bossy" described negatively	Past supervision not viewed positively
	Decisions based on experience, knowledge, and education
Attitudes toward change	
Unenthusiastic	Receptive: want purpose, rationale, and supporting research presented
	View selves as collaborative
Four words to describe unit	
Supporting	Meticulous
Challenging	Collaborative
Stressful	Intelligent
Chaotic	Shared governance

Courtesy of Sioux Valley Hospital, Sioux Falls, South Dakota.

COMPETENCE

> *It is not only what we do, but also what we do not do, for which we are accountable.*
>
> Molière

Competence is an essential component of professional nursing and is a distinct value of the nursing practice at Sioux Valley Hospital. Some may question why competence deserves mention when culture is being described. After all, isn't competence expected of all nurses? Isn't competence what makes a nurse adequate or sufficient to practice? We believe competence is more than just passing. Competency has come to mean a vehicle to professional growth and a pathway to career development.

Our present philosophy of competence began with the incorporation of the Performance Based Development System (PBDS), by Baxter, Inc. This is an individualized, competency-based orientation program. Dr Dorothy del Bueno, our primary consultant for this program, defined competent performance as "the effective application of knowledge and skill in the work setting."[11(p135)] She identified three dimensions of competency: technical/clerical skills, interpersonal relation skills, and critical thinking skills. These three dimensions of competency are performed within a context that may be the entire hospital or a specific unit or shift. del Bueno's model uses three intersecting circles inside a square as a visual aid to clarify this concept (Figure 2–1).

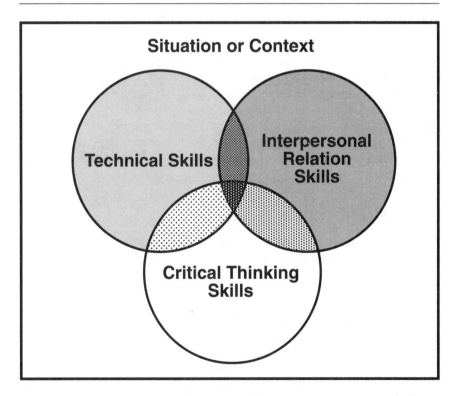

Figure 2–1 Dimensions of competent performance. *Source:* Reprinted from *Nursing Economics,* Vol 5, No 1, p 23, with permission of Jannetti Publications, Inc, © 1987.

No longer is nursing defined by task alone. Nurses use the three circles and a square concept to remind themselves of the dimensions of competency in their practice. Adult learning principles have replaced the forced-feeding techniques long applied to educational activities.[12] Self-directed learning is encouraged, with the learner's needs and experience being taken into account.

To promote competency of the novice RN, a nurse residency program for new graduate RNs was initiated. This program facilitates the transition from new graduate nurse to professional nurse. This 4- to 6-month program uses the PBDS principles as the basis for promoting competence and self-confidence. The culture of the nursing department is learned through a sharing of information and educational opportunities.

The concept of the continuum from novice to competence to expert has surfaced. The old adage "sink or swim" has finally died as staff nurses have realized the process of becoming a professional nurse. Staff nurses have adopted more realistic expectations of new employees. They have realized that it does no good to eat the young and have joined in efforts to precept new nurses. The preceptor program has fostered this commitment by offering learning experiences and rewards for preceptors.

Levels of competency and expertise are valued and respected. No longer does one have to be an expert to do something. For example, a clinical nurse specialist is not required to do all the inservicing for his or her unit. Staff nurses are continually encouraged to gain new skills or try new roles. With increased competence, professional growth results. Those who choose to stay at their present level are equally valued and respected for their ongoing contributions.

Competency is continually evaluated by peer review, meeting of credentialing standards, and portfolios (see Chapter 4 for more discussion about peer review, credentialing, and portfolios). It is an ongoing growth process, not a one-time expectation. Through this, the staff stay current and grow in their professional practice.

ADAPTABILITY TO CHANGE

> *The issue is no longer that of change or continuity*
> *but rather the nature of change. Is it to be the*
> *change of consent, or the change of coercion?*
> BISHOP G. BROMLEY OXNAM

Along with competence, the ability to adapt to change was highly valued as a norm in our culture study. Change is often not the chosen path but rather is forced upon us throughout life.

We change physically from an infant to a child to an adult to an elder, and we need to adapt to the new experiences and expectations as we grow. Seasons change, and with each change comes preparation for the next phase. Our entire world changes constantly. Change is the norm of life.

The outcomes of change are not always positive or reversible. Some are debilitating and permanent. It is the lack of choice in change and the unknown outcomes that often cause stress and fear. Yet without change, advancement would not be possible.

The health care industry is fraught with constant change. New techniques, new knowledge, and new restrictions are almost daily occurrences. In the health care industry there is often no choice. Regardless of who you are or what your role is, you will need to adapt to change.

> *The world hates change, yet it is the only thing that has brought progress.*
>
> CHARLES F. KETTERING

Changes are sometimes seen as necessary and at other times as a nuisance. We have all heard the saying "If it isn't broke, don't fix it." Yet maintenance is required on a regular basis, or break it will. Maintenance of any item is basically a change.

Change can be welcomed or resisted, light or burdensome, difficult or easy. The effect that change will have is often not known until it is attempted, but the outcome can be influenced by the attitude of the group involved in the process. If one undertakes a change with the attitude that one will prove "it won't work," typically one is correct: It won't. The persons involved in change need to be vested in the effort by being aware of the hoped for outcomes and objectives or by being aware of the reason a change is needed. Without this information, the effort may fail. This is true in health care as in all industry. Changing the way you do anything will be more positively received if the outcomes or reasons for change are shared.

Changes at Sioux Valley Hospital have been shared through a variety of avenues. For special projects, a communication notebook is used on each unit. Any bits of news on the project are shared through this route. Each nurse assumes the responsibility to keep himself or herself updated. "Seek and find" has replaced "wait to be told." Other routes of sharing information have included open forums, unit meetings, newsletters, personal letters, and committees. The people involved have been included in the decision-making process, at all levels, throughout the endeavor.

The profession of nursing is continually undergoing change. There are changes in expectations, roles, patient populations, and myriad other items. Health care research has assisted nursing in seeing the value of change. Accepting and adapting to change have become necessary qualities of the professional nurse today.

Although change causes disruption and at times conflict with old ideas, changes are often needed to provide improved quality of care. In times of decreasing resources, change is needed to meet even basic requirements. As the world changes, all are affected. As health care changes, all are affected. As professionals, nurses need to accept change and use the experience to grow.

DECISION MAKING

*If you choose to not make a decision and deal with
what comes along, be prepared for anything.*

NARCY RECKER

Flipping a coin to make a decision is appropriate when you are trying to decide something such as which flavor of ice cream to order. The choices one needs to make in health care require much more effort. These choices need clear, conscious deliberation before a decision is made. Who does the deliberation and who makes the final decision regarding the variety of problems encountered in health care have changed.

Originally, administrators of health care institutions made all decisions. Most of the original nursing schools were in the hospital setting with a physician as administrator. During this century, nursing has developed into a health care profession. As this happened, administrative positions became available for nurses, such as the director of nursing positions common to most health care institutions.

During the 1980s, a new arena for the use of nursing expertise developed in the corporate business world. The health care industry began using nurse executives in corporate decision making. The advantages of having a nursing professional involved with corporate decisions were noted. Business decisions regarding nursing were no longer being made without nursing input and leadership.

*In sharing the opportunity to decide, you also
share the responsibility for the outcome.*

NARCY RECKER

As nursing shared its expertise in the corporate arena, nursing leaders also began to seek input for decision making from staff nurses at the bedside. Participatory management, as this was called, allowed the staff to voice their opinion, to use creativity, and to be a part of the solution. Ownership of the decision was still often the responsibility of the unit or divisional nursing manager.

Presently the movement is toward shared governance. In this system the staff nurses not only are a part of the discussion but also take on the ownership of the decision. Nurses at the bedside are given the needed information, resources, and authority to deliberate the issue and make a decision. Patient care decisions are made by the staff involved whenever possible. The bedside nurse is accountable and responsible, having the authority to make decisions that affect the care of the patient. For instance, the primary nurse will consult with other members of the health care team without seeking permission from the unit manager.

In shared governance, issues involving only a particular unit are debated and resolved at the unit council. In so doing, the nurses own the decision they make. The norm is to reward critical thinking and common sense decision making. The goal is to have decisions made by the people who are affected by them. Therefore, decisions are often made by a group rather than by one individual. Inevitably, some decisions will take longer to make in this system than in the traditional hierarchy.

Management has not been eliminated, just redefined. Before the implementation of differentiated practice, most unit managers followed either the "leadership as benevolent maternalism" style or the "efficient management" style, as described by Hall and Rosen.[13] With the implementation of differentiated practice and the permission to innovate and experiment, staff learned that risks could be taken, mistakes could be made, and their commitment to try would still be supported. Managers learned to delegate and soon moved into the "leadership as enabler" style, helping staff grow.[13]

Transition periods are difficult times. The transition period will include the working of parallel systems: one beginning to take on a responsibility, one learning to relinquish a responsibility. Perplexing situations will arise. It is helpful, in working through transitional times, to reaffirm roles and responsibilities in both systems. Also, all communications must be consistent. In times of change, conflicting stories will only limit the advances that can be made.

In this difficult time of rapid change, support systems at Sioux Valley Hospital facilitated continued growth of the managers. Some managers are now following the "charismatic leadership" style.[13] Managers continue to be involved in the decision-making process of their unit councils and participate in the housewide management council, but their responsibilities have changed.

> *A decision made without the input of those involved*
> *becomes a dictatorial decree, sure to be resisted.*
> NARCY RECKER

The professional nursing staff now make the decisions regarding their practice. Peer reviews are done by the staff. Management released these duties to the staff and now concentrate on the procurement of needed resources and on advising and mentoring the professional staff in their decision making.

Decisions in a group are made by consensus rather than by vote. It takes time to reach consensus because everyone must have the same understanding. Once consensus is reached, however, much of the education has been done, and because everyone can live with the decision the power behind it is greater. The possibility of sabotage and noncompliance is diminished (see Chapter 3 for more information about consensus).

DIVERSITY

> *A clash of doctrines is not a disaster—it is an*
> *opportunity.*
> ALFRED NORTH WHITEHEAD

As culture is discussed, we repeatedly hear terms such as *shared values, beliefs, traditions,* and *social consensus.* These all connote an expected sameness. As we examine our culture, however, we discover that diversity is a key value of the culture. This is almost paradoxic, but differences and diversity are truly valued at Sioux Valley Hospital and are the building blocks of teamwork.

How does an organization come to realize the importance of differences and recognize their worth? At Sioux Valley Hospital the process began with the Ecology of Excellence philosophy.[14] The classes offered to employees were designed to assist employees in developing skills necessary to work together as business partners in a healthy, productive work environment. It was a process of empowerment, and it promoted team building.

To build a team, we recognized that it was necessary to know ourselves and to recognize and accept others for their unique contributions. Employees determined their role preference. They came to recognize what roles were needed in teams and the roles in which they preferred to function.

The Myers-Briggs Type Indicator was used to offer individuals insight into themselves and others. The Myers-Briggs is a preference indicator that makes the theory of psychologic types described by Jung understandable and useful in people's lives:

> The essence of the theory is that much seemingly random variation in behavior is actually quite orderly and consistent, being due to basic differences in the way individuals prefer to use their perception and judgment. . . . Perception involves all the ways of becoming aware of things, people, happenings, or ideas. Judgment involves all the ways of coming to conclusions about what has been perceived. If people differ systematically in what they perceive and in how they reach conclusions, then it is only reasonable for them to differ correspondingly in their reactions, interests, values, motivations, skills and interests (sic).[15(p1)]

The Myers-Briggs Type Indicator is now administered to every new employee with an explanation of what the results indicate. In keeping with the ethical standards of the tool, all results are confidential, and no records of individual type preferences are saved. The Myers-Briggs concepts are to foster team building and to assist in understanding the differences among individuals. For instance, Myers-Briggs may be useful in pairing preceptors with orientees. Although there are no magic pairs, completely opposite ways of learning and teaching can increase stress if they are not understood by both preceptor and preceptee. Differences should be used to enhance learning, not destroy it.

Most nursing committees and councils currently undergo a team type analysis. This involves each member volunteering information about his or her individual type to be used to recognize the team's strengths and potential blind spots. For instance, a team whose strength is extroversion will need to recognize its blind spot of introversion and allow time to ensure internal processing and reflection on ideas before any quick vote is taken (extroversion). If a team's strength is introversion, then the blind spot of extroversion will need to be addressed. In these two scenarios, therefore, adequate time to discuss issues aloud (external processing) and taking action quickly enough need to be addressed.

> *Culture is always a product of mixing.*
> FRIEDRICH HERTZ

Diversity within groups is welcomed. Nurses have recognized that a blend of personalities and role types assists in completing tasks. No longer does everyone have to feel that he or she needs to be able to do it all or fit into a designated carbon copy or mold. Staff can focus on the pieces they know they do well. It is okay to have someone else finish a project for you.

Not only is it evident at Sioux Valley Hospital that differences among individuals are valued, but it has been recognized that allowing for differences among groups is important. With identified outcomes and a common vision, individual units are left to decide how to obtain desired outcomes. For example, as Integrated Care was implemented nurses established ground rules. They were then allowed to be creative and to develop the idea in whatever fashion would work for their unit (see Appendix 2-A). It is only when we disclose those things that make us different from each other that we can mix our contrasting characteristics to enhance the flavor of our culture.

COMMUNICATION

> *Two may talk together under the same roof for*
> *many years, yet never really meet; and two others*
> *at first speech are old friends.*
> MARY HARTWELL CATHERWOOD

Communication is the basis for all endeavors. The need to communicate has existed since more than one individual was present on Earth. As long as the need to communicate has existed, so have problems with the process. As technology increased and the world's inhabitants became more mobile, communication challenges began to skyrocket.

Now a variety of languages can be found in any area of the world. As language has varied among countries and geographic areas, language variations among different areas of study also have developed. The business world has its own unique language, as does science, the arts, psychology, and the various other areas of human study. Health care is no exception.

The unique language common to the health care system can be frightening to an individual who enters into the system in need of help. Because of the variety of people with whom health care professionals work and see as clients, communication skills are a major area of concern. A health care professional must be able to use a variety of means to communicate. The written and spoken word as well as visual aids must be available for use.

Evaluating a client's or fellow professional's understanding is also a part of the communication process. Asking for feedback or verbalized understanding should be done to ensure that one person understands the message the other person is trying to convey. Verbal and nonverbal feedback are expected with true communication. Good, clear feedback is necessary.[16] Disagreeing and differences in opinion are accepted.

Even if the message is understood, total compliance cannot be expected. Besides communicating an idea, the message must be meaningful for the individual or group listening. Unless the idea communicated is meaningful, nothing may transpire from the experience, and the effort may be wasted.

One of the aspects of a culture is the language used. With a change in the culture, some of the words change also. A key term used when staff at Sioux Valley Hospital were learning the new differentiated practice roles was *mentor.* The new key word is now *dialogue,* which combines the best of networking and consulting where both parties involved in the dialogue have expertise and opportunities for growth.

Recognizing one's strengths builds self-esteem. Discussing challenges and opportunities for growth rather than weaknesses or problems creates a positive attitude and greater commitment to effect change.

In increasing our awareness of how people learn, we utilize the whole brain learning theory. People differ in the ways in which they gain meaning from the messages received. Therefore, we try to give the same message in more than one way. Some people are more visual; others learn by listening. Some learn by reading; others learn by doing (Figures 2–2 and 2–3).

> *Put it before them briefly so they will read it,*
> *clearly so they will appreciate it, picturesquely so*
> *they will remember it and, above all, accurately so*
> *they will be guided by its light.*
>
> Joseph Pulitzer

In making communication meaningful, one has to shift from a communication style where the communicator's needs are met to an opposite communication style, where the communicated idea's importance to all involved is identified. The shift from one communication style to the other involves the skill of negotiation.

To negotiate, one needs to balance the opportunities and consequences for all parties concerned. Trust is necessary to negotiate honestly. In negotiation, no one person may achieve all that is hoped for, but items of agreement can be derived through the shared effort. Negotiation is often employed to reach consensus.

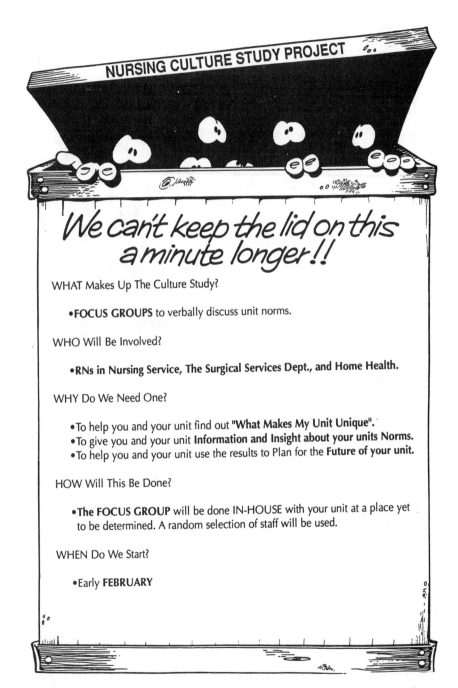

Figure 2–2 Poster in left brain language. Courtesy of Sioux Valley Hospital, Sioux Falls, South Dakota.

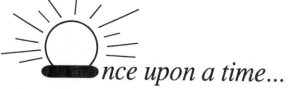

nce upon a time...

there was a Ms. Unit who wasn't sure who she was or where she was going. It was as if she was suffering from amnesia. Ms. Unit felt very distraught. "How can I know which way to go into the future if I don't know who I am or how I got this way!"

After many days of turmoil, Ms. Unit went to see the Wizard of Culture to ask for assistance. The masterful and wise Wizard of Culture explained to Ms. Unit that the solution was simple. "I will help you gain insight into yourself." The masterful Wizard continued, some of your angels in white will be asked to verbally discuss how their unit functions, and reveal its norms and values.

Ms. Unit would have to look hard and truthfully at who she was. The Wizard warned that at times the truth may be painful. But the Wizard continued - "Only when you discover the TRUE you, will the truth open you up for new possibilities and organismic harmony."

Figure 2–3 Poster in right brain language. Courtesy of Sioux Valley Hospital, Sioux Falls, South Dakota.

First party communication is expected. If staff member A has a complaint about staff member B, rather than telling everyone else about it A is expected to confront B to discuss the concern in private. If A discusses the matter with staff member C, it is C's responsibility to point out to A that the concern should be discussed with B.

Initially this is difficult to do, particularly when staff view confrontation negatively. Staff member C, a head nurse or other mentor can role play with staff member A. In particularly difficult situations, such as when staff member A is intimidated by staff member B, the mentor might accompany staff member A when confronting B.

Skillful communication is of primary importance in health care. The health care team members need to be able to communicate with each other and with the variety of clients and other individuals with whom they come in contact. Without true communication, each member of the health care team could function independently, trying to communicate his or her particular piece of information to the client. The entire team needs to communicate and negotiate among the different disciplines to fully care for the client. With a combined effort, true communication will be possible.

The nursing professionals who care for the client provide the opportunity for this combined effort by using communication skills with all individuals involved. Nurses, through their consistent contact with the client, are the pivotal communicators. Nurses who involve the client and the entire health care team in the communication process will assist the client in meeting his or her health care needs in the most efficient and effective manner possible.

RISK TAKING

> *Behold the turtle. He makes progress only when*
> *he sticks his neck out.*
>
> JAMES BRYANT CONANT

Change often involves risk. Risk taking is a specific action that may lead to change. To take a risk is to take a chance or venture to new territory. Some form of jeopardy is present.

When, why, and how people take risks are often learned from their family. Some are comfortable with risk. They understand that there may be a gain, a loss, or nothing at all obtained from the risk, but they are still willing to undertake the effort.

When to take a chance is a puzzling question. Do you only take a risk when you are forced to, or do you engage in risk routinely, knowing the possibility of failure exists? Why do people engage in risk taking? Why not stay safe and secure? Typically people take risks to increase a positive asset such as wealth, health, or happiness. They may also take a risk if another is in danger, as in the case of the person who dives into a raging river to save another person from drowning.

What may be too risky for one may not be so for another. Some people engage in risky events for a thrill. Jumping off a high bridge into a moving river can be dangerous. Yet if you make it, the thrill of the free fall and surviving is for some a positive outcome, worth the risk. It depends on your values.

The risk one is willing to take and the reasons for taking a risk are tied closely with one's values and beliefs or, in other words, one's culture. In health care, your personal culture and your professional culture merge to create a new dimension. What you would risk outside your professional environment may not be the same as what you would risk within your professional environment.

In any arena, taking a risk is taking a chance. The element of risk can prevent some individuals from trying. Nothing new is possible without some risk. If people did not take risks, Columbus would not have crossed the ocean, new vaccines would not be found, the democratic government would not be possible, and progress might come to a grinding halt. Modern health care would not exist today without those who are willing to take a risk.

To make risk taking less risky, professionals need to create an accepting, growth-oriented environment. If an environment will accept risk takers and support their efforts, whether there are positive or negative outcomes the fear of losing will be decreased. Risk taking, regardless of outcome, can be beneficial. Valuable information is often learned in failed attempts.

The process of creating such an environment at Sioux Valley Hospital was established by upper management. Failure was defined explicitly to staff as not having tried. The Ecology of Excellence philosophy helped foster this environment through the use of the Myers-Briggs Type Indicator, team building, encouraging and rewarding creativity, and focusing on growth. Differentiated practice was undertaken with the knowledge of risks involved; outcomes could be positive or negative, but a safe, accepting environment was present. More risk taking is possible in an accepting and supportive environment. Fewer risks, or more dramatic risks, may be visible in less accepting environments.

It is better to have tried and failed than not to have tried at all. In health care, we need supportive environments that encourage and support risk takers and visionaries. Without risk, success is not possible. With risk comes possible loss or gain, but always knowledge.

SUMMARY

Culture is ubiquitous, covering all areas of group life. Without this concept, one cannot really understand change or resistance to it. Understanding the culture is a key starting point to finding out what is really occurring within a group. Culture reflects the history and patterns of the structure that holds it together. Enmeshed within it are the elements that facilitate or block adaptation and change in this transformation era.

Because of the turbulence facing the health care industry, health care professionals are forced to adapt to continual external changes. The culture study at Sioux Valley Hospital was planned to assist staff with adaptation to changes. It was designed to help people clarify their core values and practices; to discard outdated methods and practices, thereby releasing time and energy for new ways of being; and to invite staff to view change as a window of opportunity rather than as a threat.

A heightened individual and corporate awareness of values, beliefs, and habits that govern the daily affairs and general direction of the organization assists people in exercising conscious choices about how things can and should be done. Discovering one's own culture is a powerful process that can lead to spontaneous or planned changes inside the organization.

All activities that revolve around organizational design, recruitment and retention, socialization, design of roles, and rewards require an understanding of how organizational culture influences present functioning. The information generated in this study served as the foundation for the development of a strategic plan for nursing that is moving the practice beyond the walls of the hospital into the community. Such a radical departure from the traditional nursing role requires the identification and honoring of values and traditions that are the essence of nursing practice. Simultaneously, it demands the elimination of beliefs and practices that are irrelevant and binding to free up time and energy for new innovation on behalf of quality and cost-effective nursing care.

Culture is a paradox: It has the capacity stubbornly to resist change or creatively and even ingeniously to embrace it. We believe that a clear sense of our current reality will assist us with the creation of an enhanced future for the client, the staff, and the organization.

REFERENCES

1. Peters TJ, Waterman RJ. *In Search of Excellence*. New York, NY: Harper & Row; 1982.
2. McLean A, Marshall J. *Intervening in Cultures*. London, England: University of Bath; 1983.
3. Van Maanen J, Schein EH. Career development. In: Hackman JR, Suttle JL, eds. *Improving Life at Work: Behavioral Science Approaches to Organizational Change*. Santa Monica, Calif: Goodyear; 1977:30–95.
4. Baker E. Managing organizational culture. *McKinsey Q*. Autumn 1980:51–61.
5. Wilkins AL. Organizational stories as symbols which control the organization. In Pondy LR, ed. *Organizational Symbolism*. Greenwich, Conn: JAI; 1983:81–92.
6. Geertz C. Religion as a cultural system. In: Banton M, ed. *Anthropological Approaches to the Study of Religion*. London, England: Tavistock; 1966:1–46.
7. Coeling HVE, Wilcox JR. Understanding organizational culture: a key to management decision-making. *J Nurs Admin*. 1988; 18(11):16–24.
8. DesRosier MB, Zellers KC. Focus groups: a program planning technique. *J Nurs Admin*. 1989; 19(3):20–25.
9. Focus groups: valuable research tool. *Adult and Continuing Education Today*. April 15, 1991; 5.
10. Hofland SL, Karpiuk K, Honan C, Friestad C. Assisting nursing staff to learn and conduct research: an interinstitutional approach. *J Nurs Staff Dev*. 1991; 7:280–285.

11. del Bueno DJ, Griffin LR, Burke SM, Foley MA. The clinical teacher: a critical link in competence development. *J Nurs Staff Dev.* 1990; 6:135–138.

12. Knowles MS. *The Modern Practice of Adult Education: From Pedagogy to Andragogy.* New York, NY: Adult Education; 1980.

13. Hall BP, Rosen LS. *Values-based Leadership Development and an Examination of Corporate Culture.* Fond du Lac, Wis: International Values Institute.

14. Karpiuk K. Career scope—midwest: South Dakota. *Nurs Manage.* 1991; 22(6):66–68.

15. Myers IB, McCaulley MH. *Manual: A Guide to the Development and Use of the Myers-Briggs Type Indicator.* Palo Alto, Calif: Consulting Psychologists Press; 1985.

16. Recker N. Career scope: the conditional compliment—verbal manipulation. *Nurs Manage.* 1993; 24(6):72–73.

FORMULA FOR CULTURAL IDENTIFICATION

1. Choose one research consultant.
2. Add pinches of philosophy and conceptual framework periodically.
3. Let simmer for 5 to 6 years on low heat.
4. Pick a variety of 20 RNs on staff.
5. Put in same room with research consultant for 1 to 2 hours every 2 weeks for a total of 8 weeks.
6. Add carefully selected items from focus group and culture literature.
7. Blend until consensus is reached on:
   • format
   • structure
   • focus group questions
8. Separate and disperse prepared staff to gather cultural aspects of individual units.
9. After collection of unit cultures, compile and share results.
10. Fold together all unit cultures in a large container and watch for mixing.

Yields: A picture of organizational culture that is the basic ingredient for change and growth.

FORMULA FOR CHANGE

1. Gather together a brainstorm of ideas.
2. Sift through present culture.
3. Sort ideas to form a vision.
4. Defrost the old ways of doing things by challenging present norms. (*Note:* Resistance, fear, and defensiveness are normal at this point.)
5. Mix in a heap of flexibility.
6. Add generous portions of innovation and patience as needed to season.
7. Blend in reasons and outcomes until staff display a vested interest.
8. Set aside and let work.
9. Check occasionally, making sure it is rising toward the envisioned outcome. (*Note:* Do not punch down, drop, or startle.)
10. Upon reaching the rim of the container, share with all and begin a new batch.

Stability is suspect.

Change is the norm.

FORMULA FOR PROFESSIONAL GROWTH

1. Proper selection of ingredients is most important. Choose staff with the following:
   - proper state license
   - openness to learn from all avenues
   - willingness to be part of a team yet ability to function independently
   - ability to direct each team member in reaching set goals
   - skillful use of communication
   - adaptability to a variety of changes
   - ethical understanding of current problems
   - acceptance of others and ability to see each person's uniqueness and value
   - ability to incorporate knowledge base with current practice and ongoing research
   - awareness of present culture yet future orientation
2. After selecting staff, mix in the health care setting of your choice that meets these specifications:
   - accepting environment
   - administration open to listening and communicating with all
   - valuing of life-long and career-long learning efforts
   - fair and just treatment given to all
   - focus on the community's present and future needs
   - valuing of employees' individual contributions
   - knowledge sought beyond community to keep up-to-date on current trends
   - law-abiding
   - able to adjust to outside influences
   - willingness to share resources and vision for the future
3. Mixing of the staff in such an environment will lead to growth of the staff and health care facility and excellent health care for those they serve.
4. No need to bake, refrigerate, or freeze.
5. Keep at room temperature, feed, and communicate with daily.
6. Place in sunny spot with adequate ventilation and hydration and watch it grow.

Appendix 2-A
Integrated Care Committee Ground Rules

1. All clients will have equal access to a primary nurse.
2. Nursing diagnosis, using North American Nursing Diagnosis Association (NANDA) nomenclature of "problem as related to" and "evidenced by," will be used as a communication tool among nurses (eg, for focus charting, change of shift report, etc).
3. All clients will be admitted by an RN within 1 hour using the patient admission form (within first home visit for home health care or sooner as determined by unit specialties).
4. All clients will have an assessment-based screening by a primary nurse or clinical care coordinator within 24 hours of admission.
5. An RN will initiate a nursing care plan within 24 hours of admission with a comprehensive care plan to be developed by a primary nurse upon assignment.
6. Upon transfer of a client to a new nursing unit, there will be documented evidence of the client's progress toward long-term goals and need for continued primary nurse intervention.
7. Nursing orders will be followed by all caregivers:
   • Documentation will be according to the nursing orders, indicating action implemented and the client's response.
   • If an order is not followed, the rationale will be documented and/or a variance report completed.
8. Primary nurses will document in the following circumstances:
   • when screening a client
   • when establishing a discharge plan
   • when changes in client needs or plan of care occur
   • when there is progress or lack of progress toward long-term goals (if not already documented by the associate nurse).
9. Primary nurses are responsible for the following:
   • developing and coordinating a comprehensive nursing care plan to include mutually determined long-term goals

- monitoring client progress via use of the Integrated Clinical Pathway(s)
- ensuring that the client is prepared for self-care and discharge

10. Clinical care coordinators are responsible for the following:
    - coordinating unit activities
    - participating in screening of clients, especially when primary nurses are unavailable

11. Associate nurses are responsible for the following:
    - establishing mutual, short-term, within-shift goals with the client
    - documenting goals, implementation, and client responses
    - adding newly apparent, well-defined nursing diagnoses to the care plan

12. The RN will delegate aspects of care to other nursing personnel, taking into consideration the nursing orders and comprehensive care plans for their group of clients.

13. Each unit will determine its ratio of primary/associate/clinical care coordinators depending on practice patterns, acuity, and length of client stay.

14. Unit guidelines/criteria for assignment of primary cases will be determined by the unit-based Integrated Care Committee.

15. Units will be staffed with differentiated practitioners based on an identified practice pattern for the clientele served.

16. Each unit will determine and implement a system to facilitate communication and teamwork among roles.

17. Newly employed RNs may be placed into either the primary nurse or the associate nurse role.

18. Job openings will be posted through personnel for all open positions.

19. A unit-based review committee process will be used when open primary nurse and clinical care coordinator positions are filled using the following:
    - an interviewing process that identifies leadership/team-building activities
    - for primary nurse placement, either the Role Choice Tool or the Factoring Tool

20. Based upon principles of adult learning, orientation of staff to their new positions will be determined mutually by the orientee, preceptor, and nursing standards (The Primary Assessment Form may be used to assist in determining orientation needs of RNs entering the primary nurse role).

21. Each primary nurse and associate nurse will complete the Role Introduction Tool or its equivalent for each role in which the nurse works on each shift or portion thereof for the first 3 to 6 months.

22. The Role Introduction Tool or its equivalent will be used by all orientees/residents until it is mutually decided (based on the nurse's integrating the role into practice) by the orientee/resident and preceptor to discontinue its use.

23. The Chart Monitoring and Evaluation Tool will be completed monthly to reinforce the Role Introduction Tool until it is determined that the guidelines for Integrated Care are being met. Thereafter, chart audits must be utilized at least quarterly to maintain accuracy and consistency within the system.

24. Each unit will implement, through its quality assurance council, a continuing monitoring and evaluation program to ensure that practice meets these guidelines.

Courtesy of Sioux Valley Hospital Integrated Care Committee, Sioux Falls, South Dakota.

3 Consensus

Narcy Recker, Kathryn Linda Karpiuk,
JoEllen Goertz Koerner, and
Kaleen B. Santema

People are usually willing to meet each other half
way but their judgment of distances varies
considerably.

AUTHOR UNKNOWN

WHAT IS CONSENSUS?

Consensus has been defined in many ways and used in a variety of situations. Often it is misused as a means to an end, when someone tires of a discussion and asks whether the group can reach consensus on an issue and go on.

Consensus is much more than merely a way to push toward a decision. True consensus is a group sharing a common goal and reaching a decision that all agree to support. Not all members may be completely satisfied, but all do agree that it is the best decision for all concerned based on their common goal.

The root word, *consent,* means a voluntary yielding to what is proposed or desired by another, an agreement in opinion or sentiment. This typically concerns two choices, such as yes or no questions, and is used in hierarchical power structure situations. Consensus means a collective opinion or general agreement and can have an unlimited number of opinions involved. The power is equally shared among all group members. The difference is in the number of opinions and in the power structure.

Each of us has probably experienced the typical power or decision-making structures. The two main decision-making structures are autocratic and democratic. In the autocratic structure, one person makes the decisions for an entire group. There are obvious advantages, including simplicity and expediency. The major disadvantage to this structure is that only one person's judgment is relied on. In the democratic (majority rule) process, decisions are made according to which options get more than 50% of the vote. Advantages to this process include efficiency, equal voting power by all, and opportunity to share through discussion. Disadvantages include a sense of competition among differing opinions, the possibility that minorities will not be heard, the fact that usually the vote is on two choices, and the possibility that a vote will be requested too early in the discussion.

Consensus is a different way for a group to reach a decision. In consensus, each person truly does have the same power, whether he or she is part of the majority or the minority group. It only takes one person to stop or block a decision from being made. Advantages of the consensus process include equal consideration of all opinions and options, open discussion allowing for the best possible decision to be made, and an agreement by all in the choice made. Disadvantages include the time needed to reach agreement and the possibility of one person blocking agreement indefinitely.

What consensus lacks in speed it makes up for by maximizing creativity, providing a fair opportunity, and providing individual satisfaction for the group members. If the group needs an immediate decision, consensus may be a hindrance; it depends on the issue at hand. If the group needs the best decision for all concerned, consensus can provide a path to that answer. Is the goal speed or quality? Is it both? Depending on how the group is built, you may be able to have the best of both.

BUILDING A GROUP BASED ON THE CONSENSUS MODEL

As with any group process, the building of the group with the necessary structural supports is the most important step.[1] This step is often rushed or not thought through, however, so that the group may be set up for hard times, if not for failure. Is the group meeting to get information, to give information, to participate in decision making, or to make an informed decision? If there is not a common goal, the group may have difficulty reaching decisions or achieving any outcomes. Members may become frustrated and may stop attending meetings. Periodic review of the purpose of the group and/or the outcomes expected may be necessary if the group's efforts are stymied. This review may also be helpful when members repeatedly stray from the course or when the group gets distracted from the purpose. For group members who have not participated before in a group within the organization, the context and culture could be more foreign than for individuals who recently have been in other similar groups in the same organization. The orientation to the group, then, will vary depending on the group's composition.

The first step in building any group is defining the purpose of the group, or why it exists. This is especially important in consensus because of the unique power that each individual member has. The common purpose has to be known and agreed on before any further steps are taken. Without this step, individuals may focus on their own concerns, not those of the group.

Once a group of people with a common purpose meets, there are several other matters that need to be understood clearly before the group begins its tasks. It will be helpful if the group knows how it fits into the structure of the institution within which it functions. It is difficult, but not impossible, for a consensus group to function within a hierarchical system. The group needs to know the limits or boundaries within which it is allowed to function.

Once the group is aware of the power forces with which it will interact outside the group, the power structure within the group needs to be addressed. As stated before, in a consensus group each member, regardless of position or tenure, has equal power. This needs to be explained clearly to the group members.

Early in the demonstration project for differentiated practice at Sioux Valley Hospital, a list of nonnegotiables was developed by the hospital's demonstration project steering committee. These were reminders to the staff and managers. A shorter list of negotiables was also developed to guide the staff when questions arose (Exhibits 3–1 and 3–2). Perhaps other negotiables could have been added, but questions did not arise on other topics.

In conjunction with any power comes responsibility. To be responsible, a person needs to know what the expectations or norms are. These norms should be reviewed periodically and changed when needed. When norms should be developed is a sticky question. Usually a group is formed and then norms for the group are established. Depending on the norms, this may lead to members asking to be released from the group. Although this might have been avoided if norms were established before group formation, preset norms may have prevented interested individuals from joining the group. Norms developed before a group is formed are not norms decided by the group but norms decided for the group by outside forces.

Norms usually address meeting frequency, time, and length; attendance; participation in discussion; visitors; pattern of information flow; and how to bring an issue to the group. A variety of other topics may be included, depending on the group's function. If the group is composed of educators, a norm may be that everyone becomes competent in one class or topic and that each member accepts the responsibility to teach that particular course (Exhibits 3–3 and 3–4).

Some items occasionally addressed in norms will need to be more specific and complete to build a group that makes decisions by consensus. These include shifts in how people communicate and interact with others or a reframing of communication and how business is accomplished. One norm adopted at Sioux Valley Hospital was based on a norm from the Statewide Project Steering Committee: When a person speaks at a meeting, the perspective needs to be clear (ie, whether the person is referring to his or her opinion or the literature). This norm was introduced early in the process of involving staff on committees and changed how people interacted. It also changed interactions with other departments. One day the hospital's librarian

Exhibit 3–1 Nonnegotiables of Model Project

1. Nursing diagnosis, without using medical diagnosis in the statement, will be used as a communication tool among nurses.
2. All patients will be admitted within 1 hour using the Case Associate (CA) admission tool (within the first home visit for home health care).
3. All patients will have a Case Manager (CM) assigned, and the CM assessment tool completed, within 24 hours of admission to a project unit.
4. The CM will initiate a comprehensive nursing care plan within 24 hours, indicating which nursing orders are delegated to a CA.
5. Nursing orders will be followed by the caregivers.
6. Documentation will be according to the nursing orders, indicating what was implemented and the patient's response. If an order is not followed, the rationale will be documented.
7. Each CM, CA, and licensed practical nurse (LPN) working on a model project unit will complete a data collection tool for each role in which the nurse worked for each shift or portion thereof. If necessary, overtime will be paid.
8. There will be a minimum of one chart audit per CM per month during the project with at least one chart audit per CM before the project.
9. CAs will keep the collaborative problem portion of the care plan updated and add newly apparent, common, well-defined nursing diagnoses. Additions to the care plan will be signed by the CM.
10. CMs will keep the comprehensive nursing care plan and teaching plan updated, write mutually determined admission-to-discharge goals, and write a summary in reference to those goals each shift worked.
11. CAs will establish mutual, short-term, within-shift goals with the patient and will document the goals, implementation, and responses.
12. LPNs will be assigned to one or more registered nurses (RNs). RNs will delegate aspects of care to the LPNs, taking into consideration the nursing orders in the comprehensive care plans for the group of patients.
13. CAs and CMs will put the initials *CA* or *CM* before their signature when signing charts to indicate the role assumed for that patient.
14. Units will be staffed according to the predetermined patterns of differentiated positions needed.
15. Nurse managers will complete a weekly summary, tabulate the staff's data collection tools, and evaluate the need for changes. These tools will be sent regularly to the project coordinator.
16. Collaborative problems will not be on the nursing plan summary.
17. Head nurses will assist the project coordinator with compiling data on the cost of the project.
18. New staff will be placed into either the CM or the CA role. Job openings will be posted on the unit for the role(s) open.
19. Head nurses will gather data when staff leave a model project unit as to whether the nurse left because of the project.

Courtesy of the Sioux Valley Hospital Differentiated Practice Steering Committee, Sioux Valley Hospital, Sioux Falls, South Dakota.

Exhibit 3–2 Negotiables of Model Project

1. CMs will give their card to patients and to families to explain their role.
2. CM/CA assignments will be on dry-erase boards on units.
3. Stickers will be put on chart covers to indicate the CM assuming that role.
4. CMs will decide which chart they will audit each month and when it will be done.
5. CAs will determine which aspects of care/nursing orders they will delegate to an LPN that are within the LPN's job description.
6. Method of patients getting on CMs' caseloads will be unit determined.

Courtesy of the Sioux Valley Hospital Differentiated Practice Steering Committee, Sioux Valley Hospital, Sioux Falls, South Dakota.

asked why computer searches including business literature were now being requested. Copies of articles from *Forbes* and *Fortune* had been requested by a group researching compensation by salary compared to wages. When the librarian understood that staff were now expected to bring information from the literature, the library improved accessibility by expanding its business holdings.

Norms should also include behavioral expectations of members both within the group and with coworkers when discussing the work of the group. For instance, if a member disagrees with the group, will that fact be confidential to the group, or will everyone in the organization be privy to that conflict? The examples of norms included in Exhibits and 3–3 and 3–4 do not address all aspects of a person's behavior, such as using first party communication. That is an expectation in this organization. In other groups, a certain behavior may not be as much a part of the culture and therefore might need to be stated clearly in the group norms.

We typically learn first party communication in infancy but are then socially taught to not use it as we continue to grow. During the formative years, when an individual makes a mistake he or she is quickly corrected with a verbal no and possibly with an explanation of why it is not appropriate behavior. This is part of the cultural and social development of the child. Somewhere during early school years, as individuality and independence develop, it seems that a new norm emerges, and we learn that it is not socially acceptable to tell an individual directly if we have a problem with his or her actions or words. A number of uninvolved individuals may be told, but not the person around whom the conversation is focused.

Such hidden negative communication can be damaging in a variety of ways. The person under scrutiny has no way of knowing and, therefore, no way of explaining the reasons for the action or words and so is left defenseless. Other individuals told may be swayed by the one-sided information, which may continue to be passed along to others. The person being discussed may hear the comments from an uninvolved party, which may create negative feelings for the person sharing the biased information. The person being discussed, not knowing that there is a concern about his or her words or actions, may continue to practice in the same fashion.

Exhibit 3–3 Integrated Care Committee Group Norms

1. The meetings will be open.
2. There must be 15 members present to have a quorum.
3. Voting will be done by show of hands. An amendment can be made at any time asking for role call vote.
4. Units will be allowed to select their own membership.
5. Alternates will be allowed to attend meetings. The alternate will not be designated but left as an open position. The alternate should be informed of the agenda before the meeting.
6. The meetings will be on a monthly basis. This can be changed (by vote) to a different schedule.
7. Meeting minutes should be distributed and posted on each unit within seven working days of the meeting.
8. An agenda for the next meeting should be included at the end of the minutes. The final agenda will be sent to the member's home address 5 days before the next meeting.
9. Debates, issues, and written recommendations are to be placed on the agenda. Either the member or a speaker recommended by the member will present the issue. Twelve members (75%) must be present to pass a voting issue. If an issue does not pass a vote, it may be reviewed at the next meeting provided that new information can be added to support the issue. A member of the committee must approve if an issue is to be reviewed more than twice.
10. Decisions can be communicated back to the unit by either the minutes or the member.

Courtesy of Sioux Valley Hospital, Sioux Falls, South Dakota.

As the outcomes are identified, it becomes obvious that such a mode of communication would not fit into a professional practice model. For that reason, first party communication, which is speaking directly with the person concerned and no one else, is an expected norm. For this to be done effectively, training in confrontation techniques is helpful. Your willingness to share concerns with another about his or her practice means that you are then opening yourself up for the same scrutiny. In confrontation training, the handling of these situations is taught and practiced.

A topic that should be part of confrontation classes is the issue of exactly what is open to the scrutiny of professional colleagues and what is none of their concern. Ground rules on what is and is not appropriate as an area of concern should be clear to all professionals. For example, an individual's personality preferences should not be under scrutiny. Whether one is an introvert or an extrovert is not an area that should be of concern to colleagues. The same individual's job performance, however, according to meeting the set standards, is of concern and open to

Exhibit 3–4 Integrated Clinical Pathways Task Force Group Norms

1. Should the meeting be open or closed?
   The meeting will be open to all nurses as well as to students and other disciplines. Any member can invite a guest speaker to address a specific issue on the agenda. The task force reserves the privilege to close meetings for confidential issues.
2. How should decisions be made?
   Decisions will be made by a group vote. Voting will not be sought until all members have had an opportunity to speak on the issue. Voting will be done by consensus of the group. If consensus is unattainable, voting will be postponed until the next meeting, where a decision will be reached.
3. If a member is not able to attend, should a substitute be allowed?
   Substitutes will be allowed to attend a meeting in the absence of a task force member. Substitutes will be given the authority to speak for task force members in their absence. Members are asked to contact the chair or nursing administrative secretary before the meeting to inform him or her of their absence and who their alternate will be.
4. What is expected of members?
   All members are expected to be in attendance at each meeting. Every member present must be given the opportunity to express his or her views.
5. How will the agenda be determined?
   Meetings will be conducted informally utilizing an agenda that is prepared at the end of the previous meeting. Each agenda item will have a specified time frame, which will be listed on the agenda. Members can add items to the agenda by contacting the chair. The chair may add additional agenda items. The agenda will be sent to the members 1 week before the meeting.
6. Should minutes be taken?
   Role call and minutes will be taken by the nursing administrative secretary. Minutes will be read at the meeting and summarized for *Nursing Speaks.*
7. How will decisions and discussion be conducted?
   All members will support decisions made by this council. Discussion is acceptable outside the meetings. No minority opinions will be identified outside the task force.
8. How will meetings be conducted?
   The chair reserves the right to cancel a meeting, reschedule a meeting, or schedule special meetings.
9. Who will facilitate the meeting when the chair is absent?
   The chair will select a member to assume responsibility of chairing the meeting.
10. How will evaluations be performed?
    Evaluation of decisions made by the task force will be an ongoing process.
11. How can members change/add to group norms?
    To change or add to group norms, the issue must be included on the agenda for discussion by the entire group.

Courtesy of Sioux Valley Hospital, Sioux Falls, South Dakota.

comments from professional colleagues. The mode in which one operates, as long as it is within legal and ethical bounds, is not necessarily open for professional scrutiny, but meeting set standards is. Clearly, one needs to know exactly what is expected of a person in a specific role, and the meeting of these expectations should be the grounds on which one is judged by colleagues.

Another requirement for effective confrontation is the ability to resist accepting second-hand information or complaints from others. If first party communication is the norm, second-hand information or gossip needs to be refused and not reinforced.

If first party communication is practiced, the participants will be more empowered concerning their practice, more aware of how their own actions and words affect others, and more trusting of their colleagues who use the same practice. No backstabbing, finger pointing, or surprises on performance evaluations should occur. Constant positive feedback and reinforcement on each other's words and actions will be the norm.[2]

Consensus will work best if there is shared trust by all members of the group. This means that each individual must look inward at his or her own attitudes and develop an openness to others. There are individual traits or gifts that are needed for certain tasks, but no personality type is right or correct for one to be a group member. Focusing on the common goal is the key factor. Openness to and acceptance of each person as unique and important are required in a consensus group.

Understanding the "Pygmalion effect" may be of benefit to groups using consensus for making decisions. Pygmalion, a character in Greek mythology, was an artist whose quest was to sculpt the perfect woman. So good was his attempt that he fell in love with his finished work. The goddess Aphrodite felt pity for him and brought the carved figure to life. The point of this story is that belief can create reality. Whatever you think of a person is typically what you will see as reality, although this may not be true.

Another example is the musical *My Fair Lady*. In this story, Higgins sees possibilities in a young working woman and changes her into a woman who could be mistaken for royalty. If one person believes another person can become more, it may become a reality. Unfortunately, the converse is also true. If you label someone as unable to communicate, regardless of what communication skills he or she learns to use you may always only see the negative side. Labels, prejudices, and assumptions need to be put aside and replaced with openness.

In a consensus group there should also be a shared sense of growth in developing communication skills. Each member must assist others in the process for the whole to benefit. As the old adage says, a chain is only as strong as its weakest link. Communication is the chain holding all together.

The *Abilene Paradox*[3] illustrates the importance of communication. In this story a family group member proposes a possible diversion for a hot afternoon simply as a means to open up conversation. Each of the other family members, although thinking the idea is poor, decides not to rock the boat, so that each heartily agrees. The suggestion is that they get into a hot, unairconditioned car and travel more than 50 miles to eat. This occurs, and all are miserable throughout the whole ordeal. Upon returning home, the person who initially suggested the outing complains that they should not have gone. The others chime in in agreement. They realize that open, honest communication, even at the risk of upsetting someone else, is the only way to decide what is best for all concerned.

Unlike other decision-making methods, consensus will take more time and will depend on how the group reaches its decision. These need to be addressed in norms. As in any group, but more so in consensus groups, some topics can take an unusually long time for the members to understand all the factors and reach a decision. See the case study in Exhibit 3–5 for an illustration of the effect that time can have on reaching consensus. In a consensus group, the members need to understand that the time needed will be taken. Without this commitment to allowing time, consensus may not be reached.

> *Take time to deliberate, but when the time for*
> *action has arrived, stop thinking and go in.*
> NAPOLEON BONAPARTE

In some consensus groups, the necessary structures that allow for ample time and prevent wasted time are built into the norms. By devising norms in this fashion, the time needed is taken, but beating the issue to death is not allowed. Two examples of such norms are those that prevent repeating past discussions for members who were absent and setting deadlines for all concerns to be voiced. Even with such structuring, reaching consensus will possibly take longer than other decision-making models, but decisions reached will be agreed on by all. When decisions are fully supported, implementation proceeds more smoothly without the consequences of the disgruntled minority sabotaging the efforts of the majority.

Finally, the process used to reach a decision needs to be addressed. How is the decision made? Is it researched and presented by the chair with discussion following? Is information obtained on a voluntary basis? Is the person who is bringing the item to the attention of the group also responsible for explaining it to the group? How does the process start, move toward conclusion, and finally reach an end point? What is done with the decision? How is it communicated, implemented, and followed up on, and who is accountable for each piece? Without a consistent process, the outcome may vary wildly from time to time. If any issue can be dropped on a group at any instant, valuable time can be wasted and hasty decisions made without needed research or discussion. The process needs to be clear to all.

Any group that is formed and assigned work without the required preparation may face a difficult future. The more clear a picture of who, what, when, where,

Exhibit 3–5 Case Study: Corporate

Consensus can be reached within a group or among groups. Nursing leadership is often called upon to assist two different groups with common goals to come to an agreement on the same outcome. When the nursing practice at Sioux Valley Hospital moved further into differentiated practice, a number of patients fell through the cracks. These individuals had unmet health care needs at discharge but did not meet the stringent requirements for home health care services. As the staff reviewed the literature and dialogued with colleagues from around the country, the notion of case management became a potential solution to the issue. A major stumbling block for this innovation, however, was the fact that South Dakota did not have any managed care. Thus the organization was not interested in case management because it would negatively affect the revenue stream in a hospital with a Medicare population approaching 50%.

The nursing administrators assisted a group of clinical nurse specialists to manage a small group of patients who were outliers, costing the institution many lost dollars. This group kept careful record of their activities and the effects they had on both quality and cost. At the same time a series of articles on nursing case management was routed to the executive management team to introduce them to the concept and the successful outcomes experienced by colleagues across the country who were living in heavily managed care environments. When appropriate in strategic planning dialogue, the nurse executive shared examples of the work of nurses in general, or of Sioux Valley Hospital nurses in particular, to illustrate further the efficacy of this model of care delivery.

At last, the wave of managed care crashed into the state, and executive management was faced with a need to take a corporate stand on the concept. By this time the small group of clinical nurse specialists had a history of experience and some expertise with this care delivery system. Furthermore, they had developed meaningful relationships with personnel in medical records, finance, and data processing and a small core of physicians. When the chief executive officer began to look for answers to manage the new force within the state, nursing came forward with examples and a proposal for nursing case management that had the support and interest of other departments within the organization.

The result of bringing together the needs of the organization and the skills of a group of staff was the establishment of the Center for Case Management managed by advanced nursing practice at Sioux Valley Hospital. Understanding all the contributing factors took time. It also was necessary for the climate to be right for this decision. Once these components were present, consensus was reached quickly.

why, and how a group will function, the easier it will be for the group to reach its goals. Start with why, because without a clear understanding of the purpose the rest of the questions are meaningless. See Exhibit 3–6 for an illustration of a committee that uses consensus for decision making.

Exhibit 3–6 Case Study: Committee

The Staffing/Scheduling Committee was established in 1986. This marked the beginning of a cultural shift in consensus-building management style. Rather than orders being sent down from on high without staff being consulted, decisions would now be made after input was received from the team. Using this participative management style was the first step in preparing staff for making decisions by consensus.

Previously the staffing/scheduling standard operating procedure was reviewed and/or revised by nursing administration annually. This task was now given to the committee for making recommendations to nursing administration. Other purposes of this committee were to oversee the implementation of the acuity-based scheduling program, to develop scheduling policy alternatives, and to develop a nursing staffing and scheduling management information system.

The entire first year of the committee was spent in revising and standardizing the staffing/scheduling standard operating procedure. The members were willing to be open to express their viewpoints, opinions, and thoughts relative to alternative solutions. Discussion, debate, and feedback occurred. Many discussions produced conflicts and differing points of view; these were necessary components of this decision-making process. There was a great deal of eagerness and commitment on the part of the committee members to produce. They felt consulted and informed and experienced a sense of connectedness. The attendance at committee meetings was high as a result of this interest and commitment.

After a year of working together and reaching consensus on the staffing/scheduling standard operating procedure, the group members had a real sense of accomplishment and empowerment. The members began to seek other alternatives to the existing scheduling system. The concept of self-scheduling was explored. Self-scheduling is the process by which staff on a unit collectively decide and implement the monthly work schedule. The committee believed that self-scheduling would increase the autonomy of the staff nurses by giving them control and responsibility for their work schedules.

The process to reach consensus to have self-scheduling was unit specific. Each unit formulated an action committee to develop unit policies. Ninety percent of the staff needed to be in favor of trialing self-scheduling before beginning. Seventy-five percent acceptance was needed to continue self-scheduling. By the end of 1987, two units were trialing self-scheduling. Five years later, the entire professional nursing practice was utilizing self-scheduling.

Careful explanation was given to the committee members initially that they were a recommending body, not a decision-making body. The original composition of this committee was a unit manager from each of the three nursing divisions, one nursing supervisor, one special projects coordinator, one professional nurse practice council member (staff nurse) from each of the three nursing divisions, and a nursing administrator, who chaired the committee. In 1988, the membership expanded to include three more staff members from each nursing division.

It did not take the group long to recognize that practicing nurses were essential to accomplishing the work of the committee. In 1991, the membership was

continues

Exhibit 3–6 continued

expanded to include three float nurses. The people whose lives were affected by these decisions needed to participate in the decision-making process to achieve acceptance and compliance. Every registered nurse job role needed to be represented. The membership of the committee changed from primarily one of management representation to that of staff.

In 1990 the nursing practice moved toward a shared governance model, as discussed in Chapter 7. The Staffing/Scheduling Committee became an ad hoc committee of the Management Council and now makes recommendations to that council rather than to nursing administration. Also in 1991 the chair was elected from the membership, with the nursing administrator serving in an advisory capacity only.

This was the first Sioux Valley Hospital committee to establish norms. Because this committee was different from any other in composition and task, a great deal of effort was spent on purpose and structure. The norms adopted by the committee were patterned after the norms of the steering committee for the Statewide Project for Nursing and Nursing Education. The original group norms of the Staffing/Scheduling Committee were primarily unchanged with the exception of the decision-making process. See Appendix 3-A for the norms of this committee.

Initially decisions were made by majority vote. During the revision and standardization of the staffing/scheduling standard operating procedure, discussion of a section continued until agreement was reached before that section was considered finished. Making decisions by consensus was accomplished much more easily after the first year because this committee was accustomed to dialoguing on issues in depth and problem solving. Therefore, when the nursing practice moved toward a shared governance model and consensus became the way decisions were made, this committee in essence had already evolved to this decision-making process by the management style of the committee chair. The norms, however, needed to be revised to reflect this change in decision-making style. It is obvious that consensus requires more time and commitment to the process.

Today, the purpose of the Staffing/Scheduling Committee is to serve as a consultant to the nursing practice regarding staffing and scheduling alternatives and issues. It also has the responsibility to develop strategies that are responsive to nursing care delivery yet appropriate given current economic constraints.

ROLES FOR A CONSENSUS GROUP

When using a consensus model for decision making, the members need to understand the group structure and the roles of the group members. Although the members fulfilling these roles may vary from meeting to meeting, the primary roles are facilitator and recorder. Other roles that may be present are norms keeper, mediator, timekeeper, process watcher, vibes watcher, and devil's advocate. The presence of these roles depends on the size, formality, and sophistication of the group in making decisions by consensus.

The facilitator is responsible for organizing the agenda before the meeting, reviewing the agenda at the beginning of the meeting with the group, following the set agenda, and helping the group determine whether consensus can be achieved. This person may often paraphrase members' ideas to help the group identify common themes and diverse ideas. When consensus does not appear possible in the time frame proposed on the agenda, the facilitator should bring that to the group's awareness. The group may then decide to postpone the decision, set up a task force to explore the topic further, or defer the decision to another meeting.

The recorder takes minutes of the main discussion points and all decisions made. The recorder must identify when consensus has been reached. This may require reading what has been recorded in the minutes to identify whether the recorder's perceptions are correct. Waiting a month or more until the next meeting to determine whether the minutes are correct on a hot topic may be too long.

The norms keeper is responsible for identifying when the group's norms are not being followed. For instance, a norm may be that everyone will have the opportunity to address an issue before a member speaks for a second time. If one member is monopolizing the discussion, the norms keeper reminds the group about the adopted norms. After the first reminder to a group, the norms keeper may merely need to say, "Norms!"

> *Many people in business—and in life in general—*
> *live by win/lose: If someone wins, then someone*
> *else must lose. Besides win/lose strategies, there*
> *are also strategies for negotiation and for win/*
> *win. Win/win means we are both in the same boat.*
> *You have an oar and so do I and we want to go to*
> *the same place.*
>
> GEORGE PEABODY

The mediator is responsible for intervening when the discussion is polarized and consensus appears impossible. The mediator may try asking this question of the group: "Can you live with ___ ?" It may not be what anyone really prefers, but it may be the compromise that is necessary for the group to move forward. In some cases it may be a temporary measure until more information can be obtained. The mediator is not necessarily an assigned role but can be assumed by any group member who sees the possibility for compromise.

The timekeeper is necessary for groups that have difficulty staying within the time frames established for the agenda. The person must be able to interrupt the group to remind the members that the time allowed for the discussion is almost or entirely over. This is a cue for the group members as well as for the facilitator that a decision must be made quickly or that the group must determine another course of action, as discussed earlier in this section.

*There are no new truths, but only truths that have
not been recognized by those who have perceived
them without noticing.*

MARY MCCARTHY

The process watcher is responsible for identifying problems in the group's processing. For instance, if the group has made several assumptions about a topic and now appears ready to make a decision, the process watcher needs to help the group understand that the assumptions may be erroneous and that the group may not have all the necessary information. Another example is when the group is making a decision on an emotional level rather than on a factual level; the process watcher should identify this response to the situation. When these difficulties are brought to the attention of the group, action can then be taken.

The vibes watcher, often an easier role for a perceptive person, is cognizant of the group's emotional climate. When individual or group feelings are not expressed but are perceived by someone watching for these feelings, the vibes watcher has two choices: Do nothing, or intervene. Bringing the feelings to the group's attention is not always necessary; an intervention may just be getting the group back on the topic. Clearing the air, however, is sometimes the best intervention, particularly if the feelings are interfering with reaching consensus.

The devil's advocate is responsible for raising the questions necessary for the group to discuss the worst scenario. These "What if . . . ?" questions will also assist the group to consider the positions of those people affected by the decision but not represented by the group.

*Self-expression must pass into communication for
its fulfillment.*

PEARL S. BUCK

All group members also have responsibilities in a consensus decision-making model. Members are expected to add items to the agenda when needed and to come prepared to the meeting. They are expected to follow the group's norms and focus on the group's purpose rather than on their own agenda. Members are expected to communicate with the group and listen to others' opinions. This may include changing their stance as more information is available to them so that consensus can be reached. When new members join the group, everyone should help orient them. Group members who represent a constituency, such as a senator, are expected to communicate with those represented. The group member must also express the views of his or her constituency, when relevant, and consider the views when making a decision.

BLOCKING IN DECISION MAKING

The equality of power in the consensus model is unique. In the majority rules process each person has an equal vote, but it is the majority of the group that decides, not the entire group. History is replete with examples of majority rule decisions with less than humanitarian outcomes. Exceptional leaders can entice individuals to join in causes without the individuals considering the consequences of the decision for the minority. Examples are slavery in the early history of the United States and the tactics of Nazi Germany. Majority rule does not always lead to the best decision for all concerned.

The unique power in the consensus model is referred to as the right to block. Blocking is a safeguard to protect the minority views and to assist in providing the highest-quality decisions for all concerned. Even though the term *blocking* may have negative connotations, this power exists to provide a positive outcome for all.

Trying to define or describe this power without using this term is difficult. Blocking is not just the ability of a person to block consensus from happening. Blocking can be defined as the withholding of a group member's consent in an effort to prevent hasty or less than adequate decisions from being made. A decision is not made in a consensus group as long as one member does not agree. That is powerful, and it is at the center of the consensus model.

Unless this concept is understood, individuals who exercise this power could be seen as troublemakers or could be blamed for not being team players. If blaming occurs, it is a sign that the concept of consensus is not understood, and this lack of knowledge should be dealt with immediately. Rash decisions can be made if all the needed or relevant information is not available or shared. A group may come to a quick and easy decision on an issue only to find, when a bit more information is made known, that everything changes.

Any time a group member is aware of relevant information that may change the outcome of a decision, it is that person's responsibility to communicate that information. A group member is responsible for giving all the information as clearly and thoroughly as possible. It becomes the responsibility of the remaining group members to listen and question to reach an understanding. To do this means that they must remain open.

If the person presenting the information gives a sound reason for his or her opinion, other people will seek alternatives. All the facts and opinions are needed, not just those that satisfy the majority. Blocking is not only a right but a major responsibility of each group member.

If a group member feels that a decision is wrong on moral, personal, or other grounds, it is his or her responsibility to act. The individual should act when the concern is noted, bringing the reasons into discussion as soon as possible. If a group member is not sure about blocking consensus, the individual should answer the questions listed in Exhibit 3–7. The answers to these questions can guide the group member's decision to block or agree. It is not always an easy decision to make.

What does a group member do if he or she cannot agree with the decision and is unable to persuade other group members to change their minds? Is the group blocked forever? In such situations, two options are available. A time out can be called, during which the group can reflect upon the information. If this does not lead to consensus, then the person blocking may choose to have his or her concerns recorded in the minutes and may ask not to be directly involved in the implementation of the decision.

An escape clause built into the structure of the group may also be a good idea in situations where a decision is needed immediately. The escape clause could allow the group to revert to a majority rule decision-making process in instances where an immediate decision is needed.[1] For example, suppose a group is no longer able to continue renting its current building. For several months alternative locations have been sought. The lease ends at the end of the week, however, and consensus on a new location has not been reached. The group may use majority rule to decide on temporary quarters. Another option is to go with the decision of the majority with an automatic review of the decision within a certain time after implementation. This will allow for reflection on outcomes based on the group's decision.

PITFALLS AND COMMON PROBLEMS

There are a variety of problems that occur with group activities. It is no different with a consensus group. Factioning, for example, is the situation where the group divides into two or more factions. If this happens consistently, a problem exists. Two reasons may lead to this behavior. One is long-term unresolved conflict, and the other is a philosophic difference between the two groups.[1] When factioning occurs, it is time to discuss the problem.

Exhibit 3–7 Questions To Facilitate Decision Concerning Blocking Consensus

Will the information I have change people's minds? Is it relevant?
Has it been discussed to the extent it should be, or are there still unknowns?
Have the reasons been stated before but may not be understood?
What will the outcomes be if this decision goes through?
Is there an immediate need to make a decision that supersedes these reasons?

Source: Information from *Building United Judgment: A Handbook for Consensus Decision Making* by Avery M, Auvine B, Streibel B, Weiss L, pp. 30-31, Center for Conflict Resolution, Madison, Wisconsin, © 1981.

If the difference is philosophic, a meeting to identify common goals and to discuss roadblocks and frustrations may help resolve the situation. Group members might also be reminded to accept differences as a given and to focus on the common goal of the group. If the factioning is related to unresolved conflict, then it is definitely time to bring these conflicts out into the open and to deal with the issues. Facts should be shared and feelings discussed as calmly as possible. A mediator may be helpful in keeping the discussion focused on the issues. Whatever the conflict, deal with it immediately and in a fair fashion for all concerned.

Another common problem can be the length of discussion time. Either extreme can be a cause for concern. Hasty decisions may be the result of insufficient information, unclear goals, or poor facilitation. Unending discussions may result from individual goals, unclear goals, or poor facilitation. If either extreme is noted, analyze the cause and direct attention to its solution. An experienced facilitator and guidelines on the group's norms can be of assistance in preventing these problems.

If the group discussion is frequently dominated by one or a few members, another problem must be addressed. Possibly this communication pattern is a part of the dominating person's style. If so, it is up to the group members to assist this member to modify the behavior. Reminding the group of the norms is not the only solution. Clarifying or summarizing what the person is attempting to say are two other possible ways to do this. This imbalance in speaking time may also be the result of an imbalance in power. In this case it is best to acknowledge the problem and work together to change it. The dominating person may need to let go and allow less experienced individuals the opportunity to express ideas.

A group that sees issues resurfacing after decisions are made has another problem. Returning to the same issues repeatedly is a sign that the decisions being made are of low quality. Several possible reasons for this exist: Group members are not voicing concerns during the discussion phase of the process, all the needed information was not available, the final decision was not clearly stated, or decisions were made on issues without implementation or accountability being decided. Analyzing why the decision was rejected so quickly may help pinpoint where attention needs to be focused.

A serious situation may arise if a member does not follow the norms, such as breaking confidentiality or attacking individuals in the group when speaking to constituents. When a member does not adhere to the norms, the member must be removed from the group. Trust has been broken, and the member's presence is disruptive to the group's functioning.

The last problem discussed here is a group member being considered uncooperative. This is probably the most difficult problem to face. This problem, like conflict management of group factions, needs to be dealt with immediately. The first step is to analyze why the person is viewed as uncooperative. Ask the individual whether he or she is committed to cooperating and to accepting differences. If the person is committed, the problem may not be the person but the group's ability to accept differences. Supporting the member in question while analyzing this problem is imperative. The person labeled as uncooperative will feel alienated and alone already.

A variety of possible solutions exists. Third party mediation is again an option. If possible, a change in the person's role may be in order until the issues are settled. For instance, a staff nurse may be voluntarily relocated to another unit for a specified time. This would necessitate having available resources to fill the person's role until he or she returns. During this time, assessment of both the original group's working relationship and the individual's new group involvement would be accomplished by an objective individual, not a member of either group. A leave of absence from the group may be necessary as a last resort. The important factor is to address the problem. Rarely does a group come to the best decision possible if different types of people are not involved in the process. Too much sameness in a group can be deadly to all who do not fit.

If all efforts toward eliciting cooperation between an individual and a group fail, then the possibility of a truly uncooperative member exists. In identifying this, it is also important to understand that the reason for the lack of cooperation is still unknown. When the point is reached where no hope of cooperation exists, however, the person may have to be asked respectfully to leave the group.

What is needed for consensus is a group willing to work together toward a common goal. With support, guidance, and the needed resources, the possibilities, although endless, will always have the best interests of all concerned as their focus.

> *May we always have the patience to listen and the courage to speak.*
>
> FACILITATION COMMITTEE,
> FEDERATION OF OHIO RIVER COOPERATIVES

REFERENCES

1. Avery M, Auvine B, Streibel B, Weiss L. *Building United Judgment: A Handbook for Consensus Decision Making*. Madison, Wis: Center for Conflict Resolution; 1981.
2. Recker N. Career scope: the conditional compliment—verbal manipulation. *Nurs Manage*. 1993; 24(6):72–73.
3. Reynolds JM. *The Abilene Paradox* [Videotape]. New York, NY: McGraw-Hill Training Systems; 1984.

EXERCISE 3–1: GROUP ACTIVITY—REFLECTIONS[1]

For this game you need to divide into pairs, which can work separately or with another pair. Begin by having the facilitator ask a simple but personal question (eg, What do you most value in this institution?).

The work of the pairs begins with one member answering the question the way he or she thinks his or her partner would answer the question, not how the person would himself or herself. The partner listens and comments on how the answer is the same or different from what the answer really would have been. The pair or pairs can then continue sharing why answers were chosen, how each felt about what the other said, and so on. Then reverse roles, and have the partner respond as he or she thinks the first person would have answered the same question.

Using this exercise can help each person gain a better understanding of the other and also can identify problem areas.

EXERCISE 3–2: GROUP ACTIVITY—DYADIC RISK TAKING[1]

For this exercise you divide into pairs. Seating can be a side-by-side arrangement, to regulate eye contact as the pair wishes, or with the partners across from each other. Each partner is asked to tell the other partner something personal about himself or herself. It can be whatever the person would like to share (eg, I don't like to eat mushrooms; my checking account has $2300 in it; I have been diagnosed as diabetic; I like the color blue).

After the statement, the partner is asked to rate the statement as to how risky it was to make (0, no risk; 1, minimal risk; 2, mild risk; and 3, a pretty big risk). The partner writes down the score but does not show it to the other person. The person should not respond to the statement, only score the response and then make a statement of his or her own.

When five statements have been made and judged by each person, the partners then share the scores with each other. Discussion is held as to why ratings were what they were and how the partners came to the conclusions they did. Also discussed is whether there are any differences in how each rated the other's statements. If there were differences, why? Did the type of statement each made change in any way?

Through this, perceptions, judgments, trust, and risk taking can be discovered.

EXERCISE 3–3: GROUP ACTIVITY—MOST PRECIOUS POSSESSION[1]

To begin this exercise, each member must come prepared by bringing along a precious possession, one that will fit in a box. Each person brings the item and, without letting anyone else see it, puts it in the designated box.

After all members have placed their possessions in the box, the facilitator begins by picking an item out of the box. Discussion begins as to whom the group thinks the item belongs to and why they think that.

When all items have been displayed and all guesses made, the owners come forward, one by one, to retrieve their possession and explain why the object means so much to them. Other members are then asked to share their feelings and what they have learned about themselves and the other members of the group.

Appendix 3-A
Sioux Valley Hospital Staffing/Scheduling Committee Group Norms, November 1992-November 1993

1. Should this committee be opened or closed?

   Closed and open by invitation or request only. It will be decided by the chair when someone can attend for the purpose of speaking about an agenda item. If there is an agenda item, the committee member is to contact the chair or secretary of this committee.

2. If students are following a committee member, should they be allowed to sit in on the meeting?

   Yes.

3. If a member is not able to attend, should a substitute be allowed?

   No substitutes or alternates. It was felt that this meeting would be confusing if not attended on a regular basis.

4. What should be done when a member of the committee does not attend regularly?

   The nursing administrative secretary will keep track of how many times each member misses a meeting. After four consecutive absences or six absences, the member will be contacted regarding his or her intent to continue on the committee or to discontinue. This will be discussed with the appropriate department head if the member wishes to resign.

5. What should a committee member do if he or she cannot attend a meeting?

   Members are to contact the administrative secretary before noon on the day of the meeting.

6. How many members should be present to have a working meeting and a voting meeting?

   To have a working meeting, there needs to be a committee member from each division. To have a voting meeting, there needs to be a voting member from each division. The chair will have the option to table a vote until the next meeting.

7. How often should the committee meet?

   Every first Monday of the month at 1430 to 1600 hours, unless exceptions are made.

8. Should minutes be taken?

    The nursing administrative secretary will take minutes.

9. If the nursing administrative secretary is gone, can minute taking be rotated among the group?

    Yes.

10. How should the information be communicated to others?

    Minutes will be routed at each meeting for review and returned to the administrative secretary at the end of each meeting. Minutes will be kept in each staffing coordinator's office for review by those on the units. It will be the responsibility of each committee member to share with his or her colleagues the information discussed at these meetings.

11. Are all decisions binding, and should minority votes not be discussed outside the committee?

    Yes.

12. How should the decision process be instituted?

    Voting will be held by consensus. If consensus cannot be reached, the issue will be brought back to the next meeting, and a vote will be taken by majority.

13. How should staff concerns and/or suggestions be given to the committee?

    Concerns/suggestions should be in writing and presented to one of the committee members to be read at the meeting.

14. How should meeting agendas be distributed?

    Agendas for the meeting will be sent out the Monday before the meeting. If a committee member has an item to be discussed at the meeting, he or she is to contact the administrative secretary before noon the Monday before the meeting so that it may be placed on the agenda.

15. Who should present the concern and/or suggestion to the committee?

    The member who received the concern or suggestion. If the member of the committee feels it is not appropriate for him or her to present, the secretary or chair will read it to the committee.

16. Should the concern and/or suggestion be anonymous?

    The committee felt that the concern and/or suggestion should be signed but would not need to be presented with the individual's name.

17. Will debate be kept confidential?

    Yes.

18. How should discussion outside the committee be handled?

    Discussion that occurs in this committee may be shared outside the committee. Decisions made by the committee are to be supported by all committee members.

19. How will decision making proceed?

    Decisions will not commence until all members present have had a chance to speak on the issue.

20. How often will issues be discussed?

    Committee members may speak on an issue twice but are requested to wait until all have spoken on the issue before they speak again.

21. Should a time limit be developed for presentation of an issue or comment?

    The committee felt this should be decided based on the issue and the amount of time needed to make a decision.

22. Should representatives from personnel and payroll be a part of this committee?

    The committee felt that payroll and personnel would be invited when issues are related to personnel and payroll.

23. If a committee member is replaced before the end of his or her term, should the new committee member finish the term or begin a new 3-year term?

    The new member will complete the term of the member rotating off the committee.

24. How will the committee be chaired?

    This committee will have a chair who will serve for 1 year. A chair-elect will serve 1 year as chair-elect and 1 year as chair.

25. Who will serve as liaison to nursing administration?

    Jane Doe, Nursing Administrator, will be a liaison to this committee on behalf of nursing administration.

Courtesy of Sioux Valley Hospital, Sioux Falls, South Dakota.

4 Choice

Kathryn Linda Karpiuk and Chris Nicolai

The strength, the grossness, spirit and gall of choice.
MURIEL RUKEYSER

Whether we are male or female, child or adult, rich or poor, American or Russian, everyone is in the business of making choices. Reflecting on the choices in life, most people are mainly aware of the major choices, those that have set a major direction in their life, such as marriage choices, career choices, family choices, and spiritual choices. There are thousands of smaller, unnoticed choices made each day, however, that profoundly affect an individual's life.

Each second, minute, hour, and day of life, individuals have the freedom to make choices. Choices are made about what to say, how much to eat, how to feel, what to think, and how to act; this list can continue ad infinitum. Americans have greater opportunity than some people in other countries to exert this freedom to choose. People of communist countries may feel overwhelmed when they are suddenly expected to make choices. Often choices in less controlling environments are made without much conscious thought. It would be overwhelming to count the number of choices people experience each and every day. Even hostages in captivity have internal choices that no one can take away. In essence, the freedom of choice is fundamental to the human spirit and life.

One of the cornerstones of differentiated practice at Sioux Valley Hospital is the concept of choice. This chapter explores the ideologies of choice. The choices made available to nursing through a professional practice model that includes differentiated practice and shared governance are then presented. Practical aspects of putting choice to work at Sioux Valley Hospital are also discussed.

THE POWER OF CHOICE

Readers may wonder why we have devoted a whole chapter to choice. What is so important about choice at Sioux Valley Hospital? To understand why choice is so important, the concept of choice needs to be explored.

One way to understand a concept (such as choice) is to discuss concepts related to it. One concept related to choice is autonomy. Leddy and Pepper[1] describe autonomy as an individual's ability to make rational and unconstrained choices or decisions. It is also the ability to act on those decisions. For example, a patient has the right to autonomy in making informed choices regarding medical care. Thus patients have the choice or self-determination to accept or reject any therapy that is prescribed for them.

Autonomy in the work setting consequently means that nurses have control over their own function in the hospital work environment. How this control is exercised is through the ability to make choices. Shared governance is one vehicle that can be used to bring the power of choice to a hospital. The whole essence of shared governance is the principle of letting nurses have the autonomy to make the choices and decisions in areas that affect their practice.

Another concept related to choice is power. The type of power to which this refers is called nutrient power. Miller defines nutrient power as "providing and caring for self, directing others regarding self care, and being the ultimate decision maker regarding care."[2(p3)] In simple terms, power is the ability through choices to influence what happens to oneself.

In contrast, when individuals do not have choices to control themselves, they are in a state of powerlessness. Miller's model[2] (Figure 4–1) depicts how powerlessness sets up a cycle of low self-esteem and depression, hopelessness, and immobilization with an inability to solve problems, to set goals, and to take action. Ultimately this powerlessness results in isolation and death.

Although this model was developed to apply to individual patients, it can be applied to a nursing unit or an entire hospital. When nurses have a lack of choice-making ability in their environment, this leads to a state of powerlessness. This powerlessness can then set up a self-perpetuating cycle as depicted in Figure 4–1. Interventions that give control back to the individual or nursing unit are needed to break this cycle.

Miller[2] developed defining characteristics of powerlessness: passivity; apathy; verbal expressions of having no control or influence over situations; verbal expressions of having no control or influence over outcomes; nonparticipation in care or decision making when opportunities are provided; dependence on others, which may result in irritability, resentment, anger, and guilt; hesitation to plan for the future or to set goals; and reluctance to express one's true feelings, fearing alienation.

Organizational survival into the 21st century may hinge on the ability to bring empowerment and the power of choice to the institution. Shared governance and

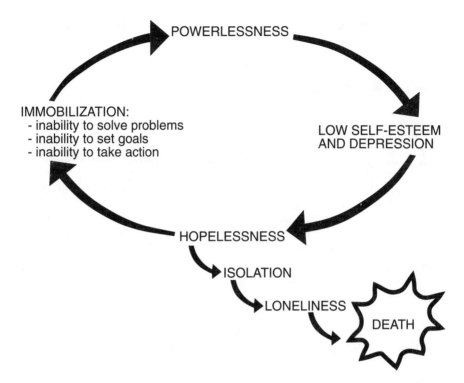

Figure 4–1 Powerlessness–hopelessness cycle. *Source:* Reprinted from *Coping with Chronic Illness: Overcoming Powerlessness,* by J.F. Miller, p. 289, with permission of F.A. Davis Company, © 1983.

differentiated practice are processes that bring the power of choice into action for the nursing practice at your institution.

CARPE DIEM

> *Other people . . . see things and say: "Why?" But I dream things that never were and I say: "Why not?"*
> PRESIDENT JOHN F. KENNEDY

In the recent movie *Dead Poet's Society,* the professor was instilling in his students an awakening to who they truly were. The professor encouraged the students to examine themselves and discover their inner dreams and ambitions. The students were then to make choices to follow their dreams and not to succumb to the pressures of other people's expectations of them. The professor's motto was *carpe diem* or "seize the day," meaning that the time was now for the students to make choices to set the course for the rest of their lives.

Seize the Day in Personal Life

It is not always easy for individuals to find out who they would most like to be and what they truly want out of life. This involves examining who they really are and who they want to be. This opens up a Pandora's box of vulnerabilities and true emotions. Such a self-examination causes people to look at their values and purpose in life. At times it seems easier to avoid this self-examination and just accept the status quo, reacting to changes as they occur in the environment.

Nurses often encourage their patients to have a thorough physical examination each year. A physical examination involves assessing each physical body system to ensure that it is working appropriately. How often do nurses recommend to themselves and their patients a good self-examination each year? This involves answering questions about one's purpose and one's endeavors. Responding to life's deepest and darkest questions can be difficult.

It is a challenge to seize the day on a personal level. The time is ripe for self-examination to look at the choices to be made now and in the future. No matter what a person's age, there are still more choices, stages, and first times awaiting.

Seize the Day Organizationally

As the health care organization is trying to survive in these economic times, how will nursing contribute to the organization's viability? At times individuals may feel paralyzed when they imagine what will happen in their organization as rumors of cutbacks and layoffs are heard. At other times individuals may assume a victim mentality and wonder what the organization will do to them next that will make life miserable.

Nurses need to seize the day and be proactive about the changes in their organizations. The time is now to do some critical and creative thinking.

Seize the Day as a Nursing Professional

The spiraling cost of health care is causing third party payers, primarily the federal government, insurance companies, and employers, to question the costs. Most of all, the nursing profession must seize the day. As the health care crisis looms large on the horizon, the time has come for the profession of nursing to look deeply and to make some hard choices.

The profession of nursing is at a critical and risky choice point. What does the profession truly want to be? What does the profession of nursing have to contribute to the nation's and world's health? How will professionals choose to solve the health care crisis? Can the community of nursing pull together to be a vital force in health care reform?

None of these questions lends itself to easy answers or quick solutions. The key, however, is to start making choices now. At a personal, professional, and organizational level, nursing cannot afford to wait. If no choices are made now, someone will be making the choices for nursing. Beware, however, because choices create change.

THE GENTLE ART OF CHOOSING

> *Since the mind is a specific bio-computer it needs*
> *specific instructions and directions. The reason*
> *most people never reach their goals is that they*
> *don't define them, learn about them or ever*
> *seriously consider them as believable or achiev-*
> *able. Winners can tell you where they are*
> *going, . . . what they plan to do along the way, and*
> *who will be sharing the adventure with them.*
>
> DENIS WAITLEY

There is nothing mystical or mysterious about the art of choosing. Yet many times making choices and plans to achieve goals are avoided. Either consciously or unconsciously, people choose not to choose, thus not participating fully in life. When people take the step to choose to choose, it will catapult them into an exhilarating, painful, exciting, confusing, and fearful state of being all at once. Specifically, choosing can be conceptualized as a three-step process.

The first step is to set a clear vision of what is to be accomplished. It is of utmost importance to become clear on the desired outcome. This is the time to ask, "What results or end product do I want?" This is the most important time of reflection and deep thought to become clear on the vision, goals, and wanted outcomes. This is the time for incubation and germinational energy.

When Sioux Valley Hospital first started thinking about changing its nursing care delivery system, we first had to be clear on what results we wanted. After much discussion and thought, consensus was reached on three desired outcomes: to increase the continuity of care for the patients, to decrease patients' lengths of stay, and to empower the nursing staff.

After the desired outcomes are clear, the second step is to formalize the choice. Once the vision is clear, it is time to decide how to obtain the goal. In essence, this is a time of planning. It may be necessary to break down the choice into several steps and to make time lines and intermediate goals. This is a time for brainstorming and looking at different processes that will help reach the vision. During this step, it is important to develop a strategic plan on how to implement the choices.

At Sioux Valley Hospital, after the desired outcomes were clear, a plan on how to reach these goals was developed. Available personnel and resources were both considered. Each unit's unique culture was also considered. Nursing units were given the autonomy (within certain guidelines) to try a strategy that would work for them. Therefore, there were various differentiated practice models that were developed on the separate units based on standard guiding principles.

After there is a clear vision and a plan to reach the vision, it is time to set the wheels in motion. The power of the choice comes when the plan is launched into action. Thus step three is the action phase, when plans are put into operation. Also in this step, progress needs to be evaluated for movement toward the desired outcomes.

At Sioux Valley Hospital, several units initiated pilot projects or trial runs of a differentiated practice model. The units were then able to compare and contrast with other pilot units what activities were working and what activities were not working. Therefore, the units were able to learn from each other's successes and failures.

One final word of wisdom: It is important for the people making the choice to become so committed to the choice that they believe it will happen and act as though it will happen. The commitment to the choice is what will help when the times become turbulent in the change process.

A LESSON FROM PSYCHE: A METAPHOR

The Greek myth of Psyche symbolizes some lessons in choice making. In the myth, Psyche wants to be reunited with her husband, whom she loves deeply. Psyche seeks the council of Aphrodite, the Goddess of love, to assist in the reunion. Aphrodite will assist Psyche, but first she must undergo four tasks set up by the Goddess for the reunion to occur: sorting seeds, acquiring some golden fleece, filling a crystal flask, and returning safely from a journey to the underworld.[3]

Task 1: Sorting the Seeds

The first task with which Psyche is challenged is to sort a huge pile of all kinds of seeds, including corn, poppy, barley, lentils, and beans. Psyche is to sort these different types of seeds into their respective piles before nightfall. To Psyche this task seems tedious and unaccomplishable. Fortunately, a group of ants come to her aid and assist in sorting each grain into the proper pile. Thus Psyche is able to achieve the first task.[3]

Similarly, when a choice must be made, there may be a huge pile of seeds to sort. This is the time to separate this from that: values, assumptions, motives, information, emotions, and intuitions. This is an important process that needs to occur when one is making choices either at a personal level or at the organizational level. It is often a time for personal and group introspection and incubation. This sorting out or time of fine discrimination needs to occur before the vision can become clear.

Often to the outsider, this may appear as a time of spinning wheels or lack of progress. Often the person or group may feel confused and overwhelmed. Feelings of wanting to abandon the project or find a cookbook answer may emerge. Nevertheless, it is important to let this time occur. Allowing this time will help with gaining a vision and finding some clarity in the quest. But just as Psyche was given a deadline of nightfall, a deadline may also need to be set for this process. Without a time frame, the individual or group risks falling into analysis paralysis and may never be able to move on a critical choice point.

Psyche in the myth had the ants to aid her. These ants can symbolize the grassroots worker in the organization. There is a need to have many nurses help when one is making choices in the care delivery system. Getting a critical mass of individuals involved can help speed the process once the plans are developed.

Task 2: Acquiring Some Golden Fleece

The second task required of Psyche is to obtain some golden fleece from the rams of the sun. These rams are huge, ferocious, horned animals that aggressively butt each other and any other creature in their sight. These fierce rams will surely hurt or even kill Psyche with their horns if she dares to pull out some of their fleece.

As Psyche is contemplating how to undertake such a dangerous task, a green reed speaks to her and advises her to wait until dark for the rams to retire. Then she can safely pick strands of fleece off the brambles against which the rams have rubbed. In this way, Psyche is able to obtain the fleece as required by Aphrodite without putting herself at risk of injury.[3]

Symbolically this teaches several lessons in the choice process. First, it is a challenge to look at the not so obvious when one is making choices. It is often said that a fish would be the last one to discover water. People are often oblivious to their surroundings. They are blinded to new ideas or ways of doing things because of the paradigm in which they are engulfed.

It is wise to look to the edges and fringes of what is happening in the world. Furthermore, do not stifle creative thinking and ideas. For the most effective thinking, differences in points of view are needed. It is said that an idea is best understood in the context of another idea.

Second, it is a challenge when one is making choices to listen to the noises in the environment and the "unnoise." Just as Psyche listened to the reed, it is important to listen to what is being said in the environment, both internally and externally. Porter-O'Grady often instructed that it is important to expect the noise and listen to it. This listening, however, needs to be extended to listening to what is unsaid as feelings uncommunicated and pains unexpressed.

Finally, just as Psyche listened to the reed, that small voice that often comes from inside must also be heard. This small voice is better known as intuition. When one is making choices, it is important to listen to the voice of inner reason and inner knowing. This involves relying on the veracity of personal intuition. At times a choice will need to be made at the gut level.

Task 3: Filling the Crystal Flask

The third task that Psyche is to accomplish involves filling a flask with water from a stream. The stream is located on a dangerous rocky cliff and is guarded by dragons. Again, Psyche feels overwhelmed and hopeless facing such a feat. This time an eagle comes to her rescue. The eagle rises above the dragons, swoops down, and fills the flask. The eagle then returns the flask to Psyche, and the third task is fulfilled.[3]

The eagle symbolizes the ability to see the world from a different perspective. Often individuals are caught closing their minds to all that cannot be viewed from their perspective. This limits their capacity to learn and grow. The mind must be open to improvement, knocking down old paradigms and respecting what at first is not seen. The world is ambiguous; there are many right answers and choices, all depending on the way things and problems are viewed. In other words, the world is not always black and white but has a rich range of hues of gray in between. At Sioux Valley Hospital, the eagles often come in the form of consultants. Consultants such as Porter-O'Grady and del Bueno have been used to bring a new perspective.

The dragons symbolize the issue of territoriallity. Often when choices are made, there will be a rippling effect that invades someone else's space. This invasion of territory may cause the dragons to rear their ugly heads and try to devour the intruder. At times, like the eagle, individuals must rise above these boundaries and not let themselves be consumed. It is wise to choose which battles are not worth fighting. In addition, Psyche was able to look at the power of the dragons. When facing great power in others, individuals may learn of their own power. Respect in the face of power is a crucial lesson. It is important to learn about personal power and how personal power status will affect the choices made in life's journey.

Task 4: The Journey to the Underworld

The final task that Psyche has to perform to be reunited with her husband is to descend to the underworld and fill a small box with beauty ointment. During her journey she encounters pathetic, needy people who desire her help. Psyche has to harden her heart against compassion and ignore these people's pleas. If she attempts to help these people, she will remain forever in the underworld.[3]

This task symbolizes the need to set the goal of the choice and stick to it even in the face of requests and distractions. There are many needy distractions that may cloud the vision at choice points in the journey of life. Often for nurses and women it is difficult to say no. Too often people get caught up in others' needs and wants, so that self-sacrifice is a risk. Until people learn to exercise the choice of saying no, they may be unable to determine the right course and may be unable to stick to it. Distractions may interfere with the primary process and the choices.

This also symbolizes that when choices that affect roles are made there will be changes that bring about a grief process. There is a giving up of the old self with a death of outworn, old knowledge. Just as Psyche had to journey through the underworld, everyone must journey through their losses and griefs. As choices are made to change the old, it may bring on a grief reaction as a deep sense of losing the status quo is felt. As Peck stated, "the pain of giving up is the pain of death, but death of the old is birth of the new."[4(p73)] It is important to recognize this grief, but do not let it stop the movement forward to the birth of a new way of practicing nursing. There will be emotional costs to transcend as the profession moves toward a new way of being.

LEVELS OF CHOICE

For an individual and an organization, there are different levels of choice that can be conceptualized. Choices can be dissected into three types: fundamental, primary, and secondary. All three levels of choices are intertwined and related to each other.

Fundamental Choices

One of the major influences on choices made is the personal value system. At some point in one's personal life or the organization's life, there has been a choice made as to what is valued. This value system helps determine the basic personal life orientation. According to Rokeach, a value system is defined as "an enduring organization of beliefs concerning preferable modes of conduct or end-states of existence along a continuum of relative importance."[5(p5)] Therefore, values are a learned set of principles and beliefs that help an individual choose among alternatives. Some go so far as to say that everything people do, every decision made, and every course of action taken are influenced by consciously or unconsciously held beliefs, attitudes, and values.

Such values could be considered the fundamental choices that set the foundation for who a person is and why a person wants something.[6] A good way to start identifying fundamental choices is by discovering the purpose of one's life. This is a simple statement explaining the purpose of one's being here on Earth. It serves as life's driving force. The purpose is used to set a person's course in life and to help guide the person when he or she is faced with making choices. In an organization, this purpose can be found in a philosophy or a mission statement. An organization's mission statement should be the driving force that directs the organization.

Primary Choices

A primary choice functions as a goal designed to reach concrete results.[6] Thus a primary choice functions as a personal intention or a desire that is held. For example, a primary choice may include such goals as wanting to be a good parent, having lots of adventure, or being successful in life.

Primary choices never stand alone. Just because a choice or goal has been formulated does not mean that it happens. Secondary choices must be made to achieve the primary choice.

Secondary Choices

A secondary choice helps the individual step toward the primary result. A secondary choice serves to support a primary choice. The secondary choices work as a team to support the primary choice. Therefore, secondary choices are made to assist the individual in reaching the goals set by the primary choice.[6]

The secondary choices are small choices in matters regarding methods or behaviors that work together to support, defend, or enhance the primary choice. An example of how these three levels of choice operate follows. An individual makes the fundamental choice to be of sound body, mind, and spirit. To support part of this fundamental value, the individual then makes the primary choice to engage in some physical exercise three times per week. This primary choice to exercise is supported by the foundational choice of being of sound body. Finally, the individual will make secondary choices such as joining a health club and buying running shoes to support the primary choice of exercising, which in turn is related to the value of having a sound body (Exhibit 4–1). All three levels of choice are intricately intertwined and related. It is important for all levels of choice to support each other if a person wants to lead a grounded and balanced life.

GENDER ISSUES AND CHOICE

> *If a man mulls over a decision, they say, "He's*
> *weighing the options." If a woman does it, they*
> *say, "She can't make up her mind."*
> BARBARA PROCTOR

Exhibit 4–1 Levels of Choice

Fundamental choice	=	To be of sound body, mind, and spirit
Primary choice	=	To exercise three times per week
Secondary choices	=	To buy running shoes
	=	To join a health club
	=	To set aside time each week for exercise
	=	To spend time with people who encourage physical activity

Source: Information from *The Path of Least Resistance: Learning To Become the Creative Force in Your Own Life* by R. Fritz, pp. 177–198, Fawcett Columbine, © 1989.

Historically, women have been oppressed by society, culture, and other forces (including themselves). This has contributed to them becoming passive victims, martyrs, or pawns moved around by other people or circumstances. Women have been expected to succumb to someone else's choices for their lives. The women's movement has made great strides over the past decade, and work continues for equality. Women's journey to such freedom has been a quest for the power to become choicemakers.

In addition, gender influences the choices made, especially choices involving relationships. Studies show that in relationships men have more of a desire for freedom and independence. Men will strive for establishing status and are comfortable telling others what to do. Therefore, men function well in a hierarchical system. Their choices in regard to relationships, whether they be work or intimate relationships, may reflect their desires for freedom and control.[7]

In contrast, women have more of a desire for interdependence and connection. In work and intimate relationships, women will try to minimize differences, will try to reach consensus, and want to avoid the appearance of superiority. The feminine approach to choices functions within contexts and gives equal legitimacy to a variety of concerns. Therefore, women will make choices in relationships that will fulfill these needs of interdependence and connection.[7]

There is value and credence in each of these orientations to choice making. In the past, however, most organizations (ie, hospitals) were set up in a hierarchical manner that did not value the feminine orientation of interdependence. The movement toward shared governance is a recognition of the need for balance in both the independent and interdependent orientations.

Individuals need to embrace both feminine and masculine polarities. Fine discernment can be used when one is faced with choices personally and professionally.

PITFALLS TO AVOID WHEN MAKING CHOICES

Pitfall 1: Choice by Limitation

Choice by limitation means that a person only chooses what seems possible or reasonable.[6] Compromises are made, and what is felt to be reasonable is chosen rather than what is truly wanted for fear of being rejected or going beyond the familiar.

It is important to escape self-imposed barriers. Settling for second best is not wanted. The choices need to be focused on the possibilities and not on the limitations.

> *Never tell people* how *to do things. Tell them* what *to do and they will surprise you with their ingenuity.*
> GEORGE S. PATTON, JR

Pitfall 2: Choice by Indirectness

Choice by indirectness involves choosing the process instead of the result.[6] If the focus is the process, wanted results will be unclear, and the chooser will not know in what direction there is movement or when the destination has been reached. Therefore, when one is making decisions about the organization's nursing delivery system, the choice should not concern only changes to the system but also the wanted results. Are decreased length of stay and continuity of care wanted? Do not put undue power in the process if the desired results are not clear. Focus on the outcome or destination rather than worrying about the process to get there.

Pitfall 3: Choice by Reaction

A choice by reaction is often made to resolve some conflict. The choice is made solely to eliminate the discomfort or some type of pressure. This choice is like a knee-jerk reaction.[6] This can also be called a Band-Aid approach.

When choices are made in a reactionary mode, the power lies in whatever is causing the discomfort. It is better to set a personal direction than to react to the direction of some other party.

Pitfall 4: Choice by Default

The choice not to make a choice is choice by default. This allows the person to think that the results or outcomes that happen are beyond his or her control. Actually the individual is giving up power to arbitrary external conditions. The individual abnegates his or her power to fate by the unwillingness to make a choice and voluntarily gives up any options.[6]

It is important to avoid passively letting circumstances dictate what happens. Life can effectively be rearranged and reorganized in ways that will bring an individual's choices into reality.

> *Security . . . does not exist in nature, nor do the*
> *children of men as a whole experience it. . . .*
> *Avoiding danger is no safer in the long run than*
> *outright exposure. . . . Life is either a daring*
> *adventure or nothing.*
>
> HELEN KELLER

Pitfall 5: Choice by Popularity Polls

The individual chooses by finding out what everyone else is willing to recommend. Power lies in the reference group. In this mode, the individual goes along with others' choices and lacks the courage to identify his or her own wants and desires. This leaves the individual feeling victimized and powerless.[6]

PERSONAL DECISION POINTS

> *Making a choice is like backing a horse—in a*
> *hundred years, they may decide you picked*
> *wrongly.*
>
> EDWARD CARPENTER

Everyone makes decisions about his or her career, whether consciously or unconsciously. A decision to be a nurse may have many factors influencing that decision. Childhood experiences, family expectations, educational opportunities, finances, peers, and previous academic courses are just a few of those factors. In the last few years there have been an increasing number of nurses who had careers in other fields before they entered nursing education. These students in particular have joined others who view nursing as a career rather than as a job.

Once the decision is made to enter the nursing field, a choice needs to be made about what kind of school to attend. Most students again have many factors to consider with this choice. The curricula most often considered are a licensed practical program, or a 2-, 3-, or 4-year registered nurse program. Other considerations are whether to attend a public or private school or a local college or distant university and the values and beliefs of the prospective student. Unfortunately, many of those factors are related to available financial resources. Therefore, the student is forced to determine what is most practical for him or her. This includes not only tuition but also distance to travel and curriculum. But then, this is true for most if not all career choices.

Presently, a basic decision for prospective nurses is the choice between a vocational or registered nurse program. In the future, prospective nurses may have another choice to make concerning education. The Healing Web is piloting basic registered nurse education of the Midwest Alliance in Nursing (MAIN) competencies.[8–10] The Healing Web is a consortium among Augustana College Department of Nursing, the University of South Dakota Department of Nursing, and the Sioux Valley Hospital Department of Patient Services. The prospective student may need to choose the education for the desired registered nurse role before school enrollment in the future.

ORGANIZATIONAL DECISION POINTS

Don't be afraid to take a big step when one is indicated. You can't cross a chasm in two small jumps.

DAVID LLOYD GEORGE

Sioux Valley Hospital's decision to participate in the South Dakota Statewide Project for Nursing and Nursing Education (Statewide Project) was necessary on two levels in the organization: administratively and on the staff level. Hospital administration needed to be committed to participation by the nursing units, as described in Chapter 1. One of the factors that was a consideration for both administration and the nurses was the fact that Sioux Valley Hospital is the largest hospital in the state. A concern was that, if future education and practice decisions were to be made as a result of the Statewide Project, Sioux Valley Hospital would not have any input into those decisions if it was not involved in the demonstration project. The nurses decided by individual patient care units whether they would commit themselves to participating in a demonstration project involving research. They made this year-long commitment by consensus with a mere 2-hour introduction to a concept that would entirely change their care delivery system. These nurses and managers were truly risk takers.

At the conclusion of the Statewide Project, the Sioux Valley Hospital Steering Committee, composed of representatives from the project units, recommended to nursing administration that differentiated nursing practice be continued on the project units and that the rest of the hospital change its care delivery system to differentiated practice. Exhibit 4–2 lists those recommendations. Nursing administration then needed to weigh the costs and benefits of changing the whole depart-

Exhibit 4–2 Recommendations of the Differentiated Practice Steering Committee

---

1. Nursing diagnosis will be used throughout the Department of Nursing at Sioux Valley Hospital.
2. Nursing process will be utilized. Delegation will occur through nursing orders.
3. Documentation will reflect nursing process and nursing diagnosis (ie, focus charting).
4. Communication will reflect nursing diagnosis (ie, change of shift report, etc).
5. Because of increasing acuity, decreasing length of stay, and the 3-day work week, the issue of continuity of care must be addressed. A form of coordinated (managed) care must be established with a registered nurse managing the care from admission to discharge.
6. Uniqueness of individual units must be maintained; standardization of certain aspects of care must be developed, however, to maintain consistency within the department.
7. Standardization must occur in the following areas:
   - terms and definitions to describe the care delivery system and competencies utilized by the various caregivers
   - elements of documentation between units that interface frequently
8. Development and maintenance of a nursing care delivery system must be staff driven.
9. Audit tools and the like must be developed to reflect Sioux Valley Hospital job descriptions and documentation process. They must be utilized frequently enough to maintain accuracy and consistency within the system.

Courtesy of the Sioux Valley Hospital Differentiated Practice Steering Committee, Sioux Valley Hospital, Sioux Falls, South Dakota.

---

ment to a differentiated nursing practice model. They were cognizant of the additional responsibility and accountability of the nurses in the case manager role. They were also aware that these nurses had agreed to fulfill this role during the project year without additional monetary compensation. This lack of additional compensation was a stipulation for participation in the Statewide Project.[11] Keeping these risk takers in this role long term and attracting additional nurses to the role, however, would be difficult without compensation.

To resolve this dilemma, nursing administration chose to form a committee to develop a clinical ladder. This committee, known as the Nursing Career Pathway Committee, was charged with developing job descriptions for nurses in a differentiated practice environment. To pay nurses differently, the job descriptions needed to demonstrate that the work was different. This criterion was mandated by the hospital's administration.

When the committee started, it struggled in sorting the seeds. It took the group five 4-hour sessions to become clear on its purpose and direction. One member commented to a colleague at the fourth meeting about the frustration that was felt because of the lack of progress that was perceived. Then, in the sixth meeting, it was a *Eureka* experience when all the pieces started to fit together and professional nursing at Sioux Valley Hospital gained clarity in the vision. It was important to take the time for sorting the seeds and incubating the creative processes.

The committee chose, after much discussion, to use the MAIN competency statements for future associate and baccalaureate graduates as the foundation for further discussion. Although the committee agreed with the intent of the MAIN job descriptions, the language was not always acceptable to this culture. Therefore, the wording of the competency statements was changed, but the format remained the same. Once consensus was reached to use the MAIN document as a starting place, the job descriptions for registered nurse in the associate role and registered nurse in the primary role (see Appendices 4-A and 4-B) were completed in just three more committee meetings. (See Chapter 3 for more information on consensus. This is an example of needing more time to reach a decision.)

By this time a year had passed since the completion of the Statewide Project. During these 2 years of differentiated practice, it became evident that another registered nurse role was needed. The neonatal intensive care unit had implemented a new role when the demonstration project began. The unit had always had a charge nurse, but this was a rotating position dependent primarily on seniority. When preparing to select nurses for the differentiated practice roles, the manager decided that a rotating charge nurse would be impractical. Therefore, permanent positions were implemented. The pediatric department had used permanent registered nurse coordinators for approximately 7 years. The coordinators work as a team on each of these units with one person in the role each shift. The role's responsibilities were a combination of traditional charge nurse and assistant head nurse roles. Staffing the unit, bed control, and making rounds with physicians were the most common tasks. Resolving conflicts interdepartmentally and intradepartmentally was the coordinator's responsibility as well, however.

Therefore, a job description for this position needed to be developed to fit the differentiated practice environment. The Nursing Career Pathway Committee tackled this additional responsibility and approved a job description for registered nurse in the clinical care coordinator role in just two meetings (see Appendix 4-C). The primary focus for this role is the patient care unit rather than the client. The responsibilities also encompass the previous divisional supervisor role and, more recently, the housewide supervisor role (see Chapter 9 for further discussion).

CAREER DECISION POINTS

> *No trumpets sound when the important decisions of our life are made. Destiny is made known silently.*
>
> AGNES DE MILLE

Career pathways are chosen by each nurse individually, and the choices are made at many different points in each career. Upon graduation, when the individual is pursuing that first position as a nurse, many choices are made: the kind of organization (clinic, long-term care, acute care, home health, rehabilitation, community health, or education, etc); public, private, or governmental (military, Indian Health, state, federal, or local); facility size; location geographically; specialized or generalist; pediatric, adult, geriatric, or all ages; full or part time; shifts and hours. Some of these choices are made deliberately. Some are ruled out without much thought or because there does not appear to be a choice (eg, relocation is not practical for those with a family business).

Some hospitals now offer a nurse residency program for new graduates.[12–19] This internship is designed to provide clinical experience with a preceptor to minimize the reality shock and to provide a transition to full clinical privileges and responsibilities. Residencies range in length from 2 to 12 months. During this time the resident has the opportunity to learn about the organizational culture. In programs that provide experience in more than one patient care unit, the resident is exposed to the various unit cultures. Near the end of the residency, when the resident interviews for a permanent position, the unit has had the opportunity to work with the applicant, and the resident has worked with the staff. The choices made are much more informed for both the unit offering the position and the nurse applicant. Most residencies are for critical care units. Some hospitals, like Sioux Valley, also have a residency for adult specialty care and women's and children's care units.

Some of the same choices are made with each new position. For example, a medical-surgical nurse may have worked in a general unit. Moving to a larger acute care facility may require choosing a particular surgical unit (eg, orthopedic, cardiac, or neurologic). When relocating, however, specialized nurses may find it more difficult to consider the range of options open to them. When continuing their education, nurses can reopen career possibilities that were formerly closed to them as well as more safely change specialties (eg, move from coronary care to maternal-child health).

Nurses at Sioux Valley Hospital have a wide range of specialties from which to choose. They also have the choice of role: registered nurse in the associate role, registered nurse in the primary role, registered nurse in the clinical care coordinator role, director of a patient care unit, clinical nurse specialist, nursing administrator, or vice president of patient services (see Appendices 4-A to 4-E for job descriptions). The choice, of course, is contingent on qualifications, competency, and job availability.

The nurses on each patient care unit choose what hours to work. The first choice made annually is whether to have 8-hour schedules, 12-hour schedules, or a combination of both options available to individual nurses. Nurses preferring the 8-hour schedule work in a team of three, so that 24 hours of care are provided. Most nurses prefer the 12-hour schedules. The units self-schedule, so that each nurse chooses which hours to work within certain unit and department guidelines.

Therefore, when a nurse wants every Tuesday night off, this is a choice that affects the schedule worked. Nevertheless, the schedule is chosen rather than dictated (see Exhibit 3–6 for more discussion about self-scheduling).

SELECTION PROCESS

During the Statewide Project, each nurse completed a Factoring Tool developed by Primm. The purpose of this tool was to help the nurse identify the preferred method of practice. Because the nurse manager also completed this tool, the appraisal of the nurse's practice could be done nonthreateningly and separate from a formal evaluation. Then the manager and the staff nurse compared the completed tools. During the ensuing discussion, the nurse chose which role would be fulfilled during the project. At the end of the first 3 months, the nurse had the option of changing roles, but few nurses chose to change roles.[20,21]

After the project was completed, the Role Choice Tool was developed (see Appendix 4-F). This tool is similar in intent to the Factoring Tool but is a Likert scale tool based on the competency statements for the registered nurse in the associate role and in the primary role. Nurses applying for the primary role complete one of these two tools. The tool chosen is determined by the unit selection committee. The selection committee completes a tool for each candidate applying for the primary role; the completed tools are then compared for each applicant.

When hired, transferred, or cross-trained, all registered nurses complete an orientation using materials selected by the staff educators to prepare them for their unit(s) of practice. The materials are from the Performance Based Development System (PBDS) management series. When nurses apply for the primary role or the clinical care coordinator role, some PBDS materials are used. The materials are chosen by the selection committee from a list of suitable options, which were determined by ad hoc committees of staff already in those roles.

In summary, the selection process for clinical II roles is unit determined with only two department guidelines: Either the Role Choice Tool or the Factoring Tool must be used by primary nurse applicants, and PBDS materials must be used for all applicants. Completion of the required PBDS materials may be done either during the interview process or at a time other than the interview.

The selection process is otherwise unit determined. Most units have elected to have a committee interview the applicants. The composition of the selection committee has varied from three to seven people; some have been entirely composed of unit staff, but most have been composed of a variety of unit and nonunit staff. Depending on the unit, some of the selection committee members may be nonnurses.

Before the interviews, the committee decides who will fulfill each role: greeter, recorder, and interviewer(s). Questions to ask each applicant and whether the question requires a written response to be submitted with the application or a verbal response during the interview are agreed upon. Some unit selection committees have used a point system to help the interviewers compare the candidates more objectively (Figure 4–2).

PROFESSIONAL ACTIVITIES

There are several professional activities among which nurses can choose. Helping staff and students as a preceptor or mentor is needed either continuously or periodically in all organizations. Participating within an employee or professional organization on committees, councils, or task forces and in peer review is often needed or required.

Nurses at Sioux Valley Hospital can choose to be a preceptor for new staff or students on their unit. This professional commitment is accepted in full knowledge that evaluation of the person is an expectation. The preceptor is rewarded by knowing that the preceptee has gained knowledge and that a professional responsibility has been fulfilled. The preceptor is also rewarded creatively, because the

Name	Education	Employment	References	Written Questions			
Myers-Briggs/ Comments	(1–5)	History (1–5)	(1–5)	#1 (1–5)	#2 (1–5)	#3 (1–10)	Subtotal (20 poss)

Interview (1–5 each)						Vignettes (1–3 each)							Grand
#1	#2	#3	#4	Overall (2 poss)	Subtotal (22 poss)	#1	#2	#3	#4	#5	#6	Subtotal (18 poss)	Total (75 poss)

Figure 4–2 Applicant evaluation form. Courtesy of Sioux Valley Hospital, Sioux Falls, South Dakota.

preceptee has been shaped somewhat by the preceptor, and monetarily for accepting this additional responsibility (see Appendix 4-G for the policy for monetary reimbursement).[22]

Participation on committees and councils is also a choice for nurses in all roles. Before the implementation of shared governance, there were many committees on unit, divisional, and departmental levels. Now there are fewer committees, but there are departmental and unit councils for which staff may be selected by their peers. The commitment for council membership is usually 2 years. Committee or task force membership usually requires a shorter time commitment, however, because once the mission or purpose has been accomplished the group dissolves.

Another professional activity pursued by nurses is membership in professional organizations. The choice of organization is usually made by specialty practice. Choices could often be made based on interest, however. For instance, the nurse could join an organization to determine whether a change in career would really be of interest. Monies gained through preceptoring can be applied to membership fees and/or to registration and other fees to attend meetings. Professional organizations present their own choices for participation.

With implementation of shared governance, peer review became a reality. The purpose of peer review is to ensure competence and to credential staff into the practice. When registered nurses apply to work at Sioux Valley Hospital, they are interviewed either by the unit on which there is an open position (for experienced nurses) or by the nursing center for a position in the residency program (for graduates with less than 6 months of experience). The credentialing review officer then determines whether the applicant is accepted as a provisional member or is not accepted. With acceptance, the applicant is assigned to a clinical service (for nursing residents, this is one of the three nursing divisions).

After 6 months as a provisional member of the nursing practice, the nurse is expected to apply for full practice privileges. The nurse submits his or her application (Exhibit 4–3) and professional portfolio for review by the credentialing officer. See Exhibit 4–4 for suggested contents of the portfolio. For residents, interviews are conducted by hiring units in the division of residency. If the person has not met the competency expected, termination will result. This could, of course, be appealed to the unit Quality Improvement Council, but there would have been counseling during this time of provisional membership.

As a full practice member, the nurse must reapply annually for continuation of practice privileges. At each decision point throughout this process, a letter of confirmation (or denial) is sent to the applicant. See Figure 4–3 for a diagram of the credentialing privileging process.

To summarize, the department guidelines are as follows: The staff person submits a professional portfolio with an application for continuing privileges by the due date, which is determined by the annual review date (so that the review can be done by the review date); and the peers use a standardized evaluation tool (see Appen-

Exhibit 4–3 Application for Membership to the Nursing Practice of the Departments of Nursing, Surgical, and Rehabilitation Services

---

Please complete the application and submit with professional portfolio.

Date: _____

Annual Review Date: _____

1. Name: _____

2. Present departmental assignment: _____

3. Present level of practice/role: _____

4. Clinical privileges carried in the following nursing specialties:

_____ _____

_____ _____

5. Application submitted for:
   ❑ same clinical privileges
   ❑ specialty practice privileges in: _____
     (submit evidence of completed orientation/PBDS)
   ❑ change in level of practice/role: _____

6. Recommendations: _____

_____

Signature: _____

Reviewer: _____

Approval: _____

Courtesy of Sioux Valley Hospital, Sioux Falls, South Dakota.

---

dices 4-H to 4-J for the generic evaluation tools for the three roles). Each unit can add more items to the evaluation. For example, flight nurses have a few additional competencies no matter what other role they fulfill on the unit.

Each unit has developed peer review to suit its culture. On some units, the reviewers are fairly constant (depending on staff turnover). On other units, names are drawn annually and therefore vary from one review to the next. The composition of the review teams also varies sometimes to include nonnurse staff. The manager has a greater or lesser role depending on the individual's management style and the experience of the staff with peer review.

CONCLUSION

By providing nursing staff with choices, staff are empowered and proactive and participate in making decisions. They make a choice by setting goals, defining the desired outcome, and finally acting on the choice made. Often there are seeds to sort, other paradigms and perspectives to consider, and the possibility of distractions when one is trying to reach a goal. Some choices require the grieving process as something cherished is relinquished.

Exhibit 4–4 Contents of Professional Portfolio

1. Table of contents
2. Professional nursing philosophy
3. Curriculum vitae, to include personal, educational, work history, professional organizations, community contributions
4. Continuing education (annual date to annual date for 1 year)
   - Inservices and workshops
   - College credits
5. Professional contributions
   - Inservices provided
   - Committee participation and sample of work done on committee
   - Presentations—in-house, community, and national
   - Research done
   - Cost analyses completed
   - Program development (small and large; eg, sibling support group)
   - Issue tracking completion (eg, self-scheduling, development of communication patterns)
   - Equipment or system evaluation (eg, product evaluation for monitors, intravenous tubing, pumps, etc; include pros and cons, recommendations)
   - Mentoring and team building issues (written out)
   - Preceptoring completed this year of new employees, one-shift students, community visitors, tours, etc
   - Governance issues: elected positions and other work
   - Consultations completed
6. Professional highlights (some might be duplicated within curriculum vitae)
   - Honors, recognition
   - Certification (eg, computers)
   - Special recognition (eg, employee of the month)
   - Letters from peers, clients, community
7. Personal assessment
   - Last year's goals (self and peers)
   - Areas for growth
8. Goals and plans for achievement for next year
9. Unit-specific criteria

Courtesy of the Sioux Valley Hospital Credentialing Committee, Sioux Valley Hospital, Sioux Falls, South Dakota.

Fundamental choices necessitate that primary and secondary choices be made. Changing a nursing care delivery system to achieve continuity of patient care is such a fundamental choice. Realizing that nursing is predominantly a female profession, nurses must also be cognizant that gender may influence how choices are made.[23]

Five pitfalls to avoid when making choices were discussed. Keeping an open mind and being proactive will help avoid these pitfalls. Also, examples of personal,

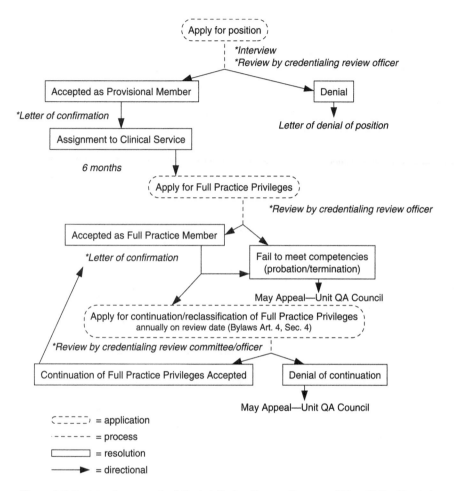

Apply for position

*Interview
*Review by credentialing review officer

Accepted as Provisional Member

Denial

*Letter of confirmation

Letter of denial of position

Assignment to Clinical Service

6 months

Apply for Full Practice Privileges

*Review by credentialing review officer

Accepted as Full Practice Member

*Letter of confirmation

Fail to meet competencies
(probation/termination)

May Appeal—Unit QA Council

Apply for continuation/reclassification of Full Practice Privileges
annually on review date (Bylaws Art. 4, Sec. 4)

*Review by credentialing review committee/officer

Continuation of Full Practice Privileges Accepted

Denial of continuation

May Appeal—Unit QA Council

= application
= process
= resolution
= directional

Figure 4–3 Registered nurse credentialing/privileging diagram. Courtesy of Sioux Valley Hospital, Sioux Falls, South Dakota.

organizational, and career decision points were discussed. At Sioux Valley Hospital, nurses have the choice not only of patient care unit and working schedule but also of the registered nurse role. The selection process for nurses interested in a clinical II role was delineated. A few examples of professional choices were also mentioned. Finally, the credentialing process using peer review was explained.

> *We did not choose the day of our birth nor may we*
> *choose the day of our death, yet choice is the*
> *sovereign faculty of the mind.*
>
> THORNTON WILDER

REFERENCES

1. Leddy S, Pepper JM. *Conceptual Bases of Professional Nursing*. New York, NY: Lippincott; 1989.

2. Miller JF. *Coping with Chronic Illness: Overcoming Powerlessness*. Philadelphia, Pa: Davis; 1983.

3. Bolen JS. *Goddesses in Every Woman: A New Psychology of Women*. New York, NY: Harper & Row; 1984.

4. Peck MS. *The Road Less Traveled: A New Psychology of Love, Traditional Values and Spiritual Growth*. New York, NY: Simon & Schuster; 1978.

5. Rokeach M. *The Nature of Human Values*. New York, NY: Free Press; 1973.

6. Fritz R. *The Path of Least Resistance: Learning to Become the Creative Force in Your Own Life*. New York, NY: Fawcett Columbine; 1989.

7. Tannen D. *You Just Don't Understand: Women and Men in Conversation*. New York, NY: Ballentine; 1990.

8. Bunkers S. The Healing Web: a transformative model for nursing. *Nurs Health Care*. 1992; 13:68–73.

9. Larson J. The Healing Web: a transformative model for nursing, part II. *Nurs Health Care*. 1992; 13:246–252.

10. Primm PL. Differentiated practice for ADN- and BSN-prepared nurses. *J Prof Nurs*. 1987; 3:218–225.

11. South Dakota Statewide Project Steering Committee. The South Dakota experience. In: Boston C, ed. *Current Issues and Perspectives on Differentiated Practice*. Chicago, Ill: American Organization of Nurse Executives; 1990:53–67.

12. Aldrich S. Neuroscience internship and graduate role conception. *J Neurosci Nurs*. 1988; 20:377–385.

13. Dear MR, Celentano DD, Weisman CS, Keen MF. Evaluating a hospital nursing internship. *J Nurs Admin*. 1982; 12(11):16–20.

14. Hartshorn JC. Evaluation of a critical care nursing internship program. *J Contin Educ Nurs*. 1992; 23:42–48.

15. Martin B. Developing retention strategies within your internship program. *Dimensions Crit Care Nurs*. 1989; 8:50–55.

16. Schempp CM, Rompre RM. Transition programs for new graduates. *J Nurs Staff Dev*. 1986; 2:150–156.

17. Stolte MM, Goss CL, Lim SSF. An oncology nursing residency program: meeting a continuing education need. *J Contin Educ Nurs*. 1988; 19:252–257.

18. Talarczyk G, Milbrandt D. A collaborative effort to facilitate role transition from student to registered nurse practitioner. *Nurs Manage*. 1988; 19(2):30–32.

19. Woodtli A, Hazzard ME, Rusch S. Senior internship: a strategy for recruitment, retention and collaboration. *Nurs Connections*. 1988; 1(3):37–50.

20. Koerner J. In South Dakota, nurses assess, then choose their practice. *Mich Hosp*. 1988; 24(3):21–24.

21. Koerner JG, Bunkers LB, Nelson B, Santema K. Implementing differentiated practice: the Sioux Valley Hospital experience. *J Nurs Admin*. 1989; 19(2):13–22.

22. Smidt V. Retaining experienced nurses: providing a bonus program for nurse preceptors. *Recruit Reten Rep*. 1993; 6(9): 1–4.

23. Reverby S. A caring dilemma: womanhood and nursing in historical perspective. *Nurs Res*. 1987; 36:5–11.

EXERCISE 4–1: INDIVIDUAL EXERCISES

1. Have you ever asked yourself what you want to accomplish in life? Ask yourself, "Why am I here on Earth?" Write your answers to this question, and this will become your own personal mission statement or life purpose. Review this from time to time to assess whether your life is on the right track.

2. Where would you like your life to be 5 years from now? What choices need to be made today for you to realize your future goals and dreams? Are you living a lifeless life?

3. Take the time to examine the fundamental choices, the primary choices, and the secondary choices in your life and your organization. Do your choices support each other? Are your life choices in balance? Do your levels of choices support each other?

EXERCISE 4–2: ORGANIZATIONAL EXERCISES

1. Look for your organization's mission statement. Do you believe that it is the driving force that directs the organization?

2. What choices in your institution need to be made by the nurses to help keep your institution on the cutting edge? How can you as nurses in your organization contribute to the challenge to be cost effective yet maintain high quality? If it is true that patients come to hospitals for nursing care, how can you make this care more affordable?

3. Think of Miller's list of defining characteristics of powerlessness in the context of the nursing unit of which you are a part. Does your nursing unit display these characteristics? Is your nursing unit ready to accept responsibility for your successes, your problems, and your professional development?

Appendix 4-A
Sioux Valley Hospital Department of Nursing Job Description: Registered Nurse in the Associate Role

JOB SUMMARY

The registered nurse in the associate role provides nursing care for clients during a specified work period. The nurse functions in structured care settings described as geographic and/or situational environments where the policies and procedures for provision of health care are established. This nurse receives assistance from the full scope of nursing expertise.

JOB RESPONSIBILITIES

1. The registered nurse in the associate role manages care of clients for a specified period of time:
   A. collects data from available resources, using established assessment format, to identify basic nursing care needs
   B. organizes and analyzes data to select pertinent nursing diagnoses and related standardized nursing care plans
   C. utilizes negotiation with the client to establish short-term goals that are consistent with the overall plan of care
   D. implements an individualized plan of care using established nursing diagnoses, policies, procedures, and Integrated Clinical Pathways
   E. evaluates client responses and modifies nursing interventions as necessary to meet client needs
   F. applies interpreted nursing research findings for nursing care
2. The registered nurse in the associate role utilizes interactive communication:
   A. assesses the client to determine immediate emotional needs and learning readiness
   B. implements goal-directed interactions to encourage expression of needs while supporting safe coping behaviors

C. modifies, implements, and evaluates a standard teaching plan to restore, maintain, or promote health

D. networks with health care team members by communicating data based on nursing diagnoses and Integrated Clinical Pathways to provide continuity of care

E. collaborates with other health care team members in interdepartmental issue recognition and resolution

3. The registered nurse in the associate role provides direct nursing care for the client for a specified time:

A. assesses and prioritizes the delivery of direct nursing care using time and resources effectively and efficiently

B. performs nursing tasks/skills both legally and safely

C. monitors and evaluates immediate patient responses to nursing/medical treatments and documents variances from Integrated Clinical Pathways

D. delegates or refers aspects of care to health care team members consistent with their roles and responsibilities

E. assumes responsibility and accountability for the direct nursing care provided

EMPLOYEE ROLE OF THE REGISTERED NURSE

1. Complies with the standards, policies, and procedures of Sioux Valley Hospital.

2. Supports staffing/scheduling policies to meet client needs.

3. Complies with departmental education requirements.

4. Promotes unit/department philosophy and goals.

5. Fosters the developmental and educational process of orientees, students, and colleagues.

6. Maintains confidentiality of information regarding clients, families, health care personnel, and the Sioux Valley Hospital network.

7. Treats others with respect and dignity, recognizing the individual uniqueness of clients and colleagues.

8. Demonstrates and reinforces professional behaviors in self and colleagues.

9. Demonstrates honest and open review of peers with an effort to influence change positively.

10. Serves as ambassador of Sioux Valley Hospital.

11. Participates in quality assurance activities.

12. Promotes efficient and effective resource utilization.

JOB SPECIFICATIONS

1. Currently licensed with South Dakota Board of Nursing to practice as a registered nurse. Works within this legal scope of practice.
2. After a formal orientation, competency in the assigned clinical area is expected within 6 months.
3. May be exposed to communicable or infectious disease, hazardous materials, and injury from performance of assigned duties. Is subject to multiple sensory and environmental stressors.

Reprinted with permission of Sioux Valley Hospital, Sioux Falls, South Dakota, © 1989.

Appendix 4-B
Sioux Valley Hospital Department of Nursing Job Description: Registered Nurse in the Primary Role

JOB SUMMARY

The registered nurse in the primary role integrates health care for clients from preadmission to postdischarge. The nurse functions in structured and unstructured health care settings described as a geographic and/or situational environment that may not have established policies and procedures. The nurse utilizes independent nursing judgment when integrating health care.

JOB RESPONSIBILITIES

1. The registered nurse in the primary role manages and integrates care of clients from preadmission to postdischarge utilizing Integrated Clinical Pathways:
   A expands the collection of data using a holistic focus to identify complex health care needs
   B. analyzes and integrates complex data to develop further nursing diagnoses
   C. uses future sight to negotiate long-term goals with the client to develop a holistic and comprehensive plan of care based on Integrated Clinical Pathways
   D. implements and/or delegates a holistic and comprehensive plan of care utilizing collaborative commitment
   E. evaluates progress toward established goals utilizing Integrated Clinical Pathways and promotes goal-directed change to meet client needs
   F. incorporates the research process to enhance nursing practice
2. The registered nurse in the primary role utilizes interactive communication:
   A. assesses the client's emotional needs and learning readiness within the client's environment to develop a holistic plan of care
   B. facilitates goal-directed interactions that are parallel to Integrated Clinical Pathways to promote effective long-term coping mechanisms and lifestyle changes

   C. designs, implements, and evaluates a holistic and comprehensive teaching plan that will maximize the client's potential for health

   D. collaborates with community resource persons by communicating comprehensive data to provide continuity of care

   E. assumes the change agent role to identify and resolve issues within the health care delivery system

3. The registered nurse in the primary role coordinates and/or provides nursing care for the client from preadmission to postdischarge:

   A. assesses and utilizes the nursing process to facilitate the delivery of holistic care using time and resources efficiently

   B. performs/delegates skills both legally and safely

   C. monitors, evaluates, and trends patient responses to nursing and medical treatments over hospital stay utilizing Integrated Clinical Pathways

   D. initiates/facilitates referrals to community resource persons to deliver services that promote quality outcomes

   E. assumes responsibility and accountability for care plan effectiveness and client outcomes

EMPLOYEE ROLE OF THE REGISTERED NURSE

1. Complies with the standards, policies, and procedures of Sioux Valley Hospital.
2. Supports staffing/scheduling policies to meet client needs.
3. Complies with departmental education requirements.
4. Promotes unit/department philosophy and goals.
5. Fosters the developmental and educational process of orientees, students, and colleagues.
6. Maintains confidentiality of information regarding clients, families, health care personnel, and the Sioux Valley Hospital network.
7. Treats others with respect and dignity, recognizing the individual uniqueness of clients and colleagues.
8. Demonstrates and reinforces professional behaviors in self and colleagues.
9. Demonstrates honest and open review of peers with an effort to influence change positively.
10. Serves as ambassador of Sioux Valley Hospital.
11. Participates in quality assurance activities.
12. Promotes efficient and effective resource utilization.

JOB SPECIFICATIONS

1. Currently licensed with South Dakota Board of Nursing to practice as a registered nurse. Works within this legal scope of practice.
2. After a formal orientation, competency in the assigned clinical area is expected within 6 months.
3. May be exposed to communicable or infectious disease, hazardous materials, and injury from performance of assigned duties. Is subject to multiple sensory and environmental stressors.

Reprinted with permission of Sioux Valley Hospital, Sioux Falls, South Dakota, © 1989.

Appendix 4-C
Sioux Valley Hospital Department of Nursing Job Description: Registered Nurse in the Clinical Care Coordinator Role

JOB SUMMARY

The registered nurse in the clinical care coordinator role facilitates health care services for clients in cooperation with the health care team. The nurse coordinates the clinical/unit nursing activities while adhering to hospital and unit philosophy, goals, and standards of care. The nurse utilizes independent and interdependent nursing judgment when integrating health care.

JOB RESPONSIBILITIES

1. The registered nurse in the clinical care coordinator role coordinates unit nursing services:
   A. assesses and efficiently allocates available resources to maintain unit standards of care
   B. mentors/delegates nursing tasks/skills both legally and safely
   C. monitors, evaluates, and trends clinical activities and unit needs and outcomes
   D. collaborates with the health care team to facilitate the referral process
   E. assumes responsibility and accountability for clinical activities and unit outcomes
2. The registered nurse in the clinical care coordinator role utilizes interactive communication:
   A. assesses the emotional climate to promote an optimal clinical environment
   B. facilitates effective communication and negotiation within the health care team
   C. evaluates and redesigns clinical activities to meet learning/teaching needs of clients/staff

   D. collaborates with community resource persons and the health care team to facilitate continuity of care

   E. functions as a change agent, advocate, and resource person for the health care team and/or clients to identify and resolve issues within the health care delivery system

3. The registered nurse in the clinical care coordinator role facilitates the integration of clients' care:

   A. focuses on the needs of the unit and proper patient assignment while keeping the interests of the division and hospital in focus, including when and where to admit and/or transfer a patient contingent upon available nursing resources

   B. uses future sight to analyze and integrate complex data to meet unit needs

   C. mentors/negotiates with the health care team to meet unit needs

   D. promotes partnership commitment to enhance the delivery of care at the unit, divisional, and hospital levels

   E. evaluates progress toward established goals and promotes change to meet unit needs

   F. incorporates the research process to enhance nursing practice

EMPLOYEE ROLE OF THE REGISTERED NURSE

1. Complies with the standards, policies, and procedures of Sioux Valley Hospital.
2. Supports staffing/scheduling policies to meet client needs.
3. Complies with department education requirements.
4. Promotes unit/department philosophy and goals.
5. Fosters the developmental and educational process of orientees, students, and colleagues.
6. Maintains confidentiality of information regarding clients, families, health care personnel, and the Sioux Valley Hospital network.
7. Treats others with respect and dignity, recognizing the individual uniqueness of clients and colleagues.
8. Demonstrates and reinforces professional behaviors in self and colleagues.
9. Demonstrates honest and open review of peers with an effort to influence change positively.
10. Serves as ambassador of Sioux Valley Hospital.
11. Participates in quality assurance activities.
12. Promotes efficient and effective resource utilization.

JOB SPECIFICATIONS

1. Currently licensed with South Dakota Board of Nursing to practice as a registered nurse. Works within this legal scope of practice.
2. After a formal orientation, competency in the assigned clinical area is expected within 6 months.
3. May be exposed to communicable or infectious disease, hazardous materials, and injury from performance of assigned duties. Is subject to multiple sensory and environmental stressors.

Reprinted with permission of Sioux Valley Hospital, Sioux Falls, South Dakota, © 1989.

Appendix 4-D
Sioux Valley Hospital Department of Nursing
Job Description: Director of ____
Care Services

JOB SUMMARY

The registered nurse in the director role is responsible for the continuous leadership of the assigned nursing service. The director ensures quality-focused and cost-effective care delivery outcomes. The director utilizes theory, research, and specialized knowledge relative to human, fiscal, and material resource management. Creative and flexible problem solving and the ability to empower others are key components of the director's leadership role.

JOB RESPONSIBILITIES

1. The registered nurse in the director role demonstrates leadership ability to achieve quality-focused and cost-effective client outcomes:
   - accepts responsibility for and empowers staff to:
     —review unit-based patient outcomes through the continuous quality improvement process
     —design new and better processes in patient care to achieve quality and superior service
     —influence organizational policy development related to patient care
   - maintains knowledge about the delivery of nursing care in the practice environment
2. The registered nurse in the director role demonstrates expertise in communication and negotiation:
   - is perceived as a leader and enhances the image of nursing within the profession, community, and organization
   - identifies, introduces, and assimilates change in the practice environment
   - supports a shared governance model of management
   - is a role model in physician and public relations

- directs and supports staff toward autonomous practice and decision making within a climate of cohesiveness and group interaction
- participates in representing the hospital and the profession of nursing organizationally, in community committees, and in task forces
- demonstrates the ability to problem solve using an analytic approach
- supports and participates in the unit peer review and credentialing process to ensure competency of staff

3. The registered nurse in the director role assumes responsibility for decisions related to human, fiscal, and material resources:
   - assists in meeting unit and organizational goals and objectives by monitoring efficient use of human resources and cost-effective material management
   - participates in strategic planning for the hospital/department
   - prepares the unit budget based on the strategic plan
   - implements the unit budget and is accountable for variations
   - influences organizational policy development

Courtesy of Sioux Valley Hospital, Sioux Falls, South Dakota.

Appendix 4-E
Sioux Valley Hospital Department of Nursing
Job Description: Clinical Nurse Specialist

DEFINITION

According to the American Nurses' Association, a clinical nurse specialist is a registered nurse who, through study and supervised practice at the graduate level (master's or doctorate), has become expert in a defined area of knowledge and practice in a selected clinical area of nursing.

JOB SUMMARY AND DESCRIPTION

The clinical nurse specialist is a registered professional nurse who demonstrates experience in a specific area of clinical nursing that has been further developed through master's preparation in nursing. A selected client population is the focus of practice. The population may be further defined according to age group; psychologic, social, cultural, or biophysical systems; or client status on the health–illness continuum. The clinical nurse specialist position is based on the needs of the client, the health care system, the nurse's expertise, and the expectations of the larger society.

The clinical nurse specialist works under the direction of a nursing administrator as a leader, innovator, and change agent in the pursuit of improved nursing practice and quality of client care. The scope of practice encompasses the use of nursing process in major areas: practice, education, consultation, and research.

Clinical Practice

1. Direct
   - Provides direct nursing care to a select client population with complex problems.
   - Utilizes a theoretical framework in providing nursing practice.
   - Initiates and applies new clinical modalities in client care based on research, expert knowledge, and technical competency.

- Assesses individual client care needs through rounds, care conferences, and communications with various health team members.
- Plans with nursing staff to identify priorities and realistic outcomes for interventions.
- Serves as a client advocate.
- Serves as a role model in providing direct client care.
- Provides case management services to select clients.

2. Indirect
   - Facilitates continuity of client care.
   - Revises and/or evaluates procedures and/or protocols.
   - Plans with nursing management/staff for the development and implementation of standards of care.
   - Advances professional nursing through publications, organizations, and other activities.
   - Collaborates with manager to develop strategic long-range plans in area of specialty.
   - Collaborates with manager regarding clinical/educational needs that affect financial planning for specialty area.
   - Promotes cost-effective client care.
   - Actively participates on organizational committees and meetings within the institution and community.
   - Supports a decentralized organization that places the responsibility and authority for decision making at the level closest to the situation.
   - Participates in peer review to evaluate own practice and involvement.

Education

1. Identifies educational needs of clients and/or families concerning health maintenance, alterations in health, the disease process, and the hospital/posthospital plan of care.
2. Plans for the education of individuals or groups of clients and families.
3. Develops or participates in the development of appropriate materials to facilitate the education of clients.
4. Plans with nursing management/staff development/nursing staff to identify educational needs of the health care team.
5. Develops and presents educational programs and conferences.
6. Facilitates the application of appropriate theories of nursing and other sciences.

7. Provides for the dissemination of current information and theories necessary for the advancement of client care.
8. Accepts responsibility for preceptoring selected students.
9. Coordinates and/or participates in community educational programs.
10. Plans and implements a program for continuing self-development.

Consultation

1. Collaborates with nursing and other health care professionals in the establishment of goals and implementation of the plan of care.
2. Collaborates with the nurse manager and staff to identify clinical activities to facilitate the professional growth of the health care team.
3. Provides leadership in the assessment, development, and implementation of policies and procedures/standards of care that are directly and indirectly related to the area of specialization.
4. Participates in the quality assurance program as related to area of specialization.
5. Facilitates nurse-to-nurse consulting process.
6. Provides client care consultation.
7. Provides consultation to other hospital departments.
8. Provides consultation to the community at large.

Research

1. Writes grants, protocols, and research study proposals.
2. Actively participates in research activities.
3. Assesses and identifies relevant researchable clinical nursing problems with staff.
4. Evaluates and disseminates research findings.
5. Evaluates the impact of various programs and interventions upon client care and nursing practice.
6. Protects the rights of research participants.

Courtesy of Sioux Valley Hospital, Sioux Falls, South Dakota.

Appendix 4-F
Role Choice Tool

Directions: Circle one number for each statement about your nursing practice. Circle 1 for "never." Circle 2 for "seldom." Circle 3 for "sometimes." Circle 4 for "usually." Circle 5 for "always."

1. Uses the nursing process to prioritize nursing care delivered.   1   2   3   4   5

2. Uses time and resources effectively and efficiently.   1   2   3   4   5

3 Attends continuing education/inservice programs to update knowledge/skills.   1   2   3   4   5

4. Treats others with respect and dignity.   1   2   3   4   5

5. Assesses patient to identify basic nursing care needs.   1   2   3   4   5

6. Negotiates long-term goals with the patient to develop a comprehensive care plan.   1   2   3   4   5

7. Follows policies and procedures while implementing an individualized care plan.   1   2   3   4   5

8. Delegates aspects of care to others on the health care team.   1   2   3   4   5

9. Selects appropriate nursing diagnoses and related standardized nursing care plans.   1   2   3   4   5

10. Evaluates the patient's immediate responses to care and treatment.   1   2   3   4   5

11. Assesses the patient's learning readiness.   1   2   3   4   5

12. Modifies nursing interventions to meet the patient's needs.   1   2   3   4   5

13. Evaluates progress toward long-term goals.   1   2   3   4   5

14. Assesses the patient's emotional needs.   1   2   3   4   5

15. Completes comprehensive assessment to identify complex nursing care needs.   1   2   3   4   5

16. Enjoys teaching patient/family about caring for self during hospitalization and after discharge.   1   2   3   4   5

1, never; 2, seldom; 3, sometimes; 4, usually; 5, always

17. Negotiates short-term goals with the patient that are
consistent with the overall care plan.   1 2 3 4 5
18. Supports safe coping behaviors.   1 2 3 4 5
19. Encourages the patient to express his or her needs. 1 2 3 4 5
20. Assesses the patient's environment to develop a
comprehensive care plan.   1 2 3 4 5
21. Prefers to work independently with patients rather
than as part of nursing care team.   1 2 3 4 5
22. Communicates data to other health team members
based on nursing diagnoses to provide continuity
of care.   1 2 3 4 5
23. Encourages lifestyle changes.   1 2 3 4 5
24. Collaborates with community resource persons to
provide continuity of care.   1 2 3 4 5
25. Uses the nursing process to facilitate delivering
comprehensive care.   1 2 3 4 5
26. Uses nursing literature to improve nursing practice
at your agency.   1 2 3 4 5
27. Delegates aspects of care to others on the health
care team appropriately.   1 2 3 4 5
28. Promotes effective long-term coping mechanisms. 1 2 3 4 5
29. Assumes responsibility and accountability for the
direct nursing care provided.   1 2 3 4 5
30. Using the nursing process, designs comprehensive
teaching plans.   1 2 3 4 5
31. Collaborates with community resources to change
health care delivery.   1 2 3 4 5
32. Initiates referrals to community resources to promote
continuity of care.   1 2 3 4 5
33. Participates in resolving identified interdepartmental
issues.   1 2 3 4 5
34. Prefers contact with family to plan comprehensively
for patient.   1 2 3 4 5
35. Assumes responsibility and accountability for
patient outcomes.   1 2 3 4 5
36. Complies with the standards, policies, and procedures of your agency.   1 2 3 4 5

1, never; 2, seldom; 3, sometimes; 4, usually; 5, always

37. Prefers to be responsible for nursing care for the shift worked.	1	2	3	4	5
38. Delegates skills both legally and safely.	1	2	3	4	5
39. Is competent in the assigned clinical area.	1	2	3	4	5
40. Prefers primary nurse assignment to team, task, or total patient care.	1	2	3	4	5
41. Assists others with their assignments while completing own duties on time.	1	2	3	4	5
42. Monitors the patient's responses to nursing and medicine throughout the treatment period.	1	2	3	4	5
43. Assumes the change agent role to resolve identified issues in the health care delivery system.	1	2	3	4	5
44. Using the nursing process, individualizes standard teaching plans.	1	2	3	4	5
45. Uses information provided by other health care team members when developing the comprehensive care plan.	1	2	3	4	5
46. Performs nursing tasks/skills legally.	1	2	3	4	5
47. Prefers to be responsible for managing the patient's nursing care from preadmission to postdischarge.	1	2	3	4	5
48. Prefers caring for patients when family is absent.	1	2	3	4	5
49. Analyzes complex data to develop additional nursing diagnoses.	1	2	3	4	5

Developed by Kathryn Linda Karpiuk and JoEllen Goertz Koerner. Courtesy of Sioux Valley Hospital, Sioux Falls, South Dakota.

Appendix 4-G
Administrative Standard Operating Procedure for Registered Nurse Incentive Plan for Preceptoring

PURPOSE

1.1 To increase the incentives for qualified preceptors by providing additional opportunities.
1.2 To facilitate the continuity of preceptor–preceptee relationships.

POLICY

2.1 Criteria:
    2.1.1 Preceptor: A qualified clinical I or clinical II registered nurse who accepts the responsibility for the consistent, direct supervision, education, and evaluation of a preceptee in addition to regular job responsibilities.
    2.1.2 Preceptee: A novice registered nurse, student, or designated individual who is assigned to be supervised, instructed, and evaluated by the preceptor.
    2.1.3 Preceptor position requirements must be successfully completed before preceptorship.
        2.1.3.1 Preceptoring requires attendance at nursing center-approved workshop/class for beginning preceptors.
        2.1.3.2 Two credit hours of continuing education per year devoted to preceptoring. These hours are not in addition to, but are a part of, continuing education as required per nursing administrative standard operating procedure E7.
        2.1.3.3 Preceptoring for special educational programs (such as Summer E) also requires attendance at special training session(s) as outlined by the program. No credit for preceptoring hours will be given unless the designated training session(s) is (are) attended.

2.2 Credit will be earned for serving as an approved preceptor.

2.2.1 One credit will be earned for each 1 hour of a 4-hour block minimum of preceptoring completed. Exception: If a long-term relationship with a preceptee of a minimum of 36 hours is planned, periods of time less than a 4-hour block may be recognized for preceptoring credit.

2.2.2 Required evaluations by primary preceptor must be completed and submitted to designated nursing center secretary within 1 week of completing preceptorship, or no credit for preceptoring hours will be given. All evaluations should include information from others to whom the preceptee has been assigned.

2.2.3 An audit to verify preceptoring hours can be undertaken by unit education council, nursing center personnel, or designee.

2.2.4 Each credit will earn $1.00, which can be utilized toward continuing education opportunities.

2.2.5 Continuing education opportunities that you wish to attend by using preceptoring credits must be approved by your director.

2.2.6 Credits earned can be utilized for:

2.2.6.1 Workshop registration

2.2.6.2 Travel, meals, lodging for workshop

2.2.6.3 Tuition reimbursement above regular standard operating procedure

2.2.6.4 Paid hours for attendance at educational offering

2.2.6.5 Membership to professional organization

2.2.6.6 Professional certification fee (nursing license renewal is not considered a certification fee)

2.2.6.7 Professional journal subscription/textbook

2.2.6.8 Professional/educational opportunities (individual proposal submitted for approval by department head/designee; eg, clinical experience in another institution, minisabbatical)

PROCEDURE

3.1 A registered nurse preceptoring record must be completed and submitted to the designated nursing center secretary for recording of accumulated credits a minimum of twice a year, during January and July.

3.2 A registered nurse preceptoring expense voucher must be submitted to the designated nursing center secretary to determine eligible credits and then must be approved by director/designee.

3.2.1 Receipts of expenses must be submitted for any reimbursement.

3.2.2 Workshop expenses will be reimbursed as per administrative standard operating procedure E280.

3.2.3 Reimbursement checks will be written to employee only, except in the case of allowable workshop advance payments.

3.2.4 A completed registered nurse preceptoring expense voucher must be submitted to the nursing center secretary to be processed.

3.2.5 Credits must be earned before they can be used.

3.2.6 Reimbursed hours for educational offerings should be submitted on time and attendance adjustment forms and attached to the expense voucher.

    3.2.6.1 Present hourly wage must be identified on the expense voucher.

    3.2.6.2 Reimbursement for paid hours will automatically have 18% subtracted for benefits adjustment from accrued credits.

    3.2.6.3 Time and attendance adjustment form and preceptoring expense voucher for paid hours must be submitted separately from any other expense voucher.

3.2.7 All forms will be in triplicate to facilitate bookkeeping.

Courtesy of Sioux Valley Hospital, Sioux Falls, South Dakota.

Appendix 4-H
Sioux Valley Hospital Department of Nursing Job Description Standards: Registered Nurse in the Associate Role

Employee Appraisal   Annual _____ Periodic _____
Name_____   Date Hired _____
Date_____   Evaluator _____

Employee collects data twice a year; peers collect data twice a year. Minimum of one chart is reviewed at each collection. Performance standards are numbered. Measurement criteria are included, with the location of information being designated in parentheses. Number and letter in square brackets refer to a specific item listed on the job description for the role.

Directions: Circle applicable letter for each performance standard. Comment in space provided.

SCALE: M = Met
         U = Unacceptable

AMERICAN NURSES ASSOCIATION (ANA) STANDARD I

The collection of data about the health status of the client/patient
is systematic and continuous. The data are accessible,
communicated, and recorded.   M   U

SIOUX VALLEY HOSPITAL (SVH) MEASUREMENT CRITERION

Information needed to provide daily quality care is collected, recorded, and communicated. Included is incorporation of research process. (Admission form, database, flowsheets, nursing notes, portfolio)

  1. Collects data from available resources, using established assessment format, to identify basic nursing care needs. [1A]

2. Applies interpreted nursing research findings for nursing care. [1F]

_____

_____

ANA STANDARD II

Nursing diagnoses are derived from health status data.   M   U

SVH MEASUREMENT CRITERION

Completes admission form upon admit and begins database. (Admission form, database)

1. Organizes and analyzes data to select pertinent nursing diagnoses and related standardized nursing care plans. [1B]

_____

_____

_____

ANA STANDARD III

The plan of nursing care includes goals derived from the
nursing diagnoses.   M   U

SVH MEASUREMENT CRITERION

Pulls standardized care plans and incorporates into documentation system. (Care plans, Clinical Pathways)

1. Organizes and analyzes data to select pertinent nursing diagnoses and related standardized nursing care plans. [1B]
2. Monitors and evaluates immediate patient responses to nursing/medical treatments and documents variances from Integrated Clinical Pathways. [3C]

_____

_____

_____

ANA STANDARD IV

The plan of nursing care includes priorities and the prescribed nursing approaches or measures to achieve the goals derived from the nursing diagnoses.   M   U

SVH MEASUREMENT CRITERION

Individual daily needs are prioritized and acted upon or delegated. (Flowsheets, nursing notes)

1. Implements an individualized plan of care using established nursing diagnoses, policies, procedures, and Integrated Clinical Pathways. [1D]
2. Assesses the client to determine immediate emotional needs and learning readiness. [2A]
3. Delegates or refers aspects of care to health care team members consistent with their roles and responsibilities. [3D]

_____

_____

_____

ANA STANDARD V

Nursing actions provide for client/patient participation in health promotion, maintenance, and restoration.   M   U

SVH MEASUREMENT CRITERION

Client and nurse reach mutual plan of action to reach daily goals. (Flowsheets, nursing notes)

1. Utilizes negotiation with the client to establish short-term goals that are consistent with the overall plan of care. [1C]

_____

_____

_____

_____

ANA STANDARD VI

Nursing actions assist the client/patient to maximize his or her health
capabilities.   M   U

SVH MEASUREMENT CRITERION

Mutual plan of action is carried out utilizing individualized teaching plan.
(Flowsheets, nursing notes, teaching sheets)

1. Implements goal-directed interactions to encourage expression of needs while
   supporting safe coping behaviors. [2B]
2. Modifies, implements, and evaluates a standard teaching plan to restore,
   maintain, or promote health. [2C]

ANA STANDARD VII

The client's/patient's progress or lack of progress toward goal
achievement is determined by the client/patient and the nurse.   M   U

SVH MEASUREMENT CRITERION

Responsible for evaluation and documentation of achievement toward reaching
daily goals with patient. (Nursing notes)

1. Evaluates client responses and modifies nursing interventions as necessary to
   meet client needs. [1E]
2. Collaborates with other health team members in interdepartmental issue
   recognition and resolution. [2E]
3. Monitors and evaluates immediate patient responses to nursing/medical
   treatments and documents variances from Integrated Clinical Pathways. [3C]
4. Assumes responsibility and accountability for the direct nursing care provided. [3E]

ANA STANDARD VIII

The client's/patient's progress or lack of progress toward
goal achievement directs reassessment, reordering of priorities,
new goal setting, and revision of the plan of nursing care.   M   U

SVH MEASUREMENT CRITERION

Daily goals are revised, documented, and communicated to health care team
members. Obstacles to reaching goals are resolved. (Care plans, flowsheets, nursing
notes)

1. Evaluates client responses and modifies nursing interventions as necessary to
   meet client needs. [1E]
2. Networks with health care team members by communicating data based on
   nursing diagnoses and Integrated Clinical Pathways to provide continuity of
   care. [2D]
3. Collaborates with other health care team members in interdepartmental issue
   recognition and resolution. [2E]

_____

_____

_____

Signature of Employee being reviewed

_____

_____

_____

_____

Signatures of Review Team Members

Courtesy of Sioux Valley Hospital, Sioux Falls, South Dakota.

Appendix 4-I
Sioux Valley Hospital Department of Nursing
Job Description Standards: Registered Nurse
in the Primary Role

Employee Appraisal
Name _____
Date _____

Annual _____ Periodic _____
Date Hired _____
Evaluator _____

Employee collects data twice a year; peers collect data twice a year. Minimum of one chart is reviewed at each collection. Performance standards are numbered. Measurement criteria are included, with the location of information being designated in parentheses. Number and letter in square brackets refer to a specific time listed on the job description for the role.

Directions: Circle applicable letter for each performance standard. Comment in space provided.

SCALE: M = Met
U = Unacceptable

AMERICAN NURSES ASSOCIATION (ANA) STANDARD I

The collection of data about the health status of the client/patient
is systematic and continuous. The data are accessible,
communicated, and recorded.   M   U

SIOUX VALLEY HOSPITAL (SVH) MEASUREMENT CRITERION

Information needed to plan for discharge is recorded and communicated systematically. Included is the incorporation of the research process. (Admission form, database, primary summaries, portfolio)

1. Expands the collection of data using a holistic focus to identify complex health care needs. [1A]

ANA STANDARD II

Nursing diagnoses are derived from health status data.   M   U

SVH MEASUREMENT CRITERION

Database is completed within specified time allowed by unit. Includes continual reassessment of client's needs. (Database, primary summaries)

1. Expands the collection of data using a holistic focus to identify complex health care needs. [1A]
2. Analyzes and integrates complex data to develop further nursing diagnoses. [1B]

ANA STANDARD III

The plan of nursing care includes goals derived from the nursing diagnoses.   M   U

SVH MEASUREMENT CRITERION

Initial plan of care is written within 24 hours and appropriate Clinical Pathway is selected and initiated. (Initial care plan, Clinical Pathways)

1. Analyzes and integrates complex data to develop further nursing diagnoses. [1B]
2. Assesses the client's emotional needs and learning readiness within the client's environment to develop a holistic plan of care. [2A]

ANA STANDARD IV

The plan of nursing care includes priorities and the prescribed nursing approaches or measures to achieve the goals derived from the nursing diagnoses.   M   U

SVH MEASUREMENT CRITERION

Goals are prioritized to meet patient's needs. (Care plans, primary summaries)

1. Uses future sight to negotiate long-term goals with the client to develop a holistic comprehensive plan of care based on Integrated Clinical Pathways. [1C]
2. Assesses the client's emotional needs and learning readiness within the client's environment to develop a holistic plan of care. [2A]

ANA STANDARD V

Nursing actions provide for client/patient participation in health promotion, maintenance, and restoration.   M   U

SVH MEASUREMENT CRITERION

Nurse and patient negotiate to set goals to meet long-term health care needs. (Care plans, primary summaries)

1. Implements and/or delegates a holistic and comprehensive plan of care utilizing collaborative commitment. [1D]
2. Uses future sight to negotiate long-term goals with the client to develop a holistic and comprehensive plan of care based on Integrated Clinical Pathways. [1C]
3. Facilitates goal-directed interactions that are parallel to Integrated Clinical Pathways to promote effective long-term coping mechanisms and lifestyle changes. [2B]

ANA STANDARD VI

Nursing actions assist the client/patient to maximize his or her health
capabilities.   M   U

SVH MEASUREMENT CRITERION

Individual needs previously identified are addressed through teaching and with
intraagency and interagency collaboration. (Care plans, teaching forms, discharge
summaries, referrals, portfolio)

1. Designs, implements, and evaluates a holistic and comprehensive teaching
   plan that will maximize the client's potential for health. [2C]
2. Collaborates with community resource persons by communicating comprehensive data to provide continuity of care. [2D]
3. Assumes the change agent role to identify and resolve issues within the health
   care delivery system. [2E]
4. Initiates/facilitates referrals to community resource persons to deliver services that promote quality outcomes. [3D]

_____

_____

ANA STANDARD VII

The client's/patient's progress or lack of progress toward goal
achievement is determined by the client/patient and the nurse.   M   U

SVH MEASUREMENT CRITERION

Responsible for assessing progress toward meeting discharge needs with patient.
(Care plans, primary summaries)

1. Evaluates progress toward established goals utilizing Integrated Clinical
   Pathways and promotes goal-directed change to meet client needs. [1E]
2. Assumes responsibility and accountability for care plan effectiveness and
   client outcomes. [3E]

_____

_____

ANA STANDARD VIII

The client's/patient's progress or lack of progress toward goal
achievement directs reassessment, reordering of priorities, new
goal setting, and revision of the plan of nursing care.   M   U

SVH MEASUREMENT CRITERION

Trends are documented and used to revise nursing care plans, to meet goals, and
to communicate to the health care team.

1. Monitors, evaluates, and trends patient responses to nursing and medical
   treatments over hospital stay utilizing Integrated Clinical Pathways. [3C]
2. Evaluates progress toward established goals utilizing Integrated Clinical
   Pathways and promotes goal-directed change to meet client needs. [1E]

_____

_____

_____

Signature of Employee being reviewed

_____

_____

_____

_____

_____

Signatures of Review Team Members

Courtesy of Sioux Valley Hospital, Sioux Falls, South Dakota.

Appendix 4-J
Sioux Valley Hospital Department of Nursing Job Description Standards: Registered Nurse in the Clinical Care Coordinator Role

Employee Appraisal   Annual _____ Periodic _____

Name_____   Date Hired _____

Date_____   Evaluator _____

Employee collects data twice a year; peers collect data twice a year. Minimum of one chart is reviewed at each collection. Performance standards are numbered. Measurement criteria are included, with the location of information being designated in parentheses. Number and letter in square brackets refer to a specific item listed on the job description for the role.

Directions: Circle applicable letter for each performance standard. Comment in space provided.

SCALE: M = Met
        U = Unacceptable
        CE = Cannot Evaluate

AMERICAN NURSES ASSOCIATION (ANA) STANDARD I

The collection of data about the health status of the client/patient is systematic and continuous. The data are accessible, communicated, and recorded.   M   U   CE

SIOUX VALLEY HOSPITAL (SVH) MEASUREMENT CRITERION

Collects, analyzes, and integrates information about patient population and unit environment to supply needed nursing resources. (Shift-to-shift report form, unit management council minutes, memos)

1. Assesses and efficiently allocates available resources to maintain unit standards of care. [1A]

2. Assesses the emotional climate to promote an optimal clinical environment. [2A]
3. Uses future sight to analyze and integrate complex data to meet unit needs. [3B]
4. Incorporates the research process to enhance nursing practice. [3F]

_____

_____

ANA STANDARD II

Nursing diagnoses are derived from health status data.   M   U   CE

SVH MEASUREMENT CRITERION

Assists in identification of patients needing a primary nurse. (Portfolio, database, input from primary nurses)

1. Mentors/delegates nursing tasks/skills both legally and safely. [1B]

_____

_____

ANA STANDARD III

The plan of nursing care includes goals derived from the
nursing diagnoses.   M   U   CE

SVH MEASUREMENT CRITERION

Responsible for continuously evaluating and trending clinical activities and plans for optimal outcomes. (Shift-to-shift report form, unit management council minutes, portfolios, input from coworkers)

1. Mentors/delegates nursing tasks/skills both legally and safely. [1B]
2. Monitors, evaluates, and trends clinical activities and unit needs and outcomes. [1C]

3. Assumes responsibility and accountability for clinical activities and unit outcomes. [1E]

_____

_____

ANA STANDARD IV

The plan of nursing care includes priorities and the prescribed nursing approaches or measures to achieve the goals derived from the nursing diagnoses.   M   U   CE

SVH MEASUREMENT CRITERION

Collaborates with health care services in meeting clients' needs and resolving issues. (Committee work, unit management council minutes, portfolio, shift-to-shift report form)

1. Collaborates with the health care team to facilitate the referral process. [1D]
2. Facilitates effective communication and negotiation within the health care team. [2B]
3. Collaborates with community resource persons and health care team to facilitate continuity of care. [2D]
4. Functions as a change agent, advocate, and resource person for the health care team and/or clients to identify and resolve issues within the health care delivery system. [2E]

_____

_____

ANA STANDARD V

Nursing actions provide for client/patient participation in health promotion, maintenance, and restoration.   M   U   CE

SVH MEASUREMENT CRITERION

Coordinates resources to meet unit, division, and hospital goals. (Staffing office personnel, portfolio)

1. Focuses on the needs of the unit and proper patient assignment while keeping the interests of the division and hospital in focus, including when and where to admit and/or transfer a patient contingent upon available nursing resources. [3A]
2. Promotes partnership commitment to enhance the delivery of care at the unit, divisional, and hospital levels. [3D]

ANA STANDARD VI

Nursing actions assist the client/patient to maximize his or her health capabilities.   M   U   CE

SVH MEASUREMENT CRITERION

Delegates, mentors, and assists nursing staff to reach identified goals. (Portfolios, inservices taught, input from coworkers)

1. Mentors/delegates nursing tasks/skills both legally and safely. [1B]
2. Mentors/negotiates with the health care team to meet unit needs. [3C]

ANA STANDARD VII

The client's/patient's progress or lack of progress toward goal achievement is determined by the client/patient and the nurse.   M   U   CE

SVH MEASUREMENT CRITERION

Collects data on goal achievement and incorporates into resource use. (Unit management council minutes, shift-to-shift report form, portfolio)

1. Evaluates progress toward established goals and promotes change to meet unit needs. [3E]

ANA STANDARD VIII

The client's/patient's progress or lack of progress toward
goal achievement directs reassessment, reordering of priorities,
new goal setting, and revision of the plan of nursing care.   M   U   CE

SVH MEASUREMENT CRITERION

Assesses and revises resource use based on changes in unit needs. (Unit management council minutes, shift-to-shift report form, portfolio)

1. Evaluates and redesigns clinical activities to meet learning/teaching needs of clients/staff. [2C]

_____

_____

_____

Signature of Employee being reviewed

_____

_____

_____

_____

_____

Signatures of Review Team Members

Courtesy of Sioux Valley Hospital, Sioux Falls, South Dakota.

5   Continuity

Pamela A. Koepsell, Rhonda Jensen,
Joan T. Reisdorfer, Cindi Slack,
Sandy Young, Anthony Weber,
Tricia Fjerestad, S. Jo Gibson, and
Nancy J. Paulson

Seeing the same thing happen every day, we infer
from this a natural necessity, as that there will be
a to-morrow.

BLAISE PASCAL

The continuum of health care is an essential component of the care of clients within the hospital. As patient lengths of stay are declining, it becomes imperative that the plan of care be communicated to the entire multidisciplinary team. With this, the nursing administration and nursing staff at Sioux Valley Hospital identified that nursing and its roles should be redefined to meet patients' needs during their hospital journey. The nursing roles would collaborate with one another to ensure a holistic approach to patient care. Throughout this chapter, the focus of continuity of care to enhance the patient's care from preadmission to postdischarge is emphasized.

DEFINITION

Webster's New World Dictionary defines continuity as uninterrupted advance or succession. *Taber's Encyclopedic Medical Dictionary* defines continuity as the state of being continuous or intimately united. It then defines continuous as without breaks, cessation, or interruption. Applying these definitions of continuity to the delivery of health care mandates that the health care provided to the client will occur without a break even though the location or environment of the individual may change. The process of continuity as well as the mechanism by which it is maintained to deliver this health care need to be identified. Ultimately, continuity would be a concept for the nurse to internalize in designing the client's plan of care.

The authors have identified that the process of continuity has five components: communication, collaboration, collegiality, accountability, and consultation. These are explored in further detail in this chapter. The five key components that have been identified in this process of continuity are intertwined with each other and do not function as solitary elements. It is through the integration of these components that a system of client health care can be delivered in a continuous manner.

COMMUNICATION

Communication is a vital component in the process of continuity. Without communication between the health care team and the client, continuity of care would not exist. There would be no exchange of the client history, needs, or goals. The focus of the health care would be the present state, based solely on the client history and needs during that particular hospitalization and ignoring the future needs that the client may manifest at the time of discharge or beyond.

It is imperative that health care members exchange appropriate information with other team members to expand their knowledge of the client's needs, not only focusing on the present state but also looking ahead to the future needs of the client. This communication must involve all disciplines. There must be a genuine trust among the health care team members to provide a collegial and collaborative relationship.

The nursing staff at Sioux Valley Hospital have been empowered by learning and practicing interdepartmental communication. Learning was promoted by the Ecology of Excellence philosophy and shared governance principles, which are discussed further in Chapters 7 and 8. Through these philosophies, nursing units and staff were propelled to implement multidisciplinary partnerships that would benefit the client's continuity of care. With this empowerment, nurses were allowed to implement change at the grassroots level rather than from an administrative level. The nursing staff could identify what would actually benefit their staff and the client when communicating information. The nursing staff's ultimate goal was to improve the system of bedside care through effective multidisciplinary communication.

COLLABORATION

To provide continuity, the health care team must collaborate. Collaboration is the working together phase to reach an agreement. The definition suggests that two parties have differing perspectives and that a cooperative effort is made to establish a common goal. These parties may be different departments that associate with and affect the same client simultaneously without exchanging information regarding the client's needs and goals as well as how the client is progressing. Through collaborative practice, the client's needs, goals, and interventions necessary to meet the goals established are communicated with each department.

Using the analogy of an ant colony, the health care team can learn how to collaborate. Ants live in colonies with a complex division of labor. Tasks are performed by particular groups. Ants collaborate through their sense of smell. Without this sense of smell, the colony would be in chaos and would not survive. The health care team also has a complex division of labor performed by multiple groups. Rather than using the sense of smell to collaborate with each other, the health care team must communicate verbally and work with one another to survive.

Two communication mechanisms that can assist with the process of collaboration are an interface agreement and the formation of an interdisciplinary task force. An interface agreement is a departmental or multidisciplinary contract that communicates to the participants that a consensus was reached on an issue by the formulation of a specific plan. Refer to Chapter 8 for further information about the utilization of interface agreements. The formation of a multidisciplinary task force enables all individuals sharing similar concerns to work together in problem solving for a mutual decision. With this shared decision, the continuity of care can be enhanced for all individuals involved.

COLLEGIALITY

Cooperation is spelled with two letters — WE.
GEORGE M. VERITY

Webster's New World Dictionary defines collegiality as the relationship of colleagues. A colleague is defined as an associate in a profession. Inherent in the concept of collegiality is valuing the other individual's expertise and the role performed in providing health care to the client.

The nursing role overlaps with many other professional roles, such as social work and chaplaincy. The professional must determine in what situations it is appropriate for role blurring to occur without jeopardizing the continuity of care and in what situations the roles must be explicitly clear to facilitate quality client care. For example, with a terminally ill client who has just learned his or her diagnosis and desires to ventilate concerns, it may be appropriate for either a social worker or a nurse to listen. If the client is a member of a highly complex dysfunctional family, however, the situation requires greater expertise, and the social worker is more qualified to intervene.

It is through similar situations that nursing must recognize when role blurring occurs and when it becomes necessary to involve other disciplines that have the required skill and knowledge for intervening with the client. Once this recognition is achieved, the nurses can begin to value each other for the expertise each discipline brings to the client's plan of care. Through this process, nurses began to collaborate with other health care members concerning the needs of their clients, thereby promoting the continuity of care concept.

While this transition was occurring at the bedside at Sioux Valley Hospital, a similar process of role blurring and clarification was occurring among the head nurse's, divisional supervisor's, and charge nurse's roles. It was the charge nurse's role that brought on new responsibilities within this role blurring and clarification process. The charge nurse's role was calling for a broader system perspective and for a longitudinal focus across the entire organization. Crisis intervention and unit and divisional staffing responsibilities, previously managed by the supervisor, became an expansion of the charge nurse role. The charge nurse role was retitled as the registered nurse (RN) in the clinical care coordinator role. Including some managerial responsibilities in the clinical care coordinator role necessitated a change in the role of the head nurse. The head nurse position was retitled unit director, expanding responsibilities to corporate level functions as well as maintenance of unit cohesiveness. The supervisors recognized that the clinical care coordinators had reached the expanded expertise that they once carried; therefore, the supervisor positions were phased out.

As nurses began to value each other's expertise and to develop an understanding of each role, complementary role blending occurred. Through these expanded roles, collegiality became an essential component in incorporating, communicating, and maintaining the continuity of client health care.

ACCOUNTABILITY

> *Assets make things possible, but people make them*
> *happen. Everything depends on people. Give*
> *people a function and a responsibility, then hold*
> *them accountable and you will be surprised with*
> *the results you will get.*
>
> ALFRED A. MONTAPERT

In the process of differentiating roles, accountability, defined as the capability of being responsible, became important. With everyone working to meet the needs of the clients, each piece was important to the whole. The associate and primary nurses were delegated certain job responsibilities to meet the needs of the client from preadmission to postdischarge. The clinical care coordinator also assisted with the client's needs by ensuring that adequate resources (staff and equipment) were available (see Appendices 4-A to 4-C for job descriptions).

Different nursing roles provide continuity over a variety of settings within a time frame. The associate nurse role is responsible for maintaining continuity within the

12-hour shift. The associate is also held accountable for the patient care required during this shift. The role of the primary nurse has become that of providing continuity from preadmission to postdischarge throughout the client's stay in the nurse's unit. The primary nurse has 24-hour accountability and plans care for the entire hospitalization. The clinical care coordinator is responsible for maintaining the environment of the unit, including staffing, bed utilization, and coordination of client care.

The associate nurse's principal accountability lies in the time frame of the care provided. These nurses are accountable for the shift care of a client. Accountability in this position includes assessing the client's short-term goals, documenting the client's progress toward meeting these goals, and determining what steps are needed to assist the client in working toward these goals. The associate nurse is also responsible for delegating to other staff the needs of the client for that shift in an effort to work toward the client's goals. This may require delegating tasks to the nurse aide, clinical care coordinator, or primary nurse.

The primary nurse's main accountability lies in the assessment of the client's whole picture from preadmission to postdischarge. From this assessment, the primary nurse is able to identify needs with the client and to establish long-term goals with short-term objectives for how to reach these goals. The primary nurse appropriately delegates to other disciplines through the mechanisms of communication, collaboration, and consultation in an effort to accomplish the tasks to meet these goals. The primary nurse also works closely with families to assist them in providing the necessary care for their loved one.

The clinical care coordinator is responsible for unit activities while ensuring adequate staffing for the unit and division. Along with accountabilities for the shift, the coordinator must also be cognizant of the future needs of the unit. Clinical care coordinators interact with other departments to negotiate and maintain a high standard of practice in promoting client health care.

The following vignette gives examples of the work associated with the associate and primary nurse roles:

> Client A is admitted to the hospital for surgery. The preadmission information—current medications, medical history, and support person after surgery—is obtained by the RN in the AM admissions unit. Upon the client's transfer to the surgical unit, the associate nurse receiving report learns that the client lives alone and is 85 years of age. This information is shared with the clinical care coordinator, and then reported to the primary nurse. The primary nurse then discusses needs and goals with the client. Mutual goals are established, and a care plan is implemented with the use of nursing diagnoses. The associate nurse begins to work on short-term goals for the client, such as medication education, ambulation assistance, activities of daily living, and other tasks that will progress the client toward long-term goals. The primary nurse works with the client in a different

manner; this nurse communicates, collaborates, and consults with other multidisciplinary partners to ensure that the client's needs are being met and that the goals will be achieved at the time of discharge. The primary nurse may also be the communicator to outside referral agencies to facilitate the appropriate home care interventions to aid in the continuity of care from hospital to home.

CONSULTATION

Consultation is defined as the act of consulting or conferring and as providing professional or expert advice. A consultant is one who gives professional advice or services in a field of special knowledge or training.

To provide and maintain continuity of health care, it was imperative for the primary nurses at Sioux Valley Hospital to develop and refine their consultation skills. Initially, this was achieved through inservices and workshops that focused on the art of delegating and consulting. Nurses needed to reframe their thinking to reflect that they did not need to be the experts on every facet of patient care but rather the experts on what resources, both human and material, were available. The nurses also needed to know how to tap into those resources. It was at this time that nursing began to realize what a wealth of knowledge and expertise they had in their own environment that they were currently not utilizing to their maximum capacity. Nurses learned that they need to value their own nursing partners within the organization. This was a gradual process, but through this process the care of the patient was enhanced.

Another level of consultation was beginning to be established at Sioux Valley Hospital. This was the consultation between the nursing staff and the advanced practice nurse or clinical nurse specialist (CNS). The role of the advanced practice nurse is discussed and further defined in Chapter 6.

CASE MANAGEMENT

It soon became evident that a system needed to be implemented to bridge the gap between home and hospital care. Specific patients required greater follow-up to help maintain compliance with the medical/nursing plan of care. Case management was identified to be that system.

At Sioux Valley Hospital, case management is defined as a multifaceted system with many elements, including health assessment; planning; service procurement, delivery, and coordination; and monitoring of services. It is designed to optimize the patient's self-care capability and participation in health care decisions. The CNS utilizes this system to integrate, coordinate, negotiate, and advocate on a continuum for patients with complex health care needs while assisting in effective utilization of the health care dollar. The vision of case management has been nebulous for several years. The CNSs are the case managers of patients who meet the criteria of being frequently admitted to the hospital and incurring high costs when admitted. See Chapter 6 for further discussion.

INTEGRATED CARE

Integrated Care provides specific quality of care and financial benefits. Concurrent and retrospective case studies document the efficiency of integration.

In light of Florence Nightingale's goals of holistic care and the general health of patients, health care institutions are continuing to transform nursing practice into a professional model based on systems theory and interactive practice. A review of nursing practice reveals many efforts to focus on nursing models that delineate direct care responsibilities to patients. As Newman has written, nursing is clearly ready to move into an integrative, collaborative stage of development.[1] Furthermore, an organizational structure that makes nursing clinicians directly responsible to clients would facilitate nursing's response to clients' health concerns whenever and wherever they occur.

Integrated Care is a system of patient care delivery through the differentiation of nursing practice that integrates the allocation of resources—human, fiscal, and material—over a variety of settings within appropriate time frames. Patient care is expanded beyond physiologic needs to the entire episode of illness from preadmission to postdischarge. The Integrated Care delivery system was implemented at Sioux Valley Hospital for enhanced continuity of patient care, increased professionalism, and improved efficiency in patient care. This care delivery model facilitates the patient's participation in self-care as well as family involvement.

After the completion of the South Dakota Statewide Project for Nursing and Nursing Education in 1988, the Integrated Care Committee was formulated in 1989 to provide assistance in the development, implementation, and evaluation of a nursing managed care system with differentiated practice roles. The term *integrated care* was selected to describe the nursing care delivered, focusing on a cooperative and collaborative environment. Differentiation implies variance among nurses in skills, attitudes, values, behaviors, and beliefs in four different domains: time frame, interpersonal scope and focus, structure (environment), and the orientation to lifelong learning. This nursing care delivery model is based on differences in nurse experience, competence, and individual preference. There is a difference in orientation to particular goals and behavior. The nurse's practice level depends on demonstrated competency. The operationalization is discussed later in this chapter.

The success of this system is the nurse's understanding of the mutually valued roles of the associate nurse, primary nurse, and clinical care coordinator. Equally important is the mutual respect and the knowledge of the roles and responsibilities of the unit nursing director, nursing assistants, and health unit coordinator. Inherent in this nurse valuing must be an organizational climate that supports nursing leadership and practice along with a unifying vision for growth and development.

The American Hospital Association (AHA) and the American Organization of Nurse Executives (AONE) have consistently advocated organizational redesign to meet the complex and transforming needs of the American public. In support of the need to differentiate nursing practice roles, the AHA and the AONE formulated a position paper that sought to advance the following[2]:

- identification of care delivery systems with nursing staffing models that recognize and appropriately utilize the different levels of competence, education, experience, and skill among registered nurses, as well as between registered nurses, and other nursing personnel responsible to registered nurses
- distribution of successful strategies that facilitate the differentiation of nursing practice roles
- collaboration between nursing service and nursing education in order to facilitate the development of nursing education curricula that support the differentiation of nursing practice roles required to ensure the delivery of cost-effective, quality patient care
- evaluation, facilitation, support, and implementation of the difference of nursing practice roles in organized health care settings

In accordance with the views of Porter-O'Grady,[3] the organizational structure must be devised in such a way that nursing activities and the time necessary to perform them are a portion of the delivery system. Being involved in nursing activities without supporting the processes essential to nursing practice is like constructing a building on sand. The Integrated Care delivery model at Sioux Valley Hospital has demonstrated significant quality and resource outcomes, improved nurse satisfaction, and an increased focus on the continuity of patient care throughout the lifespan or an episode of illness.

BENEFITS OF INTEGRATED CARE

A continuum of patient care is provided through an Integrated Care delivery system based on differentiated practice roles. This model improves health care delivery through the integration of patient care services while maintaining quality and maximizing efficiency in resource allocation and utilization. A systematic approach to delivery of patient care ensures coordination of care, which is of higher value than fragmented care for patients with complex, ongoing health care needs. Primary nursing of the 1990s and beyond will ensure that patients have a primary nurse responsible for their well-being throughout hospitalization.[4] Nurses are accountable for patient care outcomes and become the coordinators of care.

The benefits of the Integrated Care model are significant and divided into the following categories: patient/family, physician, nursing, hospital, and community. These benefits are addressed briefly below.

Patient questionnaires have consistently been commendatory concerning nursing care at Sioux Valley Hospital. There has been a difference noted in the qualitative responses on the surveys beginning with the demonstration project up to the present Integrated Care delivery system. The patients and families remember the full names of nurses who have spent time with them, especially the primary nurse. If readmitted, the patient often requests to be placed on the unit where care was previously received because of familiarity with the primary nurse. Before the present delivery system, patients would remark nonspecifically about nursing care, such as "the blonde nurse on nights spent extra time with me" and "the charge nurse was special." The patients and families provide more descriptive feedback that includes the benefits that they have received, such as:

- greater participation in care and goal setting
- greater focus on self-care
- timely education
- preparation of the caregiver for discharge/care of the client
- greater ability to anticipate events (decreased anxiety)
- greater confidence and respect for caregiver roles

Physician-perceived benefits to our nursing care delivery system have evolved for some and for others have been apparent from the onset. The physicians have verbally shared among themselves the benefits of this nursing model, which overall has been to everyone's benefit. The physicians have been most satisfied with the ability to find a knowledgeable nurse readily when they arrive on a patient care unit. Along with this nurse presence, the primary nurse or clinical care coordinator provides a nursing summary of the patient's condition for the previous 24 hours along with plans for discharge. The physician input into discharge planning is sought on day 1 or 2 after admission, so that appropriate patient placement is done in the most timely manner. The following observations have occurred relating to physicians and nursing:

- greater collaboration and problem solving
- increased respect and confidence
- strengthened professional behaviors
- mutual valuing of roles and responsibilities

Many patient care units completed physician surveys to substantiate the results demonstrated. A copy of a physician survey is included in Appendix 5-A. The survey was centered on the continuity of nursing care, discharge planning, and documentation of nursing information. Some patient care units have attributed an increase in patient volume to physician satisfaction with the differentiated nursing roles.

Nursing satisfaction with the Integrated Care delivery system has been high. As part of the Statewide Project, a job satisfaction tool was distributed to employees in the Department of Patient Services before implementation and after project completion. The tool, Nurses and Work Satisfaction,[5] showed that there was increased job satisfaction on all the patient care units surveyed. The actual results and analysis of the findings have been published previously.[6]

The Integrated Care committees on each unit distributed surveys to the nurses assigned on each unit to evaluate the nursing care delivered with the requirement of suggestions for improvements. In addition, the nursing units completed a survey that quantified the strengths, weaknesses, opportunities, and threats (SWOT) of the care delivered to patients. The components of this survey included the following: technical, business, hotel and services, case management, relations with support services, and nurse satisfaction. These SWOT surveys were distributed and evaluated on a yearly basis by the Integrated Care Committee. Recommendations for changes were discussed at the unit level and then were shared with the hospital Integrated Care Committee.

Some observable benefits from the Integrated Care delivery system for nurses include:

- stronger focus on care planning and nursing diagnosis
- greater accountability to the specific role of the professional nurse
- valuing of others' expertise and differences
- teamwork enhanced among all job categories (especially with responsibilities understood)
- greater individual and group self-esteem along with strengthened relationships
- changing career expectations for job responsibilities and opportunities
- nurses seeking decision-making authority on issues that affect their practice
- greater focus on personal education and career goals
- personal fulfillment acknowledged as a result of positive patient outcomes and feedback
- perception of greater valuing of the nurse role by administration along with qualitative and quantitative data on patient outcomes, especially patient length of stay information
- ability to affect patient outcomes more positively with multidisciplinary collaboration
- greater nursing unit ownership and pride in meeting holistic patient care needs

The vacancy rate for RNs has been less than 5% since 1990. The clinical care coordinator and primary nurse vacancy rates are extremely low. Many nursing units have retained the original nurses who began with the Integrated Care system, especially for the clinical II nurse category, which includes the RN roles of the primary nurse and clinical care coordinator. Presently, positions are filled as soon as the application and interview process is completed for either the primary nurse or the clinical care coordinator role. Nursing students and colleagues have shared positive comments relative to the clearly defined and operational practice roles. Most favorably, nursing staff have been empowered to become involved in practice issues and in redefining nursing's role in today's health care environment along with a future plan. A major component of this redefinition is maintaining the continuum of patient care to include prehospitalization and postdischarge. The financial benefits of integration have been documented in the home health and hospice division of Sioux Valley Hospital (Exhibit 5–1).

In late 1992, RNs in the advanced practice role began gathering baseline cost data to determine the financial benefits of case management. This will provide the advanced practice group with the information upon which to base bids for preferred provider status on health maintenance organization contracts. Financial outcomes are identified in Chapter 8.

> *Happiness lies . . . in the joy of achievement, in the thrill of creative effort.*
>
> FRANKLIN D. ROOSEVELT

OPERATIONALIZATION OF INTEGRATED CARE

The concept of Integrated Care at Sioux Valley Hospital was established to meet the complex needs of patients by utilizing nursing roles that capitalized upon different levels of practice. Differences in practice include levels of competence, education, experience, and skill.

Integrated Care was allowed to grow and develop differently in each area in a way that would best serve the needs of the different patient populations and cultures of the units. The housewide Integrated Care Committee provided the guidelines by which the same framework among areas was maintained (see Appendix 2-A). These guidelines included job descriptions for the roles and use of the Role Choice Tool (see Appendices 4-A, 4-B, and 4-F). Utilizing the guidelines, each unit established its own committee to identify how the roles of Integrated Care would be implemented in the area.

Maternal–Child Health

Implementing differentiated practice within the maternal-child health (MCH) division brought new challenges and changes for the nursing staff. Although it may have been a time of turmoil and frustration for the staff, it also brought a new perspective to the nursing profession. Nurses were expected to practice independ-

Exhibit 5–1 Case Study: Reducing Costs in Hospice

History: Hospice at Sioux Valley Hospital is a Medicare-certified program accredited by the Joint Commission on Accreditation of Healthcare Organizations. As such, the charges for the program are based on an established per diem rate with capitated payment on the aggregate. Tables 5–1 to 5–3 provide documentation of the decreased spending in the program at the onset of Integrated Care and the benefits of the advanced practice nurse in monitoring ongoing controls through the use of case management.

Discussion: In 1987, differentiated practice was implemented in the hospice division. The information in Table 5–1 documents baseline data; $n = 18$ patients for September 1987 to August 1988 and $n = 30$ patients for September 1988 to August 1989. In September 1988 to August 1989, the addition of a clinical nurse specialist (CNS) and the shift of the nurses in differentiated practice from novice to expert provided noticeable controls related to spending for medical supplies, laboratory testing, radiology, and home medical equipment. Pharmaceuticals were the one area that experienced increased costs in the program. This increase was related to a 56% increase in the cost of pharmaceuticals to the hospital, and at the same time the CNS advocated liberal use of pain medications. Also, expanding to 30 patients may have increased the validity of the data.

The data for September 1989 to August 1990 and September 1991 to August 1992 (Tables 5–2 and 5–3) indicate a further decrease in costs associated with medical supplies, laboratory, durable medical equipment, and radiology. By this time, Integrated Care was practiced at a relatively expert level by all three roles within the hospice program. Also, the CNS had advocated on behalf of clients for donations of medical supplies and home medical equipment. The CNS had become expert in the use of community resources to facilitate this cost savings to the program through a better understanding of available resources and medical supplies.

Through the entire implementation process, quality of care was monitored by the Quality Assurance Council of the hospice. This monitoring had many facets, but two of the significant ones were family/significant other satisfaction questionnaires and physician satisfaction questionnaires. In addition, results documented 100% effectiveness in pain management and symptom control.

Methods: To duplicate this study, the administrator of the hospice needs a strong interdepartmental relationship with the admissions, medical record, and billing departments. Hospice patients need to be identified within the overall hospital system such that their medical record and the billing process from admission to the program through receipt of payment from Medicare can be easily identified. This author decentralized the billing function to the hospice team. The volunteer coordinator was cross-trained to the billing process. This individual knew the patients and all staff members. The hospice staff identified a product use tracking mechanism and provided the data to the hospice volunteer coordinator, who entered the data into the computer system. Charges may be entered and deleted just for the purpose of product use tracking. Once the billing office has completed the billing form, mailed it to Medicare, and received payment, the clerk sends a copy of the bill to the administrator indicating total dollars received and total dollars applied to the hospice program discount account.

Table 5–1 Hospice Program Funding, 1987–1989

Cost Category	1987–1988 (n = 18)	1988–1989 (n = 30)	Sept 1987– Aug 1988	Sept 1988– Aug 1989
Aggregate capitated allowance per client	$8,406.00	$9,010.00		
Average cost per client	$1,810.00	$2,584.00		
Medical supplies per client			$1.01/day	$0.58/day
Laboratory per client			$2.46/day	$0.08/day
Durable medical equipment per client			$0.53/day	$0.07/day
Pharmacy			$2.95/day ($0.13/day/ client)	$4.13/day ($0.19/day/ client)
Radiology per client (includes medical X ray)			$0.87/day	$0.40/day

Courtesy of Sioux Valley Hospital, Sioux Falls, South Dakota.

ently through the use of databases, nursing diagnoses, and client care plans; this included collaborating with other disciplines in planning care with the client.

At the time of implementation, all units were offered the opportunity to participate in the project. They had to acquire an 85% vote of support from the staff to be included in this project. Three units in this division chose to participate as demonstration units: the postpartum/normal newborn nursery unit, the neonatal intensive care unit (NICU), and the pediatric unit (with clients younger than

Table 5–2 Hospice Program Funding, 1989–1991

Cost Category	1989–1990	1990–1991	Sept 1989– Aug 1990	Sept 1990– Aug 1991
Aggregate capitated allowance per client	$9,787.00	$10,712.00		
Average cost per client	$4,004.00	$4,069.07		
Medical supplies per client			$0.04/day	$0.04/day
Laboratory per client			$0.02/day	$0.03/day
Durable medical equipment per client			$0.02/day	$0.002/day
Pharmacy			$6.08/day ($0.26/day/ client)	$5.58/day ($0.15/day/ client)
Radiology per client (includes medical X ray)			$0.002/day	$0.08/day
Nutrition per client			$0.002/day	$0.03/day

Courtesy of Sioux Valley Hospital, Sioux Falls, South Dakota.

Table 5–3 Hospice Program Funding, 1991–1992

Cost Category	Sept 1991–Aug 1992
Aggregate capitation	$11,551.00
Average cost per client	$4,769.00
Medical supplies per client	$0.15/day
Laboratory per client	$0.12/day
Durable medical equipment per client	$0.10/day
Pharmacy	$12.22/day
	($1.48/day/client)
Radiology per client (includes medical X ray)	$0.14/day
Nutrition per client	$0.02/day
Physician fees per client	$0.033/day
Other (consults, respiratory care)	$0.04/day/client

Courtesy of Sioux Valley Hospital, Sioux Falls, South Dakota.

adolescents). During this demonstration project, it became evident that the vital component in the client's recovery and progress toward discharge was the continuity of nursing care. This continuity of nursing care was facilitated by the primary nurse, the associate nurse, and the clinical care coordinator roles, as identified earlier.

When the concept of differentiated practice was operationalized in this division, a number of factors were taken into account: identification of the primary nurses, associate nurses, and clinical care coordinators; the number of primary nurses and clinical care coordinators each unit would have; the patients' lengths of stay; the patient population; the patient needs; the working schedule of the primary nurse (8-hour or 12-hour shifts); and the intradivisional communication necessary to promote continuity of care. Each of these factors is discussed below.

Each unit determined the number of positions available for the primary nurse and the clinical care coordinator roles. In this determination, the positions available were based on the number of full-time equivalent employees hired into that unit. Through this development of the roles, it was determined that 33% to 35% of the nursing staff on the units would fulfill the primary nurse and clinical care coordinator roles to meet the patient needs. Initially, the primary nurses within this division were assigned to 12-hour shifts, covering both the day and the night shifts. The primary nurse was also scheduled to work weekends and holidays. In this role, the primary nurse provided hands-on patient care and communicated to colleagues the needs, the identified nursing diagnoses, and the plan of care pertinent to each patient. Hands-on care refers to the technical skills of nursing: physiologic monitoring, medication administration, mobilization, hygiene, and the like.

Over the course of the evolution of differentiated practice, the units needed to refocus on the primary nurse role and its purpose and intent. When evaluating this role, some units, depending upon the patient population and needs, identified that the primary nurse should be more available, providing the client with teaching materials and making referrals for follow-up care. This meant allowing some primary nurses to work 8-hour shifts or to cease providing hands-on patient care. This allowed them to become the client integrator of patient care, teaching, referrals, communication, and so forth. Those working primarily on weekdays facilitated interagency and intradivisional communication to meet the clients' needs and goals. Reevaluation of this role allowed the primary nurse to become more flexible for patients and staff when planning care and arranging discharge with possible home care.

The wide diversity of clients seen in this nursing division necessitated that each unit establish its own process for screening clients and identifying the client's need for a primary nurse. These screening tools were devised to assist nursing staff, particularly the primary nurse and the clinical care coordinator, to determine whether patients indeed had any complex physical, psychosocial, spiritual, or social needs (Exhibit 5–2). If so, then a primary nurse was assigned.

In the NICU, a standard was determined at the initial implementation of the demonstration project that all infants would be assigned a primary nurse. This determination came forth because of the unexpected preterm delivery, which raises

---

Exhibit 5–2 Initial Screen for an Obstetric Patient

Please check the following criteria that apply:

1. _____ Single—no support system
2. _____ Single—not keeping
3. _____ Known or suspected substance abuse
4. _____ Complications of pregnancy and/or delivery (prolonged antepartum stay, magnesium sulfate after delivery, pregnancy-induced hypertension, surgical intervention postdelivery such as dilation and curettage or hysterectomy)
5. _____ Poor or limited coping mechanisms (limited cognitive functioning, low pain tolerance, stress such as infant anomaly or illness)
6. _____ History of depression
7. _____ Multiple physical and/or technical needs (cerebral palsy, tracheotomy, insulin pump, etc)
8. _____ Previous social services involvement (Medicaid; Women, Infants, and Children nutrition program; history of child abuse; children in foster care; etc)
9. _____ Comprehensive teaching needs
10. _____ Primary nurse not indicated

Courtesy of Sioux Valley Hospital, Sioux Falls, South Dakota.

the possibility of prolonged hospitalization, unexpected outcome, and emotional strains that families might encounter while the child is hospitalized. At the onset of differentiated practice within this unit, and by focusing primarily on continuity of care, nursing teams were organized. In the 40-bed NICU, there are 100 RNs on staff who work three 12-hour shifts per week. To provide continuity of caregivers to the infants and families, a system needed to be implemented. Therefore, nursing teams were developed in an effort to provide the family and infant with some familiarity and to enhance the continuity of care.

The evolution of the nursing teams in the NICU is outlined in Figures 5–1 to 5–3. These figures also outline the goals for these teams and problems that were encountered. Currently the five-team model is in place, with the primary nurses on each team working schedules opposite each other. Primary nurses within the NICU provide hands-on patient care and work 12-hour shifts, covering weekends, nights, and holidays. The associate nurses also provide a vital component in the delivery of care to the infants on each team. When the associate nurse is the first person to have contact with the infant/family, it is his or her responsibility to place this infant onto the team and to communicate this to the primary nurses, an identified accountability and responsibility of this role.

Through this team process, continuity of care for the infant and family can be maintained. With a team concept, a trusting and working relationship can be established with the family and the nursing team (Exhibit 5–3). It is the clinical care coordinator and the primary nurse who facilitate the team member assignments to the infants on their team. Therefore, the clinical care coordinators and primary

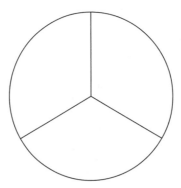

Figure 5–1 Initial arrangement of nursing teams. There were three teams consisting of 6 full-time primary nurses and 10 to 12 associate nurses. The team goal was to develop a consistent approach to nursing care for infants and an organized teaching plan for parents. The problem encountered was that infants received inconsistent care because of increased nursing staff on each team. Courtesy of Pamela A. Koepsell, Sioux Valley Hospital, Sioux Falls, South Dakota.

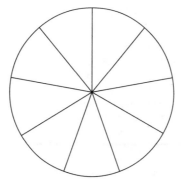

Figure 5–2 Intermediate arrangement of nursing teams. There were nine teams consisting of two full-time primary nurses and four to five associate nurses. The team goal was to improve consistency and continuity of care given to infants by each team. The problems encountered were that 12-hour shifts restricted primary nurse coverage to six 12-hour shifts per week and that primary nurses sometimes chose to work part-time but remained in the primary nurse role. Courtesy of Pamela A. Koepsell, Sioux Valley Hospital, Sioux Falls, South Dakota.

nurses are accountable for keeping the team communication board (Figure 5–4) current.

Not only is there communication regarding the continuity of care within these units, but there is intradivisional and interdivisional communication as well. Primary nurses from each of these units on occasion consult with one another when

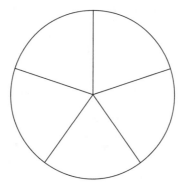

Figure 5–3 Current arrangement of nursing teams (as of May 1, 1993). There are five teams consisting of 2 to 3 full-time or job-sharing primary nurse positions and 8 to 10 associate nurse positions. The team goal is to improve further the consistency of care given to infants by each team. Courtesy of Pamela A. Koepsell, Sioux Valley Hospital, Sioux Falls, South Dakota.

Exhibit 5–3 Case Study: Premature Infant

Mrs Smith is a 25-year-old white woman (gravida 5, para 4) who was transferred to this tertiary care center from a smaller community hospital for further evaluation of early labor, breech presentation, and fetal distress. Attempts to stop labor were unsuccessful. As a result of these prenatal complications and extreme prematurity of the fetus, a cesarean section was performed. Sam was born at gestation week 24 weighing only 730 g (1 lb 10 oz). Sam was admitted to the NICU for medical management. He required vigorous ventilatory support and at 4 months of age a tracheostomy for respiratory management. Over the course of his hospitalization, numerous complications associated with his extreme prematurity occurred that prolonged his hospitalization. Sam was hospitalized in the NICU and the extended care nursery for 18 months for bronchopulmonary dysplasia. He was oxygen dependent and had the tracheostomy at discharge.

Sam's family resides in a rural community with little access to medical services except for a local community rescue squad and a physician's assistant located several miles away. The clinic in the area had been forced to close as a result of financial constraints and lack of a medical doctor several years before Sam's birth. The nearest hospital was approximately 45 miles away, where a pediatrician was on staff.

Sam's father was employed, and the family did have medical insurance. During Sam's hospitalization, his father's medical insurance company changed, and the new insurer did not agree to assume coverage for Sam's preexisting condition. This left Sam's family strained financially. The hospital social worker involved in Sam's case assisted the family with their financial burdens and helped them complete the appropriate forms for federal assistance.

With Sam's premature delivery and prolonged hospitalization, the family was faced with many struggles and obstacles. There were financial concerns as mentioned above, altered parent and family bonding, ineffective family coping, and unfamiliar medical terminology. Eventually, in-depth discharge teaching was provided not only for the family but also for the community of residence, the emergency department personnel, and his pediatrician at the nearest hospital.

Sam was assigned to a primary nurse when he was admitted to the NICU. It was the primary nurse's responsibility to complete the family database and to identify and prioritize concerns that would be associated with Sam's hospitalization. The primary nurse and physicians communicated with the family on a routine basis as to Sam's progress and condition. The primary nurse established a close and trusting relationship with Sam's extended family during his hospitalization.

Within the NICU, the nursing staff worked in teams, and the primary nurse communicated to her team Sam's needs and the family's needs. It became apparent that some of the nursing staff on the team had a difficult time caring for a long-term infant such as Sam, and these concerns were expressed to the primary nurse. It was then that the primary nurse's ultimate decision to develop a core group of nurses (which included some nurses on other nursing teams to meet the scheduling needs) who were willing to care for Sam on a routine basis. With this approach to nursing care, the family could identify who Sam's nurses were and

continues

Exhibit 5–3 continued

could develop a special bond with them. Sam began to know his nurses and responded to them in his own special way. This system also allowed the family to address concerns to the nurses when issues arose. For this approach to be effective, the primary nurse needed to make a continuity calendar that included all the caregivers for Sam. The primary nurse then assigned nurses to Sam utilizing this calendar to ensure that all the nursing shifts were covered. This continuity calendar proved to be an essential component in Sam's care.

Throughout Sam's hospitalization, his family visited routinely. Initially only his parents and grandparents were allowed to visit, but as his hospitalization became prolonged the primary nurse confronted the physicians and asked whether it would be possible for his siblings to visit. The physicians approved of this visitation request and permitted his siblings to visit as long as they were asymptomatic of any illness. With this less stringent visiting policy, family unity was supported. Sam was able to interact with his older siblings, and his siblings were able to learn more about why Sam required hospitalization. On several occasions, the unit offered a sibling support group, which Sam's siblings were allowed to attend; this placed them with other children who had a sibling in the NICU. Now the primary nurse was focusing on the entire family rather than just on Sam.

Multiple care conferences were held to discuss Sam's medical needs and conditions. These conferences were multidisciplinary: Not only were physicians and nurses present, but ancillary staff were also present to discuss developmental needs for Sam and financial needs for the family. The parents were also encouraged to participate and share their concerns during these conferences. From these conferences, the primary nurse formulated and revised Sam's nursing care plan and communicated issues with Sam's caregivers.

As time progressed, it became apparent that Sam would be well enough to be discharged to his home. The primary nurse recognized the need to organize and coordinate Sam's discharge with the neonatal nurse practitioner who had been working closely with the physician managing Sam's medical care. The primary nurse collaborated with the nurse practitioner and the social worker in an effort to provide a smooth transition from hospital to home. It required numerous referrals to accomplish this transition. It was at this time that the responsibilities of the primary nurse became crucial.

At an earlier care conference, it became evident that Sam would require home nursing care secondary to his chronic lung disease and medical needs. With the need for home nursing care, it was imperative to include the home health care department in Sam's discharge planning. With limited nursing personnel in Sam's home community, it became necessary for Sioux Valley Hospital's home health care department to provide the nursing care for him. It was the primary nurse's responsibility to work with the hospital's home health care department in educating these nurses about Sam's unique needs.

With the implementation of home care nursing, a nurse case manager was assigned to Sam. In this situation, Sam's primary nurse was willing to expand her nursing to the exteriors of the hospital to provide home nursing coverage in addition

continues

Exhibit 5–3 continued

to her present staff position. This allowed the primary nurse to continue caring for Sam after discharge. With this expanded role as case manager, the nurse was required to travel to Sam's residence several times throughout the month to evaluate and assess his nursing and medical needs and to update his plan of care.

As Sam's primary nurse took on this new role of case manager for home care, it was her responsibility to assess the home environment. This involved evaluating the home for accessibility to electrical outlets and safety measures that would be necessary for Sam. This environmental assessment provided information about items/equipment that the home would need before Sam's discharge.

Because Sam had a chronic respiratory condition, the weather and temperature were critical in his health care. It was noted that the home in which he would be residing had no air conditioning. It was important that Sam not be exposed to extreme weather changes such as high humidity and temperatures; thus the need for an air conditioner was evident. Through Sam's church and community, funds were raised, and an air conditioner was purchased for the family before Sam's arrival home.

Parental and community education was essential to Sam's care. Throughout Sam's stay at the hospital, the family became adept at providing the necessary care that Sam required, so that little education was left to do at the time of discharge. Community education about Sam's care was crucial, however. It would be the local rescue squad that would respond in an emergency. They needed to be instructed on tracheostomy care and insertion should that become necessary. The primary nurse/case manager and the neonatal nurse practitioner involved in Sam's care arranged to go to Sam's community and provide an educational inservice for these individuals. These individuals responded to this need and identified that, should an emergency call come in for Sam, it would be paged out as a "Sam Call," and all personnel would respond directly to his home.

To assist in an emergency situation, Sam's parents had access to a LifeLine button. This Lifeline button provided a means for direct access to Sioux Valley Hospital's home health care department and the local nursing home should a crisis arise. This button enabled the parents or caregivers to notify the appropriate personnel should an emergency occur. Pressing the button activated an alarm at the local nursing home, which alerted the rescue squad. An intercom device was a part of this Lifeline system. Should an emergency occur, health personnel could communicate with Sam's parents or caregivers regarding the situation until medical help arrived at the home.

Because Sam's community was without a hospital, arrangements were also made with the helicopter air ambulance service based out of the tertiary care center to respond if necessary. It was approved that the local rescue squad could initiate this service if indicated.

On the same day that the primary nurse/case manager and the neonatal nurse practitioner inserviced the local rescue squad, the nurses also traveled to the community where Sam would probably be hospitalized should he become ill. The primary nurse/case manager and the neonatal nurse practitioner met with the

continues

Exhibit 5–3 continued

emergency department personnel and shared with them the history of Sam and his medical needs. An inservice was given on pediatric tracheostomies. That same day, a visit was made to the pediatrician who would be seeing Sam upon discharge. Medical information was shared, and a list of medical supplies that would be necessary for Sam was exchanged. The pediatrician took the initiative to have the hospital obtain all necessary supplies should they be needed.

With this thorough educational approach to the community, hospital personnel, and pediatrician, the transitional period from the hospital to the home indeed went smoothly. The nursing personnel who cared for Sam in the home were also educated about Sam's needs before caring for him alone. After Sam's discharge, the case manager communicated with the pediatrician on a routine basis to discuss Sam's medical and nursing needs.

Sam required hospitalization that first week after discharge for an upper respiratory infection and was discharged to his home 3 days later. The next hospitalization occurred 6 months later, when his tracheostomy tube decannulated. Unable to reinsert the tracheostomy tube, his parents activated the Lifeline button. They assessed his respiratory status and then applied oxygen per mask and monitored his oxygenation level with the use of the home oximeter. Within minutes, the rescue squad arrived. Sam was then transported via ambulance to the hospital 45 miles from his home for medical attention. The pediatrician assessed Sam, and the decision to transport him to the tertiary acute care center was made.

Sam arrived at Sioux Valley Hospital for further evaluation. It was apparent that he was in no immediate respiratory distress without his tracheostomy tube, so that the decision was made to leave the tracheostomy tube out and observe him closely. Sam remained on minimal oxygen therapy. He was discharged several days later to his home without any further complications. Home health nursing care continued for several weeks after this incident to ensure that his respiratory status did not deteriorate.

Looking back on this situation, the primary nurse was an essential figure in the care of this child. Not only did she recognize the needs that Sam and his family encountered during his hospitalization, but she also assisted with the referral processes to provide continuity of care from hospital to home. It became obvious when Sam required emergency interventions when his tracheostomy tube became decannulated that the outreach education was valuable and effective, as evidenced by the response time of the rescue squad.

As a primary nurse within the walls of the hospital expanding to encompass the role of the case manager outside the walls of the hospital, the same nurse was able to provide continuous care to Sam. Integrating care among the hospital personnel, the home health care personnel, the rescue squad, and the pediatrician was a rewarding and positive experience for this primary nurse. The primary nurse continues to be in contact with Sam's family and visits them periodically. A special relationship developed with this family and Sam's primary nurse during his hospitalization.

PRIMARY NURSE	PATIENT CASELOAD	ANTEPARTUM	NURSING CARE TEAM
Mary Jones	Baby Boy Blue Baby Girl Smith		Nancy Johnson Julie Nelson Kari Hill Ann Miller Sarah Anderson
Patsy Miller	Baby Boy Sand Baby Boy Mills	Alice Jones	Ruth Parks Ellen Roberts John Allen Laurie Dickerson Ann Oakley
Carol Olson	Baby Girl James Baby Boy Tom		Del Small Bob Stevens Emilie Richards Karen Woods Katie Christenson

Figure 5–4 Integrated Care delivery NICU assignment board. Courtesy of Sioux Valley Hospital, Sioux Falls, South Dakota.

Exhibit 5–4 Case Study: Transcultural Perinatal Nursing

Chin Lei was a young woman, with dwarfism, in her childbearing years who was expecting her first child in several weeks. Chin Lei had come to the United States with her family from Asia and had been in the United States for nearly 10 years but had a limited command of the English language. During these past 10 years, she had resided with her father and stepmother before her marriage. The marriage had been prearranged by her family in Asia and was conducted by proxy. Just 2 weeks after the marriage, the husband left, and Chin Lei faced living alone and was filing for a divorce. She was able to stay with friends and acquaintances, but with the infant's arrival she would have to find her own housing. It was learned that her family would not assist her because of her failed marriage.

Chin Lei was introduced to the labor and delivery/antepartum staff by the childbirth educator, who had been working with Chin Lei regarding the labor and delivery process. The childbirth educator had consulted one of the primary nurses to work with Chin Lei, to provide a tour of the labor and delivery unit, and to discuss routines and expectations for expectant mothers.

On the first encounter with Chin Lei, the primary nurse identified that this would be a challenging client. The primary nurse gathered initial assessment data (this was before the implementation of the perinatal database). With the information obtained, the primary nurse recognized a number of concerns and barriers that

continues

Exhibit 5–4 continued

would complicate Chin Lei's care. From these data, the primary nurse realized the need to communicate, consult, and collaborate with other health team members in providing the care Chin Lei would need.

It became apparent that a multidisciplinary care conference was needed to address each of the anticipated problems encountered during the primary nurse's initial assessment of Chin Lei. In preparation for this conference, the primary nurse contacted the divisional social worker, the childbirth educator, the perinatal CNS, and a primary nurse from the postpartum/normal newborn nursery. Each of these concerns was addressed, and an identified plan was created for each.

Primary and ultimate concerns were Chin Lei's impaired communication skills and the fact that she had limited knowledge of the birth process. At this care conference, the staff determined the best communicative approach to use with Chin Lei. Through this discussion, it was determined that Chin Lei would benefit by attending childbirth classes. Staff were also to address Chin Lei with slow, carefully worded sentences and demonstrative gestures.

Another concern was alteration in parenting skills. Again, the team felt that it would be advantageous for Chin Lei to attend the childbirth and parenting classes. It would be imperative for staff to become role models in the infant's care and to provide simple terminology and pictures to demonstrate appropriate parenting skills with Chin Lei.

Another obstacle identified was Chin Lei's altered and ineffective individual and family coping process. With no family support after her failed marriage, Chin Lei needed to find new mechanisms for coping and surviving on her own. The social worker shared with the team that Chin Lei was eligible to receive financial aid through various federal programs. Chin Lei met the social worker and completed the application process for these assistance programs.

A concern relating to Chin Lei's altered growth and development was addressed. With Chin Lei being diagnosed with dwarfism, there was a great deal of concern that her child might also have dwarfism. This information was shared with Chin Lei's physician, and follow-up evaluations would occur as needed. Staff were encouraged to allow Chin Lei to express her fears regarding the possibility of her child having dwarfism and to be supportive of her needs.

Finally, because of Chin Lei's physical size, hospital clothing would be a problem at the time of delivery. The primary nurse began to problem solve as to what type of patient gown should be used during her hospitalization. It would be necessary to hem a patient gown by 2 ft to attire Chin Lei adequately. This task was accomplished by the primary nurse.

One month after the first encounter with Chin Lei, she was admitted as an outpatient for a scheduled amniocentesis with the possibility of a scheduled cesarean section secondary to her dwarfism later that same day. The primary nurse who had been working closely with Chin Lei was not scheduled to work that day, but she chose to rearrange her work schedule to be there during this time because a trusting relationship between the two had developed. During the course of this admission, the primary nurse and Chin Lei became more acquainted. Chin

continues

Exhibit 5–4 continued

Lei relaxed and shared some valuable information with her primary nurse. Chin Lei confided that her former living arrangement with her father and stepmother would not be emotionally suitable upon the birth of the child. She would not be permitted to return to her father's home because of her failed marriage; she was now a member of the growing population of homeless people in this community. At Chin Lei's request, the primary nurse investigated the possibility of Chin Lei staying at an adult day care facility, a supervised center for adults with special needs, after her discharge.

By late afternoon, the results of the amniocentesis indicated that the fetus was mature and that the cesarean section should be performed. Chin Lei gave birth to a healthy, normal infant. Later that shift, Chin Lei was transferred to the postpartum/ normal newborn nursery unit. The postpartum primary nurse who had been involved in the multidisciplinary care conference now assumed the care of Chin Lei. The labor and delivery primary nurse continued to visit Chin Lei and provided the postpartum primary nurse with valuable information during Chin Lei's hospitalization. Before Chin Lei's discharge, another multidisciplinary care conference was held to address discharge needs and follow-up care programs. Again, all team members from the first care conference were involved.

The social worker had been working closely with Chin Lei throughout this time. With Chin Lei's situation, she was moved to the top of the county's list for subsidized housing. Two nurses from a physician's office offered to have Chin Lei and her infant live with them during the interim pending the county's subsidized housing arrangements.

Chin Lei's discharge planning became the efforts of the entire hospital staff and community. The primary nurse began receiving offers for infant clothes, furniture, household items, and other forms of assistance. The social worker was able to arrange assistance programs for both mother and infant care and nutrition support.

Once Chin Lei was discharged, the labor and delivery primary nurse continued to stay in close contact with her through phone calls and home visits. Two months after Chin Lei's discharge from the hospital, she and her infant moved into their own apartment. Chin Lei invited her labor and delivery primary nurse to come for tea one afternoon. Chin Lei shared with the primary nurse on this visit that in the 10 years she had been in the United States no one had taken the time to get to know her and help her as this primary nurse had. Those few words, no matter how broken they were spoken, made the primary nurse realize what nursing was all about. It clarified how important the role of a primary nurse is to the structure of Integrated Care.

the care of the client overlaps, ensuring that all aspects of care and the needs of the client are addressed and met before discharge. For example, a primary nurse from the labor and delivery/antepartum unit may consult a primary nurse from the NICU to educate a mother in early labor about the NICU environment and what she may expect should she deliver prematurely or if complications should arise. In another situation, a referral to a pediatric primary nurse may be pertinent for an infant who is being discharged from the NICU. During this referral process, a brief history of the infant's hospitalization is exchanged, and a tour of the pediatric unit is made available for families to become familiar with the unit and the staff should a readmission become necessary. See Exhibit 5-4 for a case study involving three departments.

Whenever continuity of care is necessary after discharge, the home health care department may be consulted to follow through with the needed nursing or medical interventions. Again, nursing's focus is the continuity of care for the client.

Also during the development of differentiated practice within this division, the labor and delivery/antepartum unit, the postpartum/normal newborn nursery, and the NICU recognized that a vital component to this practice was absent. This component was a patient communication tool that could be used throughout these units. Once identified, a MCH Integrated Care Committee was established to develop a tool that would address the patient's history and needs during hospitalization and from which all units could benefit.

This communication tool became known as the perinatal database (Appendix 5-B). In implementing this medical record form, expectant mothers were given the form to complete when attending Sioux Valley Hospital's expectant childbirth classes. Once the forms were completed, the childbirth educator and a primary nurse from each of the units reviewed the tool to determine whether the patient required a primary nurse during this admission. The completed form was placed on file in the labor and delivery unit until the patient's admission.

A few months after implementation of the perinatal database, it was given to expectant mothers in the physician's office at the request of some physicians. With shortened maternity stays, the physician's office staff have assumed responsibility not only for much of the prenatal education, but also some of the postnatal care. This database provides the physician with information about the patient's needs and concerns before hospitalization.

Once the patient delivers, the database accompanies the patient's medical record to the postpartum/normal newborn nursery unit, and the nursing staff review this information rather than ask the patient repetitive questions. Should the infant of this patient be admitted to the NICU, a copy of the perinatal database is sent to the NICU and placed on the infant's medical record, so that all information can be shared with the infant's primary nurse. This database has become an effective communication tool for all staff within these units.

This form has proven to be beneficial and a time saver for the nursing staff. Nurses are able to address the patient's needs quickly and effectively from the information that the patient provided on the database. The patient needs are readily identified, and care plans are established based on the information gathered from this tool.

Home Health Care

In 1987, with the advent of differentiated practice, the home health care department at Sioux Valley Hospital volunteered to be included in the demonstration project. Providing continuity through a continuum of care was a primary goal of the home health care department. It was thought that the concept of a primary nurse managing the care of patients discharged from the hospital and following the patient from home back to the hospital would facilitate this goal.

The home health care staff numbers were small, which made the education and mentoring process less difficult. The staff were also highly motivated and were proponents of the need for life-long learning. All these factors enabled the home health care department to incorporate the concepts of differentiated practice readily into their nursing practice.

With the facilitation of differentiated practice in the home health care department, the link to nursing care in the home and the community was enhanced. Patients were able to leave the hospital and continue to receive the necessary care in their home through the coordinated efforts of the nursing staff in the hospital as well as of the nursing staff of the home health care department.

The implementation of this process was rather simple. A case manager within the home health care department assumed the primary nurse role responsibility of managing the patient's care should there be home nursing and medical needs at the time the patient was discharged from the hospital. The home health care case manager collaborated with the patient's assigned primary nurse in the hospital to coordinate the patient's care before discharge and assisted in the management of care beyond discharge. This process facilitated the continuity of care from the hospital to the home and, if necessary, back into the hospital.

The utilization of the home health care department in the demonstration project proved to be valuable. The patient's care was enhanced and maintained in the home setting with little disruption.

Critical Care

The intensive care unit (ICU) consisted of two geographically different units with 8 and 11 beds, respectively. The ICU started integrating care by establishing a primary nurse role with 12 pioneers who applied and interviewed for these positions. The primary nurses worked 12-hour shifts, provided hands-on client care, and carried a one- to two-client caseload. As the trial period progressed, it was apparent that the goal of continuity was unattainable with this format. The client population was such that their medical status changed daily. Medical and nursing plans could change drastically in the 4 days that the primary nurse was not scheduled to work. Frequently the primary nurse was not available during critical incidents.

To increase day-to-day continuity, the number of primary nurses decreased to six, and their shift schedule changed. The role progressed to one person working 8-hour shifts to improve continuity. This 8-hour position rotated among the remaining primary nurses. This was an improvement, but it did not provide coverage for enough patients.

This phase did, however, establish the importance of 8-hour shifts in providing continuity in the ICU. It was clear that a person working 8-hour shifts could increase the continuity of family care, provide for a consistent knowledge base on complex clients, and provide the overall picture for both nursing and medical staff. From this role, a demonstration project was developed using five primary nurses on 8-hour days. At this time, it was recognized that an important piece of this role would be continuity throughout the weekends, when nursing and medical staff continuity was diminished. Weekend coverage was established with one primary nurse working and one on-call for busy weekends. The major focus for the primary nurse on the weekend was to provide continuity within the care plan by rounding with the physicians and collaborating with nursing staff regarding the plan of care.

To allocate resources best, criteria were established for which patients would receive the expertise of a primary nurse. Each patient was screened by a primary nurse, but only those patients who fit the criteria of dysfunctional family dynamics, multiple diagnoses, extended length of stay, actual/potential alteration in lifestyle, or deviation from an Integrated Clinical Pathway were assigned to a primary nurse. Assignments were made on the basis of caseload, and stickers were placed on the medical record to indicate who the primary nurse was. At the completion of the demonstration project, the outcomes showed cost containment, increased family and physician satisfaction, increased continuity of care, and early preventive interventions (Exhibit 5–5).

Exhibit 5–5 Case Study: Adult Accident Victim

Janet, age 42, was admitted to the ICU on May 10 as a result of injuries sustained in a motor vehicle accident. Her injuries included a fracture of C1–2, an acute abdomen, and a left frontal subdural hematoma necessitating intubation, exploratory laparotomy with splenectomy and gastrostomy tube placement, and a craniotomy with halo vest placement. Janet spent the next month in the ICU, during which her medical course was complicated by a liver laceration, continuous fevers of unknown origin, pneumonia with respiratory complications, intolerance to gastrostomy tube feedings, deep vein thrombosis of her right arm, and slow neurologic progress.

Because Janet's condition was so complex, she was assigned to a primary nurse. The primary nurse recognized a number of nursing goals for Janet while she was in the ICU: increasing family satisfaction, providing family support, facilitating physician practice, coordinating care through collaboration, assisting nursing staff, improving continuity of care in complex situations, and monitoring unnecessary cost expenditures.

continues

Exhibit 5–5 continued

Nursing support became important as Janet's husband tried to cope with her condition. During the first 2 weeks, the primary nurse was a main support for him whenever a crisis occurred. The primary nurse met with him daily for 30 to 60 minutes to answer questions, address concerns, and allow him time to express his feelings. From the conversations that occurred, Janet's husband expressed interest in her care and demonstrated strong support of her. This supporting relationship was maximized through negotiation of visiting hours and educating him about the most effective way to interact with his wife. As the weeks passed in the ICU, the primary nurse continually reinforced the idea that Janet's progress would be slow. As Janet improved and moved toward discharge from the ICU, the primary nurse encouraged Janet's husband to look toward the future by visiting the transfer unit to meet the staff and by talking about her discharge.

In the first 2 weeks, the complexity of Janet's case escalated. The primary nurse identified the need for and suggested consultation with various medical specialists. As each new physician was consulted, the primary nurse was able to facilitate their practice by providing them with a history of Janet's hospital stay. She then coordinated the many specialists on the case and facilitated their practice and communication by relaying messages and plans among the physicians. Continuous records were kept to assist each specialist with treatment. For the infectious disease physician, the primary nurse kept records of culture reports, sequential white blood counts, antibiotic usage, and invasive line changes. For the pulmonologist, records of arterial blood gases and ventilatory weaning efforts were kept. Orders were also obtained to initiate rehabilitation measures early in Janet's ICU stay to maximize her recovery. Through close monitoring of her fluid status, the primary nurse identified and obtained treatment for subtle changes to prevent fluid overload. When Janet's temperature rose and her husband mentioned a previously abscessed tooth to the primary nurse, she alerted the physicians and gathered information about Janet's dental history from her local dentist.

Throughout Janet's stay in the ICU, the primary nurse became a frequent resource for the nursing staff. Janet required a unique bed for several days to meet her medical needs. During this time she required tests that necessitated a complex process of repositioning her on this bed. The primary nurse became the expert practitioner in utilizing this therapy and assisted the nursing staff with this process. The primary nurse also assisted the nursing staff with crisis situations as they occurred.

Although not all cost savings could be proved, the primary nurse speculated that early interventions to identify fluid overload, to facilitate aggressive respiratory treatment, and to establish early rehabilitation shortened Janet's stay in the ICU. The primary nurse also was able to coordinate and trend laboratory values and to prevent repetitive laboratory tests from being done. Through this effort, a savings of $2265 in laboratory work was documented.

Janet transferred to the orthopedic unit on June 10 and was transferred to the rehabilitation unit on July 23. She was able to be discharged to her home 3 months after her accident and continues to make progress there through the supportive efforts of her husband.

As the primary nurse role developed, the role of the associate nurse became clear. Frequently in this setting, the focus of care is short term. Medical and nursing objectives may be met in 1- and 2-hour time frames. The associate nurses were able to focus on interventions to meet the goals. Minute to minute, hour to hour, accountability was their focus. They were able to collaborate with the primary nurse regarding long-term goals, day-to-day changes, and the medical focus of care.

The role of the clinical care coordinator was developed about 1 year after the primary nurse role. The role of the charge nurse in the unit had undergone a change during the preceding year. The role before the implementation of Integrated Care included noting all the orders and making all the physician contacts. It became apparent that, as the ICU added beds and the patient population changed with increased complexity and acuity, these expectations would become unrealistic and would fragment care. The decision was made to move the responsibility for noting orders and calling physicians into the associate nurse role. This change decreased fragmentation of care and shifted the accountability for care to the associate role. The clinical care coordinator role encompassed the previous role of charge nurse and eventually the supervisor role along with added responsibilities for staffing, bed control, and unit leadership (see Chapter 9 for further discussion).

Adult Specialty Care Services

The medical-surgical specialties, now adult specialty care services, established Integrated Care in much the same way as the ICU. Each unit established its own committee to plan and implement the roles according to the guidelines. The initial steps were to review information and to educate those people who were interested in the subject. The committees then decided how to implement the roles. The pioneering unit chose to start out by working 8-hour shifts to provide continuity. Other units followed suit. Interested RNs interviewed for selection by the interviewing committees. Those who accepted positions as primary nurses attended workshops that expanded their knowledge of their new role. The expansion to this primary nurse system meant that several positions could be integrated into this role and that continuity would be enhanced. These roles included the discharge planners, the clinicians, and the assistant head nurses. The primary nurses provided care in areas not previously achieved. This included more family interaction, increased referrals in house and outside Sioux Valley Hospital, and client and environmental assessment. Some units chose to provide Integrated Care for all clients, whereas other units established guidelines on those clients with complex needs.

The clinical care coordinator role was established in much the same way through involvement on the unit level to coordinate selection and delineation of roles. The coordinators assumed more responsibility for staffing, interviewing, leadership, and unit activities. The associate role changed in vision but evolved at a slower rate.

The Integrated Care system enabled increased motivation. Value was placed on bedside care, but individuals were encouraged to expand their vision of the bedside nurse. As a result, the associate nurse was able to focus on how this role fit into the delivery system.

COMMUNICATION TOOLS

Not only did the nursing practice change when differentiated practice was operationalized, but it also became evident that the documentation tools would need to be altered to meet the new practice needs as well as the client's needs. Throughout the hospital, a number of communication tools evolved to enhance a consistent approach to clients' care. These tools—standards of practice, standards of care, nursing diagnosis (including standardized and individualized care plans), data-bases, and Integrated Clinical Pathways—provided practitioners with a method to communicate the client's needs and goals to other health team members. Thus a continuous and consistent plan of care for the client was established. Each of the communication tools is discussed and their relationship to continuity of care addressed below.

> *A thing that will help your inner life is to set up in*
> *your mind a standard of values, so that you know*
> *what is really significant, important, and valuable.*
> JOHN MILLER

Standards of Practice

Standards of practice are essential elements in the nursing profession at Sioux Valley Hospital. Although they are not documentation tools to be used with the client, these standards of practice are fundamental to the nursing profession. These tools identify the responsibilities and accountabilities of nurses caring for clients. The purpose of these standards is to identify for nurses their obligation to provide and improve nursing and to enhance the quality of care that is provided to clients and families.[7] Through the implementation of differentiated practice, the associate nurse, primary nurse, and clinical care coordinator roles were clarified and the competencies for each identified. Therefore, these standards of practice communicate to the clients and families the expectations of the nursing roles to ensure that quality care is delivered to the clients and families.

Standards of Care

Standards of care, as defined by the American Nurses' Association and accepted by Sioux Valley Hospital, are the "authoritative statements that describe a competent level of clinical nursing practice demonstrated through assessment, diagnosis, outcome identification, planning, implementation, and evaluation."[7(p21)] The term *standards of care* was not new to staff at Sioux Valley Hospital. Standards of care have been written for each of the units within the hospital, reflect the specialty of the unit, and are in accordance with the guidelines of the Joint Commission on Accreditation for Healthcare Organizations. These standards of care became an essential component of the implementation of nursing diagnosis, which was a new term for the nursing profession at Sioux Valley Hospital.

The standards of care became the foundation for units as they began to increase their understanding of nursing diagnosis and the purpose of nursing diagnosis for their client's needs. These standards of care identified nursing routines that could be incorporated into nursing orders and nursing interventions for client care. Thus the beginning concept of nursing diagnosis was defined. Later these standards of care became an essential component of the Integrated Clinical Pathways.

Nursing Diagnosis

Nursing diagnosis was a foreign term to many nurses. The question of how nurses could actually identify a diagnosis for a client was often raised. It was at the same time that differentiated practice was introduced at Sioux Valley Hospital that nursing diagnosis was introduced. Nursing diagnosis became the primary terminology for patient care plans and discharge plans. With the introduction of nursing diagnosis, there was much confusion between the concept of nursing diagnosis and patient care plans that were identified on patient Kardexes. How were these two different? Education was a key to understanding these differences.

The North American Nursing Diagnosis Association defines nursing diagnosis as "a clinical judgment about an individual, family, or community response to actual or potential health problems/life processes which provide the basis for definitive therapy toward achievement of outcomes for which the nurse is accountable."[8(p65)] Nursing diagnoses identified pertinent client problems for which nurses could safely and independently intervene (as defined by the South Dakota Board of Nursing Practice Act Scope of Practice) without a physician's order. Nurses were able to prioritize client problems through the use of nursing diagnoses. The patient care plans on Kardexes identified the nursing and medical tasks that were necessary for patient care. Often, the informal care plans reflected the standards of care that had been identified by each unit. With the understanding of nursing diagnosis, nurses were able to establish a plan of care based on the client's needs and the nurse's independent judgment without stepping outside their scope of nursing practice.

A hospital Nursing Diagnosis Committee and unit nursing diagnosis committees were formed to alleviate any misunderstanding that the term *nursing diagnosis* may have generated. These committees also became the champions and architects (refer to Chapter 7 for discussion of these roles) of this topic, and their members were designated as resource personnel to introduce, clarify, and define nursing diagnosis to all nursing units.

As nursing diagnosis became more familiar to staff, nursing diagnoses were incorporated into standardized and individualized client care plans. Individualized care plans were mutually established by the primary nurse and the client. These care plans then became the communication tools for other nursing and health care staff in providing the necessary interventions that the client required during hospitalization. Information for these care plans was gathered from a number of sources: client, family, physician, and other health care staff. From these sources, problems and needs of the client were identified and prioritized; then a mutual plan of care was established with the client.

Patients with multiple problems frequently had several actual nursing diagnoses and multiple potential diagnoses. Although the actual diagnoses were the primary concern, attention needed to focus also on prevention of problems. The primary nurses in critical care identified the need to develop a problem list to focus nursing care on priority and secondary/potential problems (Figure 5–5). This list would help the primary and associate nurses focus goals on prevention.

Databases

The critical care and adult specialty care services developed an admission database (see Appendix 5-C) to be used by the primary nurses. Databases were essential tools for identifying and prioritizing client needs. The information on these databases asked questions that encompassed the whole client. Physical, psychosocial, emotional, spiritual, environmental, educational, and other needs the client wished to share were recognized with this tool. Upon review of the information the client shared, the primary nurse was able to better understand the client's needs during hospitalization and after discharge. The database became a permanent part of the medical record. The information on this tool kept staff from repeatedly asking the client similar questions regarding health care needs at present and after discharge. Often, client databases from previous admissions were retrieved and updated with the client rather than the entire form being completed again. Thus the database was an essential communication tool for all staff to utilize when providing care to their clients.

Integrated Clinical Pathways: An Impetus for Change

The effectiveness of all communication tools has been a vital component of the implementation of differentiated practice. These tools, however, created additional

SIOUX VALLEY HOSPITAL

Nursing Plan of Care Summary

Discharge/Long Term Goal _____

_____

Referrals Consulted

_____ on _____ R/T _____

_____ on _____ R/T _____

_____ on _____ R/T _____

_____ on _____ R/T _____

Problem Number	Nursing Diagnosis (Problem Statement)	Priority Nursing Problem (Date) and Signature	Identified But Not a Priority Problem (Date)	Date of Problem Resolution (Date)

Unresolved Nursing Problems Upon DC/Tx	Date and Referral to Whom

Figure 5–5 Nursing plan of care summary. Reprinted with permission of Sioux Valley Hospital, Sioux Falls, South Dakota, © 1991.

paperwork and documentation to be completed by the nursing staff. Staff recognized that similar documentation was taking place in multiple places and that it would be more effective to consolidate documentation. Consequently, Integrated Clinical Pathways were introduced to the clinical practice at Sioux Valley Hospital.

Even within the walls of a hospital, care can become specialized to the point of fragmentation. The documentation of that care can become unwieldy as the volume of paperwork multiplies and becomes burdensome. For these reasons, the Integrated Clinical Pathway methodology was selected as the approach to enhance interdisciplinary collaboration, to streamline documentation, and to encourage patient/family participation in the plan of care.[9]

An Integrated Clinical Pathway is defined as a tool to manage a patient's care through an acute episode of illness. Clinical Pathways map or outline care on a timeline and are specific to a medical diagnosis or surgical procedure and to a physician or physician group. Certain categories are highlighted (eg, tests, treatments, consults, medication, nutrition, activity, discharge planning, nursing diagnosis/interdisciplinary focus, nursing interventions/teaching, and patient outcomes) and list the key activities that need to occur in a predictable and timely manner to achieve an appropriate length of stay with expected patient outcomes.[10,11] An interdisciplinary approach is utilized, and resources are coordinated by the associate nurse, primary nurse, and/or CNS to achieve high-quality care in a cost-effective manner.

Establishing Integrated Clinical Pathways as the model to manage patient care within the hospital walls requires judiciously sequenced organization and fully committed support from the hospital's senior administration, nursing, and medical staff leaders.[12] All departments need to be cognizant of the Pathway process and their unique roles. Ongoing evaluation with periodic educational updates of progress is essential to success. A project director is also essential to coordinate the implementation and evaluation phases of Integrated Clinical Pathways.

A nursing task force for Integrated Clinical Pathways was formed at Sioux Valley Hospital with two representatives (a primary nurse and an associate nurse) from each nursing unit. All CNSs served on the task force as consultants. Others who served on the task force included a nursing administrator, clinical nursing director, staff education representatives, quality improvement manager, nurse researcher, computer expert, and clinic nurse. The goals of the task force were to develop the following:

- Clinical Pathways for the top five medical diagnoses for each nursing unit
- guidelines and education of staff for utilization of Clinical Pathways, including streamlining of documentation
- a system to track variances and clinical outcomes and to incorporate concurrent quality improvement monitoring
- a system to trend and analyze data regarding variances, clinical outcomes, cost effectiveness, and patient/nurse/physician satisfaction

- a computerized prototype specific to Sioux Valley Hospital's Clinical Pathway format

The general surgical unit was selected as the demonstration site for implementation. Surgical patient care is more routine and follows a day-by-day timeline more readily than the medical populations. Other timelines can be used to accommodate medical populations, such as a step or stage progression. In the NICU, for example, Pathways are developed by both gestational age and diagnosis.

It is imperative that physicians are included in the development of these tools. It is helpful to start with physicians who are interested and influential and who efficiently manage patient care. Integrated Clinical Pathways are written for a specific physician or physician group to reflect personal practice patterns and to avoid the charge of cookbook medicine.[13] They are used in a descriptive rather than prescriptive manner when introduced.

Integrated Clinical Pathways are developed in collaboration with the physician or physician group and all appropriate members of the health care team to outline key activities and expected outcomes for a specific medical diagnosis or surgical procedure. For example, the coronary artery bypass Pathway was developed by the ICU and telemetry nursing staff in conjunction with the cardiovascular surgeons, cardiovascular CNS, cardiac rehabilitation staff, respiratory therapists, dietitians, social workers, diabetes resource nurse, and smoking cessation staff (see Appendix 5-D for a sample Pathway).

Retrospective chart review of five to six recent discharges with the same diagnosis and similar lengths of stay and charges is one way to develop a Clinical Pathway. The physician or physician group, the nurses, and all appropriate health care team members then edit and refine the Pathway before implementation.

Variances are deviations from the Pathway and are called exceptions. The exceptions to the Integrated Clinical Pathway are trended and examined to identify and resolve barriers to recovery and system problems. Other exceptions might be positive, leading to an early discharge for the patient. There are four types of exceptions: patient/family, hospital systems, caregiver/clinician, and community resources.[11,14] Refer to Appendix 5-E for a listing of exceptions that are tracked.

Before the Clinical Pathways were implemented, there were three major steps involved in the documentation process at Sioux Valley Hospital:

1. documentation of the individualized plan of care on standardized care plans
2. documentation of the actual care delivered on numerous flowsheets and forms and in the nursing notes
3. documentation in the computer of the actual care delivered to reflect the acuity of each patient

To introduce the Pathways into an already fragmented and cumbersome maze of paperwork, streamlining the documentation system was essential. Integrated Clinical Pathways incorporate the medical, nursing, and all other appropriate disciplines into one comprehensive plan of care. The nursing diagnoses, key nursing activities, teaching, and key patient outcomes are incorporated into the Clinical Pathway and reflect the standards of care for the particular diagnosis. Therefore, step 1 above is streamlined. Only patient-specific nursing diagnoses, interventions, and outcomes not listed on the Pathway need to be incorporated to individualize the Pathway. Integrated Clinical Pathways are part of the permanent record and eliminate the Kardex and nursing discharge summary form also. By totaling acuity points accrued for each day of the Pathway, it was identified that patients who followed the Clinical Pathway could be assigned an automatic acuity rating without the need for the time-consuming computer rating system. Therefore, step 3 above was eliminated. Streamlining step 1, and eliminating step 3 allowed more time for the nurse to be at the bedside and to focus on the actual documentation of care delivered, including physical assessments and patient responses.

Benefits and Outcomes

Integrated Clinical Pathways are valuable orientation tools for novice nurses, float nurses, students, physician residents, physician consults, physicians covering for the attending, other disciplines, and patients and families. The expectations are clearly defined to enhance quality of care. Outlining the plan of care augments continuity of care on a shift-to-shift basis as well as for patients who transfer from one unit to another. An interdisciplinary approach avoids fragmentation and duplication of services. Sequencing key events on the Pathway avoids last-minute complexities and oversights that may compromise effective discharge planning.

The most significant impact on nursing has been a paradigm shift from planning care to managing care and from completing tasks to achieving outcomes. The professional accountability and enhanced fiscal awareness have dramatically improved.

Physicians have responded favorably to Clinical Pathways because of the maximized efficiency of their time. Because the Clinical Pathway outlines the care, nurses can anticipate orders for the day and are better prepared to assist physicians with rounds. This avoids telephone calls for routine or noncritical orders in the evening or 5 minutes after the physician leaves the unit.

Physicians also experience a decrease in the amount of time spent on the telephone with insurance companies. Clinical Pathways answer the routine questions insurance companies ask about tests and treatments to be ordered and anticipated length of stay. The protocols established by Clinical Pathways provide an opportunity for physicians and hospitals to demonstrate high-quality plans of care cost efficiently as managed care and preferred providers become more prevalent.

Patients and families have also responded favorably to Clinical Pathways. The associate or primary nurse reviews the content on a daily basis, so that patients and families know the expectations and can participate actively in the plan of care. Teaching is emphasized and is spread out on a continuum rather than just before discharge.

Tracking of data and variance analysis identify inefficiencies in hospital systems that extend patients' hospital stays. For example, maintaining a wider range and greater capacity for diagnostic testing after hours and on weekends can avoid the many costs of nontherapeutic days that keep patients waiting in the hospital. The hospital benefits significantly from Integrated Clinical Pathways as the utilization of resources is coordinated to achieve a decrease in length of stay and overall charges while quality of care is maintained. Examples of the favorable impact that Clinical Pathways have had on reducing length of stay and hospitalization charges can be found in Figures 5–6 to 5–9.

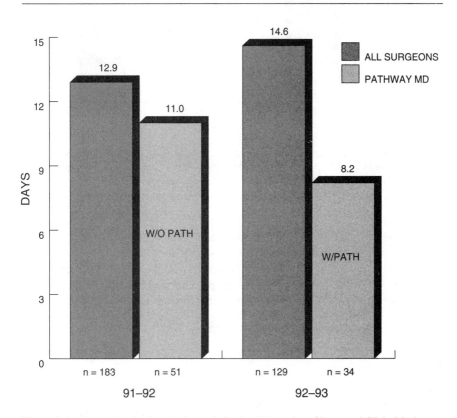

Figure 5–6 Average length of stay before and after implementation of Integrated Clinical Pathways: Comparison of data from March 1991–March 1992 and March 1992–March 1993 for DRG 148 colon resection with complications. Courtesy of Sioux Valley Hospital, Sioux Falls, South Dakota.

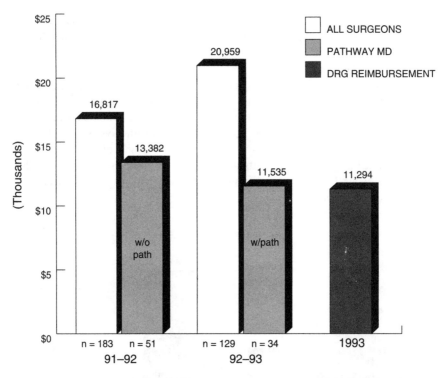

Figure 5–7 Average charge before and after implementation of Integrated Clinical Pathways: Comparison of data from March 1991–March 1992 and March 1992–March 1993 for DRG 148 colon resection with complications. Courtesy of Sioux Valley Hospital, Sioux Falls, South Dakota.

In this era of diagnosis-related groups and with the advent of managed care, dwindling reimbursement, and shortening hospitalization, Integrated Clinical Pathways offer a proactive approach to managing patient care. All processes of continuity, including communication, collaboration, collegiality, accountability, and consultation, are fulfilled by this innovative plan of care.

Success is dependent on effort.

SOPHOCLES

THE FUTURE

Integrated Clinical Pathways are an effective tool for case management of patients within the walls of a hospital. With lengths of stay shortening and the massive shift to outpatient care, Pathway development will need to expand to

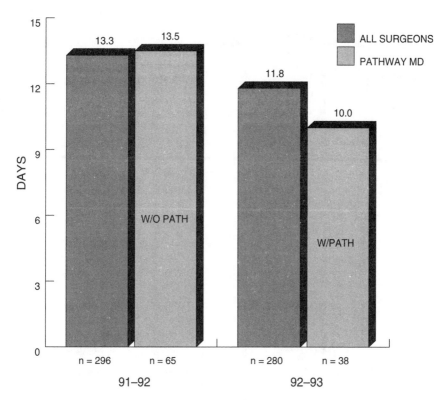

Figure 5–8 Average length of stay before and after implementation of Integrated Clinical Pathways: Comparison of data from June 1991–March 1992 and June 1992–March 1993 for DRG 106 coronary artery bypass graft with cardiac catheterization. Courtesy of Sioux Valley Hospital, Sioux Falls, South Dakota.

include outpatient, interagency, and community information. This could include home health, nursing homes, and other community support services.

For patients with chronic medical conditions causing multiple hospitalizations and emergency department visits, the role of the advanced practice nurse/CNS as case manager will need to develop more fully. Following high-risk, chronically ill patients on a continuum will allow coordination of services in the hospital with other programs across numerous health care settings. Providing this vital link will optimize quality of care on a continuum. Integrated Clinical Pathways decrease fragmentation and advocate the appropriate use of the health care dollar for these complex patients and their families.

Focusing on prevention and shifting from illness and cure to wellness and care[15] will also be essential to future health care. Establishing nurse practitioner-run wellness clinics, which emphasize the importance of empowering patients to

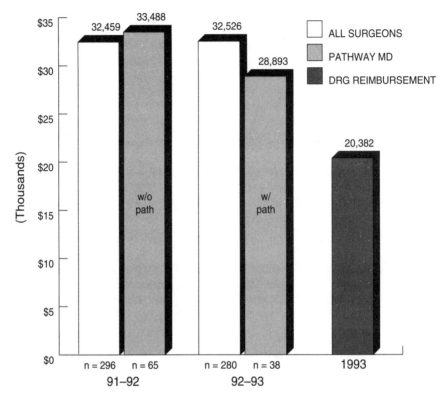

Figure 5–9 Average charge before and after implementation of Integrated Clinical Pathways: Comparison of data from June 1991–March 1992 and June 1992–March 1993 for DRG 106 coronary artery bypass graft with cardiac catheterization. Courtesy of Sioux Valley Hospital, Sioux Falls, South Dakota.

develop their potential for well-being, will appropriately place nursing in a prevention and teaching capacity.

As Sioux Valley Hospital plans for the nursing profession in the future and how to enhance further the process of continuity of care, two new concepts have been introduced to the nursing practice: computerization and work redesign. How each of these could affect the continuity process for clients entering this institution is discussed below.

Computerization

With technical advances, computerization provides a means for communication within the walls of the hospital. Computer technology would enable nursing personnel and other health care members to document their interactions with their clients and the progress their clients are making toward long-term goals. In an effort to implement documentation by means of computerization, Sioux Valley Hospital is evaluating several computer documentation systems to assist nurses to make better clinical decisions through effective management of accurate, timely, and complete information. With computerization, nurses would have more time to care for their clients, being freed from the task of documenting assessments, goals, interactions, and outcomes on multiple forms.

Work Redesign

Further focusing on continuity for patients along with improving quality and reducing costs is the initiative of work redesign. Work redesign is a process through which roles are redefined and the patient care delivery system is restructured. Work redesign of roles has developed as a complementary system to Integrated Care and in response to the unit emphasis on improved efficiency. On most units the assistive roles, such as the nurse assistant and the health unit coordinator, have been redefined. There is a common theme throughout the hospital of change and efficiency, which is stated as "work smarter, not harder." Some restructuring of roles occurred as a result of the necessity to fulfill patient care needs and expanded job responsibilities.

The unit director's role has also been redefined in view of institutional changes and national trends. The title of the head nurse changed to unit director to clarify the role further and to reflect its development. The nursing assistant responsibilities vary from unit to unit depending on clinical tasks and nonclinical task demands, unit decisions, and budgeting purposes. On many adult specialty care units, the nursing assistants are assigned aspects of patient care such as activities of daily living, obtaining vital signs, recording intake and output, and documenting care completed. Some units have cross-trained nursing assistants to function as health unit coordinators primarily for computer order entry.

Delegation of tasks to nursing assistants has been most appropriately completed with the clear delineation of roles and responsibilities. This includes an understanding of roles among all caregivers. Delegation can only be learned and practiced in an environment in which professional responsibilities are valued and quality outcomes are measurable.

In 1992, Sioux Valley Hospital focused on work redesign as an institutional process and strategic plan. The development and implementation of "patient-focused care" is currently underway. Patient-focused care will be implemented initially on two patient care units that are being constructed. There has been a paradigm shift in the terminology and process of the standard nursing care unit, which is now the patient care unit. Patient-focused care is the restructuring and redesigning of patient units, professional responsibilities, and hospital delivery systems to enhance customer value. The goal of this process is to allow health care professionals to focus their efforts on the patient and to increase the amount of time spent with the patient while avoiding unnecessary steps. Whereas the Integrated Care delivery system affected primarily nursing personnel, the patient-focused care design is a total hospital reorganization.

CONCLUSION

With the implementation of Integrated Care, the process of continuity of care for the patient has indeed been enhanced. The communication that takes place among the different roles and the other multidisciplinary caregivers allows these individuals to provide the necessary interventions to their patients in the most time- and cost-efficient manner. Through this collaborative and communicative process, a continuum of care is delivered to the patient, be it within one unit or across multiple units. The patient's hospital journey becomes more streamlined and less fragmented with the implementation of differentiated nursing roles and the utilization of the communication tools devised by the nursing staff.

Integrated Care at Sioux Valley Hospital has proven to be effective in providing a continuum of health care for its patients and families. The different roles have been mutually valued. Each role is intertwined with the others to provide the care that is required to meet each patient's needs and goals.

REFERENCES

1. Newman MA. Toward an integrative model of professional practice. *J Prof Nurs.* 1990; 6:167–173.
2. American Hospital Association and American Organization of Nurse Executives. *Joint Position Statement on Differentiated Practice.*Chicago, Ill: American Hospital Association; 1991.
3. Porter-O'Grady T, Finnigan S. *Shared Governance for Nursing: A Creative Approach to Professional Accountability.* Gaithersburg, Md: Aspen Publishers; 1984.
4. Andreoli K. Primary nursing for the 1990s and beyond. *J Prof Nurs.* 1992; 8:202.
5. Stamps PL, Piedmont EB. *Nurses and Work Satisfaction: An Index for Measurement.* Ann Arbor, Mich: Health Administration Press Perspectives; 1986.
6. Koerner JG, Bunkers L, Nelson B, Santema K. Implementing differentiated practice: the Sioux Valley Hospital experience. *J Nurs Admin.* 1989; 19(2):13–22.
7. American Nurses' Association. *Standards of Clinical Nursing Practice.* Washington, DC: American Nurses' Association; 1991.
8. Carroll-Johnson RM, ed. *Classification of Nursing Diagnoses: Proceedings of the Ninth Conference.* Philadelphia, Pa: Lippincott; 1991.
9. As case management evolves, pathways may need revision. *Hosp Case Manage.* 1993; 1(5):88,93.

10. Sinnen MT, Schifalacqua MM. Coordinated care in a community hospital. *Nurs Manage.* 1991; 22(3):38–42.

11. Zander K. Care maps: the core of cost/quality care. *The New Definition.* 1991; 6(3).

12. Guiliano KK, Poirer CE. Nursing case management: critical pathways to desirable outcomes. *Nurs Manage.* 1991; 22(3):52–55.

13. American Hospital Association. *Clinical Practice Guidelines: An Awareness Paper for Hospitals.* Chicago, Ill: American Hospital Association; 1992 (March):1–11.

14. Zander K. Quantifying, managing, and improving quality. *The New Definition.* 1993; 8(1).

15. American Nurses' Association. *Nursing's Agenda for Health Care Reform.* Kansas City, Mo: American Nurses' Association; 1990.

EXERCISE 5–1: FORMULAS FOR IMPLEMENTING INTEGRATED CARE

1. How to assess the need for Integrated Care: Assess the nursing patient unit's population, their lengths of stay, the complexity of their conditions, and the variety of patient needs. Does this assessment warrant a system to integrate and coordinate client care?
2. Planning for Integrated Care: Is it more effective to implement the three identified nursing roles of differentiated practice at the same time? Alternatively, is it more appropriate to develop two nursing roles and then expand into the clinical care coordinator role?
3. Assess the referral interactions that are necessary and take place within the unit. Are there referrals that are not being made in a timely manner? Are discharges being delayed because of these unmade referral interactions?

   To ensure that the primary nurse role will be effective and workable, the primary nurse must:
   - provide information about what this role specifically entails, how, and why (discuss how this role differs from the associate nurse and clinical care coordinator roles; provide staff education regarding this role before implementation)
   - articulate and define the job description of the primary nurse role
   - be visible to all staff to share client issues
   - have the ability to collaborate and delegate effectively and reasonably
   - recognize and assume only those responsibilities that he or she is able to keep and perform
   - recognize that consultation is an essential component and make the appropriate referrals to these consultants rather than address the issues himself or herself (identify the expertise of individuals)

EXERCISE 5–2: STEPS TO COMPLETE A FINANCIAL ANALYSIS

Financial analysis is completed by the hospice administrator and the volunteer coordinator. The data are analyzed routinely once per year. The specific steps to complete the financial analysis are as follows:

1. Calculate the total number of patients analyzed (each patient will be counted only once even if there is more than one monthly bill recorded).
2. Calculate the time span of the analysis in total patient days.
3. Review each bill for the charges that apply to each acuity level in the hospice, as defined by the Medicare Conditions of Participation, as routine home care, respite care, continuous home care, and general inpatient care.

4. Categorize each bill for the costs of each product used in each category: Medicare supplies, home medical equipment, medical X ray, medical laboratory, pharmacy, radiology, nutrition, and other.
5. Total the costs in each category for each patient.
6. Total the costs for each category for all patients.
7. Divide total costs per category by total patient days to get the per day rate.

Appendix 5-A
Sioux Valley Hospital Perception of Nursing Care Questionnaire: Physician

Please place an X in the space to the right below the word that best describes your perception of the frequency with which each event occurs. If you have any additional remarks, please use the space provided at the end of the questionnaire.

	Always	Usually	Sometimes	Seldom	Never	N/A
1. Continuity of nursing care is evidenced from admission to postdischarge.						
2. Your patients are satisfied with their nursing care.						
3. The nurses attend to your patients' families.						
4. Appropriate information is supplied to your patients' families.						
5. You are given accurate information concerning your patients.						
6. Information from the nursing notes is beneficial.						
7. Discharge planning is reflected in documentation.						
8. Nursing personnel collaborate with other departments to facilitate patient care.						
9. Patient care conferences are beneficial to patients, families, and the multidisciplinary health care team.						

	Always	Usually	Sometimes	Seldom	Never	N/A
10. Patients and their families are instructed for home care.						
11. Provisions are made by the nurses for continued care after discharge (arranging referrals, needed supplies, and equipment).						

Additional comments:

Courtesy of Sioux Valley Hospital, 3100 Unit, Sioux Falls, South Dakota.

Appendix 5-B
Perinatal Database

SIOUX VALLEY HOSPITAL

Perinatal Data Base

**Do Not Fill In Shaded Areas

Date: _____ Due Date: _____

Mother's OB Physician _____

Family Physician _____

Baby's Physician _____

Consults

Which Hospital do you plan to deliver at? _____

Mother of Infant _____ Age _____ Work _____

Address, City, State, Zip _____ Last grade completed _____

Home Phone Number _____ Work Phone Number _____

Who will be your support person in labor? _____ How are you related? _____

Home Phone Number _____ Work Phone Number _____

The Following Are Questions To Better Assist Your Physician And The Healthcare Team In Your Care:

Health ❑ This section deferred—see Perinatal Admission Record

What pregnancy is this for you ❑ 1st ❑ 2nd ❑ 3rd ❑ 4th ❑ _____   Date of 1st prenatal visit _____

Are you expecting twins? ❑ Yes ❑ No How many full-term babies have you had? _____

How many babies have been premature? (less than 37 weeks) _____

How many miscarriages/abortions have you had? _____ How many living children do you have? ___

Describe your health. _____

List any medical problems you have. _____ ❑ None

List any medical or pregnancy related problems you have had with past pregnancies. _____

_____ ❑ None

List any medical or pregnancy related problems you have had with this pregnancy. _____

_____ ❑ None

Do you plan to deliver ❑ vaginally ❑ by cesarean; reason _____ ❑ vaginal birth after cesarean?

Are you choosing adoption? ❑ Yes ❑ No ❑ Undecided.

Describe your special wishes/concerns for this birth experience. _____

_____ ❑ None

Do any members of your family have milk intolerance or milk allergies? ❑ Yes ❑ No

List any allergies you have and how you react (ie: medications, food, metals, other). _____

_____ ❑ None

Medication/Drug History ❑ None

	Type	Amount	Frequency of Use	Last Time Used
❑ Vitamins (Including prenatal vitamins)				
❑ Laxatives				
❑ Antacids				
❑ Cold Medicines				
❑ Caffeine				
❑ Aspirin				
❑ Sleeping Pills				

	Type	Amount	Frequency of Use	Last Time Used
❑ Marijuana				
❑ Cocaine				
❑ Alcohol				
❑ Nicotine				
❑ Other Medications				

Does anyone in your household smoke? ❑ Yes ❑ No

Have you ever been treated for addiction? ❑ Yes ❑ No For what?_____ When? _____

Describe any problems you have with vision, hearing, or language. List any aids or equipment you use.
_____ ❑ None

Have you been exposed to any childhood diseases during this pregnancy? ❑ Yes ❑ No

If yes, what? _____

When were you exposed?_____ Have you already had this disease? _____

ACTIVITY

What do you do for exercise now and how often? _____ ❑ No

Has your activity been limited? (If so, describe) _____ ❑ No

SLEEP

How can we help you rest or sleep while you are in the hospital? _____

_____

NUTRITIONAL   Height_____   Pre-pregnancy weight_____

Check any that apply:

Do you have any problems with ❑ your appetite? ❑ indigestion? ❑ nausea? ❑ vomiting? ❑ No

Do you have any special ❑ food restrictions? ❑ diet/nutrition concerns? _____ ❑ No

How many cups of water do you drink per day?_____ Cups of other fluids?_____

Diet history _____
_____
_____ ❑ NA

Do you plan to ❑ breastfeed ❑ bottlefeed ❑ Undecided

Would you like a lactation (breastfeeding) consultant to contact you ❑ Before delivery? ❑ While in the hospital? ❑ No

Did you ❑ breastfeed or ❑ bottlefeed your other children?_____ How long did you breastfeed? _____

Describe any problems with breast or bottlefeeding. _____ ❑ None

ELIMINATION

Do you have any problems with ❑ constipation? ❑ diarrhea? ❑ hemorrhoids? ❑ No

Describe any problems with passing urine. _____ ❑ None

Do you have any history of bladder infections? _____

Have you been treated during this pregnancy? ❑ Yes ❑ No

If so, describe. _____

SEXUALITY

Do you have a history of infertility? ❑ Yes ❑ No Number of years _____

Do you plan to use birth control after delivery? ❑ Yes ❑ No If yes, describe. _____

Have you used this method before? ❑ Yes ❑ No

Do you have any concerns about sexual intercourse ❑ before delivery ❑ after delivery ❑ No

Do you have history of any of the following (check if applies):

❑ Gonorrhea ❑ Syphillis ❑ Oral Herpes ❑ Vaginal Herpes ❑ Chlamydia ❑ Vaginal Warts
❑ Yeast Infections ❑ Trichomoniasis ❑ HIV Positive ❑ AIDS ❑ None

PERCEPTIONS/EDUCATION

Describe your concerns/fears about pain during labor. _____

_____ ❑ No Fears

What helps you deal with pain? _____

_____ ❑ Don't Know

Describe your type of pain and rate your level of pain (scale 1 = minimum; 10 = maximum)

before delivery _____

labor & delivery _____

after delivery _____

Check the items you would like to learn more about related to:

Care During Pregnancy	**Care After Delivery**	**Health Care Follow-up**
❑ Prenatal tests:_____	❑ Recovery & care after	❑ Routine physical exams
❑ Pain management in labor	childbirth	❑ Immunizations
❑ Preterm labor	❑ Emotions and adjustments	❑ Nutrition
❑ Gestational diabetes	❑ Sibling adjustments	❑ Sexually transmitted diseases
❑ Toxemia/High Blood Pressure	❑ Feeding your baby	❑ Contraception
❑ Twins	❑ Infant bathing	❑ Infant car seats/seat belts
❑ Exercise in pregnancy	❑ Care of umbilical cord	❑ Infant/child CPR
❑ Smoking in pregnancy/after delivery	❑ Circumcision	❑ Selecting child care
❑ Alcohol/drug use in pregnancy	❑ Coping with a fussy baby	❑ Breast self-exam
❑ Sexuality in pregnancy	❑ Taking baby's temperature	❑ Pap smears
❑ Vaginal birth after cesarean	❑ When your child is ill	
❑ Cesarean birth		

What would you **most** like to learn about during your hospitalization:

_____

_____

Would you like a childbirth educator to contact you ❑ during your antepartum hospitalization? ❑ No
Would you like to be added to the Women and Children's Health mailing list for program information?
❑ Yes ❑ No

PP Booklet given_____ (date) ICN booklet given_____ (date)

EMOTIONAL RESPONSES

Describe any major changes/stresses in your life (divorce, family, finances, grief, illness, job, marriage, recent move, other). _____

_____

What do you do when you are tense or under stress (ie: problem-solve, eat, sleep, take medication, seek help)? _____

_____

To whom do you turn in time of need? _____

What would you like to change in your life? _____

_____

Check if applies:

❑ History of baby blues   When?_____ Duration: _____

❑ History of depression   When?_____ Duration: _____

Prioritize how you want to use your time during your Postpartum hospital stay (Rank 1–4 with 1 being the most important): ❑ Sleep/Rest ❑ Time for Self/Immediate Family ❑ Teaching ❑ Visitors

HOME PLANNING

Marital Status: ❑ Single ❑ Married ❑ Widowed ❑ Divorced ❑ Separated

Ages of children living with you. _____

Do you have other dependents living with you? (If so, what is their relationship to you?) _____

_____ ❑ None

Which of the following do you have: ❑ Insurance ❑ Medicaid ❑ Baby Care ❑ Self-pay cash? ❑ None
Do you have concerns about your financial expenses for this pregnancy? ❑ Yes ❑ No
Would you like someone from the business office to contact you to help determine your insurance
coverage or payment options? ❑ Before delivery ❑ While in the hospital ❑ No
Would you like to visit with Social Services about financial or community services available to you?
❑ Before delivery ❑ While in hospital ❑ No

Will you be discharged to ❑ Home ❑ Relative's Home ❑ Other: _____
Do you plan to return to work?_____ (If so, when) _____
Are you using any programs/agencies in your community (ie: baby care, food stamps, WIC, etc.)
❑ Yes ❑ No

Services needed upon discharge (ie: WIC, etc) _____❑ None
Equipment needed upon discharge (ie: car seat, bili-lites, monitors, pumps, etc.) _____
_____ ❑ None
Would you like a visit by a nurse at your home after discharge from ❑ Antepartum? ❑ PP? ❑ ICN?
Reason: _____

RELIGION
Religious preference _____
Would you like to visit with a hospital chaplain during your hospitalization? ❑ Yes ❑ No
Any religious or ethnic concerns that may influence your care while hospitalized? _____
_____

Infant baptism while hospitalized ❑ Yes ❑ No ❑ Done

OTHER
Is there anything else you would like to share about yourself which may be helpful to us in caring for you.
_____

Date:_____ Signature of Patient _____
Thank you for completing this Perinatal Data Base.
◆◆
Comments _____

Primary Nurse to follow ❑ yes ❑ no Unit_____ RN Signature _____ Date_____
Primary Nurse to follow ❑ yes ❑ no Unit_____ RN Signature _____ Date_____
Primary Nurse to follow ❑ yes ❑ no Unit_____ RN Signature _____ Date_____
Reviewed by Primary Nurse/Clinical Care Coordinator _____ ❑ NA Date_____
READMISSION UPDATE
Summary of changes in patient needs/problems Date_____
_____
_____
_____

Reprinted with permission of Sioux Valley Hospital, Sioux Falls, South Dakota, © 1991.

Appendix 5-C
Admission Database

SIOUX VALLEY HOSPITAL

Admission Database

The following questions have been designed to gather information about you and your family. From this we will work with you to develop a plan of nursing care.

HEALTH AND ILLNESS

How long do you expect to be in the hospital? ___

_____

Do you rate your health as ❏good ❏fair ❏poor?
Do you have any problems/questions concerning your medications? _____
What would you like to know about your illness/surgery?

_____

ACTIVITY

	Yes	No
Can you bathe yourself?	____	____
Can you dress yourself?	____	____
Do you drive?	____	____
Can you do your own housework?	____	____
Do you need assistance with moving about?	____	____
Can you prepare meals?	____	____
Can you do your shopping?	____	____

Comments _____

_____

VALUES-BELIEFS

Are there any religious/ethnic activities, restrictions that may influence your care while hospitalized?
❏ yes ❏ no
Comments _____

_____

ROLE RELATIONSHIPS/HOME PLANNING

Significant other _____
Who do you live with? _____
Do you anticipate needing help after leaving the hospital? _____
What family/friends can help you if needed? ____

_____

Where do you plan on living after you are discharged? _____

_____

Is there anyone at home dependent on you? ____

_____

Who in your family helps you make decisions regarding your care? _____
Have you used community services in the past (Meals-on-Wheels, Home Aid)? _____

_____

Who can assist with transportation if needed? ___

_____

Do you have stairs at your home? _____
Are the bathroom and bedroom on the main floor?

_____

Are there equipment/services you would like/need upon discharge? _____
Will you need or want a visit by a nurse after discharge? _____
Comments _____

_____

COPING/INDEPENDENCE

Do you have financial concerns? _____
What concerns or stresses are you having in relationship to being in the hospital? _____

_____

Has your family ever had a crisis/situation like this happen before? _____
How did you cope? _____

_____

SEXUALITY/REPRODUCTIVE

List any questions or concerns you have about:

Sexual activity _____

_____

Body image _____

_____

PATIENT REQUESTS

What else would you like to share which may be
helpful to us in caring for you? _____

_____

_____

What information do you need or want to know?

	Yes	No
Parking	____	____
Visiting Hours	____	____
Sleeping Accommodations	____	____
Financial Concerns	____	____
Community Support Groups	____	____
Emotional Support	____	____
Medicare/Insurance Coverage	____	____

Information from _____

(signature)

Date_____ _____

relationship to patient

HEALTH MAINTENANCE

What do you do to keep healthy and prevent
health problems?

Routine physical exam

❑ Yearly ❑ Sometimes ❑ Never

Weight

❑ Ideal ❑ Overweight ❑ Underweight

Exercise

❑ Regularly ❑ Sometimes ❑ Never

Monthly self breast/testicular exam

❑ Usually ❑ Sometimes ❑ Never

Routine eye exam

❑ Yearly ❑ Sometimes ❑ Never

Dental exam

❑ Yearly ❑ Sometimes ❑ Never

Immunizations/last date

____ Flu ____ Tetanus ____ Other

Use seatbelt

❑ Usually ❑ Sometimes ❑ Never

Would you like information/assistance on any of
these topics? ❑ Yes ❑ No

Please specify: _____

Information given: _____

Thank you for taking time to complete this form. The remainder of this form is for nursing staff only.

◆◆

Additional Comments _____

Primary Nurse to follow ❑yes ❑no Unit____ RN Signature _____Date____
Primary Nurse to follow ❑yes ❑no Unit____ RN Signature _____Date____
Primary Nurse to follow ❑yes ❑no Unit____ RN Signature _____Date____
Reviewed by Primary Nurse/Clinical Care Coordinator _____ Date____

READMISSION UPDATE

Summary of changes in patient needs/problems Date_____

_____

_____

_____

_____

Signature of patient/family _____ Signature of Nurse _____

Date_____ ❑Primary Nurse to follow ❑Does not need Primary Nurse at this time

Reprinted with permission of Sioux Valley Hospital, Sioux Falls, South Dakota, © 1990.

Appendix 5-D
Sample Integrated Clinical Pathway

	SIOUX VALLEY HOSPITAL	**Integrated Clinical Pathway**

COLON RESECTION
DRG #149
Physician Group:
Attending MD: **Dr. E. Rolfsmeyer**
Primary RN: _____
Date Reviewed by MD/RN/Patient: _____
Advance Directive: Yes_____ No_____
Code Status: _____

MEDICAL HISTORY

Admit Date	ICU Date	Transfer Date	Allergies:

Present Problem: _____

Surgical & Special Procedures: _____

Past History: _____

Physician Consults:

Date	Physician	Reason	First Visit	Signed Off

Phone Numbers:
Name _____
Relationship _____
Home _____
Work _____
Name _____
Relationship _____
Home _____
Work _____

DISCHARGE PLANNING

Discharge Destination	Date	Initial	Community Services	Date	Initial	Transportation	Date	Initial
Home			Meals on Wheels			Family		
Home w/VNA			Hospice			Wheelchair Service		
Home w/Home Health ___			Respite Care			Paratransit		
Home w/Public Health Nurse			HEARTH			Ambulance		
Nursing Home, Skilled			Dept. Social Services			Indian Health Services		
Nursing Home, Intermediate			Senior Companion			State Penitentiary		
Nursing Home,			Homemaker			Other _____		
Assisted Living			Lifeline					
Rehab			Wellness Center: _____			**Equipment**	**Date**	**Initial**
Swing Bed: _____			Cardiac Rehab			Home Oxygen		
VA Hospital			Vascular Rehab			Home IV Therapy _____		
Hospice Cottage			Support Group: _____			Assistive Devices _____		
State Penitentiary								
Motel: _____			Other: _____			Other: _____		
Other: _____								

Initials/Signature:
____/_____   ____/_____
____/_____   ____/_____   ____/_____

01 OFF PATHWAY ☐ YES
DATE___/___/___

DAY/DATE	Admit: Pre-op Date_____	Day 1: OR Date_____	Day 2: POD 1 Date_____	Day 3: POD 2 Date_____	Day 4: POD 3 Date_____
CONSULTS	Anesthesia RT (AM Admission/PAT)				
LABS	H&H, Lytes CEA PT, PTT		Chem I H&H		Chem I H&H
X-RAY	Type & Screen CXR				
OTHER	EKG				
TREATMENTS/ PULMONARY	1. Volurex (if smoker or resp. history) RT to instruct	1. NG to L/MCS, check patency Q4H, irrigate w/30cc NS Q4H PRN 2. Dressing 3. JP 4. Foley care Q shift	1. NG to LCS, check patency Q4H, irrigate w/30cc NS Q4H PRN 2. Dressing 3. JP 4. Foley care Q shift	1. NG to LCS, check patency Q4H, irrigate w/30cc NS Q4H PRN 2. DC drsg 3. JP site care w/ H202/gauze drsg Q day _____ 4. Foley care Q shift	1. NG to LCS, check patency Q4H, irrigage w/30cc NS Q4H PRN 2. JP site care w/ H202/gauze drsg Qday _____ 3. DC foley
MEDICATIONS/ IVs	Bowel prep Colyte_____ Neomycin 1 gm po x3 Flagyl po x3 Check for pre-op antibiotic order	IV: D5 1/2 NS w/ 20KCl at 125 cc/hr PCA (IV antibiotic in OR holding)	IV at 125cc/hr PCA	IV at 125 cc/hr PCA	IV at 125 cc/hr PCA
NUTRITION	Clear liquid, then NPO after MN	NPO/Ice Chips	NPO/Ice Chips	NPO/Ice Chips	NPO/Ice Chips
ACTIVITY/PT SAFETY	Up as ordered: _____	Dangle/ambuate in p.m.	Chair TID: _____ Walk QID w/assist:	Chair TID: _____ Walk QID w/assist:	Chair TID: _____ Walk QID w/assist:
DISCHARGE PLANNING	Complete Assessment Tool	Review Assessment Tool	Assess needs; make referrals as appropriate	Review plans; revise as needed	Review plans; revise as needed
NURSING DX/ INTERDISCI- PLINARY FOCUS	1. Knowledge	1. Knowledge 2. Comfort 3. Potential infection 4. Nutrition 5. Activity	1. Knowledge 2. Comfort 3. Potential infection 4. Nutrition 5. Activity	1. Knowledge 2. Comfort 3. Potential infection 4. Nutrition 5. Activity	1. Knowledge 2. Comfort 3. Potential infection 4. Nutrition 5. Activity
KEY NURSING ACTIVITIES/ TEACHING	1. Routine VS 2. Provide Surgical Awareness handout & video; SVH instructions for Colon Resection 3. Instruct: bowel prep, IV, NG, JP, foley catheter, pain control w/PCA, NPO, I&O, TCDB, incision, early ambulation, frequent monitoring post-op 4. Review pathway w/pt/family	1. PACU Standards 2. VS: Post-op then Q4H 3. I&O Q 6 hours 4. TCDB Q2H 5. Dangle/ambulate in p.m. 6. Assess lungs, bowel sounds Q4H 7. Inspect drsg, drains 8. Instruct to report sputum production 9. Reinforce teaching for Volurex, PCA, NPO	1. VS: QID 2. I&O Q 6 hours 3. TCDB Q2H 4. Assist w/ADLs 5. Assess lungs, bowel sounds, drsg, drains Q 4 hours 6. Instruct to report sputum production 7. Reinforce post-op teaching 8. Monitor PCA pain control	1. VS: QID 2. I&O Q 6 hours 3. TCDB Q2H W/A; assist w/ADLs 4. Assess lungs, bowel sounds, wound, drains QID and prn 5. Reinforce post-op teaching 6. Monitor PCA pain control	1. VS routine; 2. I&O Q 6 hours 3. Encourage effective TCDB & Volurex 4. Assist w/ADLs 5. Assess lungs, bowel sounds, wound, drain QID and prn 6. Teach importance of passing flatus/ having BM & reason for cont'd I&O
KEY PATIENT OUTCOMES	1. Demonstrates use of Volurex 2. Verbalizes understanding of pre-op teaching 3. Complies w/NPO status 4. Verbalizes under- standing of pathway progression 5. OR permit obtained	1. PACU Standards resolved or referred 2. VSS, I&O stable 3. No N/V 4. Pain controlled 5. Demonstrates effective TCDB 6. Tolerates activity w/o complications	1. VSS, I&O stable 2. Demonstrates effective TCDB, use of Volurex 3. Tolerates activity w/o complications 4. Pain controlled w/o N/V 5. Verbalizes understanding of post-op teaching	1. VSS, I&O stable 2. Demonstrates effective TCDB, use of Volurex 3. Tolerates activity w/o complications 4. Pain controlled w/o N/V 5. Verbalizes understanding of post-op teaching	1. VSS, I&O stable 2. Demonstrates effective TCDB, use of Volurex 3. Tolerates activity 4. Pain controlled w/o N/V 5. Voids w/o difficulty 6. Verbalizes understanding of teaching
SHIFT RN SIGNATURE	AM Admit: D. N.	PACU: D. N.	D. N.	D. N.	D. N.
INITIALS/ SIGNATURE	____/_____ ____/_____		_____	____/_____ ____/_____	

Day 5: POD 4 Date_____	Day 6: POD 5 Date_____	Day 7: POD 6 Date_____	Day 8: POD 7 Date_____	
				KEY 1. Initialed in Red = Ordered 2. Black Line = Not Ordered 3. Pinked Out = Completed 4. Circle in Black = Exception 5. DC = Discontinue 6. D/C = Discharge
1. DC NG (when bowel sounds x4 quads and passing flatus) 2. JP site care w/H202/ gauze drsg every day	1. JP site care w/H202/ gauze drsg every day	1. DC JP. Site care w/ H202 and 4x4 gauze drsg 2. DC staples, steri-strip w/benzoine	1. Check drsg 2. Check wound	
IV at 75 cc/hr DC PCA PO pain med Check home meds	DC IV PO pain med Home meds	PO pain med Home meds	PO pain med Home meds	**Special Orders**
Clear liq 1st meal; full liq 2nd meal (toast OK); advance to soft 3rd meal	Soft or regular	Regular	Regular	
Chair TID: _____ Walk QID w/assist:	Up ad lib	Up ad lib May shower after JP out x2 hours	Up ad lib May shower	
Discuss home arrangements; include family Begin D/C Teaching Form	Confirm home arrangements Continue D/C Teaching Form	MD writes D/C instructions and Rx for home meds Complete D/C Teaching Form	Review/reinforce D/C Teaching Form	
1. Knowledge 2. Comfort 3. Potential infection 4. Nutrition 5. Activity	1. Knowledge 2. Comfort; resolve 3. Potential infection 4. Nutrition: Resolve 5. Activity: resolve/refer	1. Knowledge 2. Potential infection	1. Knowledge: resolve/ refer 2. Potential infection: resolve/refer	
1. VS routine 2. I&O every 6 hours 3. Encourage effective TCDB and Volurex 4. Assist w/ADLs 5. Assess lungs, bowel sounds, wound, drains, flatus every shift 6. Teach possibility of gas pains 7. Encourage PO intake 8. Instruct PO pain meds 9. Instruct pt/family on home meds, diet, activity, bowel care and wound infections	1. VS routine 2. I&O every 6 hours 3. Encourage independence w/ADLs, TCDB, Volurex 4. Assess lungs, bowel sounds, wound, drains, flatus every shift 5. Encourage PO intake 6. Instruct PO pain meds 7. Review D/C Teaching Form	1. VS routine 2. DC I&O 3. Encourage independence w/ADLs, TCDB, Volurex 4. Assess lungs, bowel sounds, wound, drains, flatus every shift 5. Encourage PO intake 6. Instruct PO pain meds 7. Review D/C Teaching Form	1. VS routine 2. Assess lungs, bowel sounds, wound, drsg, flatus/BM every shift 3. Assess tolerance to activity and diet 4. Provide Colon Resection Discharge Teaching Form	
1. VSS, I&O stable 2. Demonstrates effective TCDB 3. Tolerates activity 4. Pain controlled w/PCA or PO pain med 5. Passing flatus 6. Tolerates diet w/o N/V 7. Verbalizes understanding of teaching	1. VSS, I&O stable 2. Demonstrates effective TCDB 3. Tolerates diet, activity w/o complications 4. Pain controlled w/PO pain med 5. Verbalizes understanding of teaching	1. VSS, I&O stable 2. Demonstrates independence w/ADLs, TCDB 3. Tolerates diet, activity w/o complications 4. Verbalizes understanding of D/C teaching	1. VSS 2. Demonstrates independence w/ADLs 3. Tolerates diet, activity 4. Verbalizes understanding of D/C instructions	D/C Date:___/___/___ D/C Time: _____ Actual LOS: _____
D. N.	D. N.	D. N.	D. N.	
_____/_____	_____/_____	_____/_____		
_____/_____	_____/_____	_____/_____		

Reprinted with permission of Sioux Valley Hospital, Sioux Falls, South Dakota, © 1992.

Appendix 5-E
Sioux Valley Hospital Exceptions to Clinical Pathway Codes

P. PATIENT/FAMILY
Patient complication (this admission)
- P1   Suspected/confirmed infection
- P2   Bleeding/hematoma/back to OR/GI Bleed
- P3   Respiratory failure/ventilator dependent
- P4   Heart failure/IABP support
- P5   Renal failure/insufficiency
- P6   Cardiac rhythm disturbance/temporary pacer
- P7   Hypotension/hypertension/CO/CI
- P8   DVT/PE
- P9   CVA/Neuro Deficit
- P10   Pain Control
- P11   Other (N/V, activity intolerance, hypoglycemia, etc.)
- P12   Ileus

Preexisting condition
- P21   Diabetes
- P22   COPD/Respiratory History
- P23   CHF
- P24   Renal failure/insufficiency
- P25   CVA/Neuro deficit
- P26   GI ulcers
- P27   Cardiac/CAD/CABG/MI/PPM
- P28   Cancer (list type)
- P29   Psychosocial
- P30   Other

Other
- P31   Undecided about therapy
- P32   Refuses test, therapy or discharge plan
- P33   Family not available
- P34   Patient achieved intervention earlier than anticipated
- P35   Miscellaneous

C. CAREGIVER/CLINICIAN

Related to physicians

C1   Test/procedure ordered by Clinical Path MD not on pathway
C2   Test/procedure ordered by other MD not on pathway
C3   Test/procedure not ordered that is on pathway
C4   Surgery done that is not on pathway
C5   Abnormal diagnostic/lab test not followed up
C6   Rounds not made (specify day of week)
C7   Rounds late in day
C8   Rounds late in day delaying discharge
C9   Consult made but patient not seen within 24 hours (specify day of week)
C10   Hospital bed (prolonged/inapppropriate use)
C11   Telemetry bed (prolonged/inappropriate use)
C12   Critical care bed (prolonged/inappropriate use)
C13   Admitted the night before surgery
C14   Order intervention earlier than anticipated
C15   Order intervention later than anticipated
C16   Other

Related to nursing

C21   MD order not followed through
C22   Nursing order not followed through
C23   Wrong ordering of tests
C24   Lack of discharge planning causing delay
C25   Lack of patient education causing delay
C26   Order intervention earlier than anticipated
C27   Order intervention later than anticipated
C28   Other

Communication

C31   Breakdown with other department

Other

C41   Miscellaneous

S. HOSPITAL SYSTEMS

Related to test/treatment/procedure scheduling

S1   Incorrect sequencing of tests
S2   Ordering process incorrect
S3   Busy schedule, no openings
S4   Done late in day, delaying discharge
S5   Scheduling not done on weekends
S6   Not done on weekend
S7   Not done on evening or night shift
S8   Could be done as outpatient
S9   Awaiting test results, causing delay in discharge
S10   Other

Related to surgery
    S21 Busy schedule, no openings
    S22 Not done on weekends
    S23 Delayed, other
    S24 Could be done as outpatient
    S25 Other
Awaiting another hospital bed
    S31 No telemetry bed available
    S32 No pulmonary bed available
    S33 No neuro acute bed available
    S34 No renal bed available
    S35 No observation bed available
    S36 No rehab bed available
    S37 Other
Equipment/supplies
    S41 Not available
    S42 Out of order
Other
    S51 Miscellaneous

R. RESOURCES/ COMMUNITY

Skilled nursing facility
    R1 No bed available in area
    R2 Accepted but no bed
    R3 Does not accept on weekends/holidays/after hours
    R4 Bed available; would not accept patient (list reason)
    R5 Other
Home services
    R21 Home health care services not available
    R22 Home equipment not available
    R23 Home IV/TPN not available
    R24 Supplies/medications not available
    R25 Other
Appropriate facility/bed
    R31 Not available
    R32 Available earlier than anticipated
    R33 Other
Communication
    R41 Breakdown with other agency
    R42 Other
Other
    R51 Miscellaneous

6 Consultation

Rebecca Johnson Blue, Linda Birch Bunkers,
Carol McGinnis, Lois J. McMahon,
and Phyllis Newstrom

The camera has been transformed in the past century from the simple black box used to photograph posed, quiet subjects to the high-tech instruments that can catch complex action from any distance. Those simple black boxes met the needs of most people whose desire was to capture a simple pose. For those who wanted a clearer, wider view or who dreamed of capturing the complexities of their subject, however, the simple black box needed to be improved. So it is in professional nursing practice. At one time we were satisfied with a basic level of competency that well met the needs of our patients. Today, with the higher acuity and complexity of our patients, we are faced with the need for an improved version of the black box camera. We need a model that broadens our view, deepens our depth, and sharpens our perspective. Yet we demand that it be user friendly and cost effective and still allow us to use our simple black box when that is all we need to use. A lens is needed that broadens, deepens, and sharpens nursing practice. Consultation can be that lens.

This chapter discusses consultation and its impact on nursing practice. Consultation is viewed from all roles of the differentiated practice model of nursing with an emphasis on advanced practice. For the purpose of this chapter, an advanced practice nurse is defined as one who has completed a master's degree in nursing and is functioning in an advanced role as a clinical nurse specialist (CNS), nursing educator, or nurse manager.

THE PROCESS OF KNOWING

> *A single conversation across the table with a wise*
> *[person] is better than ten years' study of books.*
> HENRY WADSWORTH LONGFELLOW

Consultation is an evolving art in nursing. It has been used throughout history every time people have asked for guidance, support, knowledge, and expertise from others. Nursing has been no different. Although nurses historically did not often use the word *consultation,* they have consulted one another, such as in team conferencing or when asking for advice or help from someone more expert. Referrals most often came during a simple discussion with a group of nurses on the nursing unit, while passing in the hall, while sharing information during meals and breaks, or while waiting in line for the copying machine. Since the implementation of differentiated practice, nurses have begun to see themselves as formal consultants. The shutter has been opened, allowing the lens to focus. A new picture has developed.

Webster defines the word *consult* as "to ask advice of; to seek an opinion from; to refer to or turn to; to talk things over in order to decide or plan something; consider; confer" and the word *consultation* as "the act of consulting; a meeting to discuss, decide or plan something." In nursing literature, consultation is described by Oda as, "a helping process . . . a form of planned change utilizing interpersonal relationships."[1(p8)] Rutherford defines consultation as "the ability of an individual to understand clients' problems and to work with them to use existing resources to a maximum."[2(p344)]

> *All experience is an arch, to build upon.*
> HENRY ADAMS

The consultant may be a nurse in any role. The associate nurse has the important responsibility of assessing and implementing interventions to meet the current needs of the patient during the shift of duty. In addition to medication administration, dressing changes, and patient teaching, the nurse acts as a consultant to others on the unit. Newly employed nurses on the unit may request an explanation of a documentation form. Those who are unfamiliar with a particular intravenous access device may also consult an associate nurse.

The primary nurse is frequently involved in the consultation process both as consultant and as consultee. The primary nurse is viewed as the gatekeeper, advocating and planning efficient and quality patient care during the length of stay on a unit. In addition to arranging family care conferences, writing home health referrals, and updating care plans, the primary nurse makes time for consultation. This may involve a phone call from another nursing unit requesting expertise in orthopedics or a physician asking for an opinion on an appropriate length of stay for a patient. The primary nurse is also the consultee when he or she is utilizing the expertise of health team members such as social workers, pharmacists, and physical therapists to assist in care planning. Consultation is occurring everywhere in health care, and for good reason. It is a process that greatly enhances an individual practitioner's capacity for providing quality patient care.

Inherent in the role of advanced practice nursing is consultation. During activities such as symptom management, program development, or conflict resolution, the advanced practice nurse is consulting. The consultee may be a nurse, another hospital department, or a patient's family. The consultation may not always occur at the bedside of the patient, but it is ultimately patient focused.

To gain a greater understanding of consultation and how it may occur within the roles of differentiated practice, Nicolai and Pitts-Wilhelm[3] working from del Bueno's[4] original work on competency, created a conceptual model for Sioux Valley Hospital's differentiated practice (Figure 6–1). As described by del Bueno[4] (see Figure 2–1), competency is based on the acquisition of three skill sets: technical/clerical, interpersonal/communication, and critical thinking/management. Nicolai and Pitts-Wilhelm,[3] in their model, describe the ties that bind the different practice roles together and indicate features that differentiate them. These three skill sets are defined by structure, process, and outcome in Figure 6–1 (see Appendices 4-A through 4-C for job descriptions).

It is the advanced practice nurse's competency in communication that enables him or her to build a successful practice. The word *build* is intended to be taken literally. Most, if not all, of the advanced practice nurses in our institution have built their own practices one consultation at a time. This consultation may be requested initially because of the advanced practitioner's technical ability or management knowledge, but consultations continue because of the consultant's communication skills.

A common characteristic of all advanced practice nurses at Sioux Valley Hospital is the fluidity of their role. The structure in which advanced practitioners function allows, but, more important, demands, access to patients from a variety of settings and enables continuity of care outside the walls of the hospital. This lack of structure enhances the nurse's ability to identify the shape, form, and patterns of a client's life. Rather than using the length of the hospital stay or the confines of a single nursing unit as the boundary, nurses frame care within the situational and contextual boundaries of each client. Each encounter may be brief. For example, the advanced practice nutrition nurse may be consulted by a physician to suggest an appropriate feeding tube for a surgical patient. That same nutrition nurse may be consulted by a home health agency to make several home visits to a patient and caregiver struggling with home parenteral nutrition. The lenses of advanced practice change frequently to allow for wide-angle views or for close-up, detailed perspectives.

The outcomes of nursing care can be placed in a hierarchical design with the foundation being comfort and physiologic stabilization. This outcome is ensured by the skilled attention of the bedside nurse practicing in the associate role. The next step, carried out by the primary nurse, is to provide continuity of care and a timely prepared discharge utilizing Integrated Clinical Pathways.

For those patients with complex physiologic and psychosocial challenges, the advanced practice nurse intervenes toward the goals of empowered decision making and transformative Integrated Care. A CNS in geriatrics at Sioux Valley Hospital describes her role as that of enabler. By providing new knowledge, role modeling

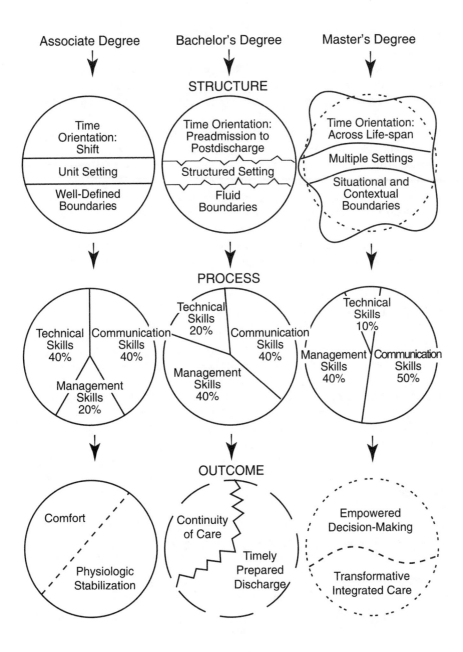

Figure 6–1 Framework for differentiating practice roles of nursing. *Source:* Reprinted from *Differentiating Nursing Practice: Into the Twenty-First Century* by I.E. Goertzen, ed., p. 86, with permission of the American Academy of Nursing, © 1991.

communication techniques, and identifying clinical strengths in the associate and primary nurses, she enables them to reach a higher level of expertise in geriatric nursing. Koerner and Bunkers identify that "transformational leadership involves change, innovation, growth, and empowerment of self and others. It occurs when one or more persons engage with others in such a way that leaders and followers raise one another to higher levels of motivation and morality."[5(p3)] It is this transformational leadership that has occurred in all areas of nursing practice at Sioux Valley Hospital. Advanced practice educators have utilized and taught adult learning principles to staff preceptors. Those preceptors in turn model the principles to empower their preceptees toward enlightened learning opportunities. Advanced practice managers have mentored staff nurses into the roles of clinical care coordinators, where their empowered decision-making skills are essential to the day-to-day management of the nursing units. Managers have been active participants and facilitators in the transformation of our governance processes. Leadership is shared and valued at all levels in our nursing practice.

CONSULTATION AT WORK: CASE STUDIES

The following case studies are a sampling of the real life stories that occur as the consultation process unfolds. They demonstrate the various settings, issues, and persons that can benefit from use of the consultation process. Exhibit 6–1 is a snapshot of consultation in the day-to-day practice of a CNS working on an antepartum unit. Exhibit 6–2 is a view of consultation through the work of an advanced practice nurse educator. Finally, Exhibit 6–3 projects the role of an advanced practice manager consulting outside the hospital. As these case studies demonstrate, consultation can occur in a variety of settings and conditions and with a variety of outcomes. Furthermore, in each case both consultee and consultant benefitted.

TEAM BUILDING THROUGH CONSULTATION

Teams are strengthened through consultation, yet team-building skills, education, and continued emphasis on individual values are essential elements of the foundation and development of a differentiated practice environment. Consultation and teams are each only as strong as the other.

> *The greatest trust, between [people], is the trust of giving counsel.*
> FRANCIS BACON

Exhibit 6–1 Case Study: Advocating for a Mother and Her Unborn Child

> A young unwed mother was experiencing a challenging pregnancy. The pregnancy was unplanned, and the woman's support system was precarious. Her mother had died when she was a child, her father was not happy about the pregnancy, her boyfriend was unwilling to be involved, and she had no close friends. In addition, her day-to-day health was uncertain as she struggled with the effects the pregnancy was having on her diabetes. In the midst of this maturational crisis of pregnancy and the superimposed crises of multiple hospital admissions for diabetic control, this woman's three physicians were pressuring her to give up her child for adoption.
>
> The perinatal CNS was asked to consult on this patient. She received two separate consultations, one from the obstetrician, who wanted the CNS to encourage the patient to give the child up for adoption, and another from the staff nurses, who believed the patient needed medication.
>
> After reviewing the case, talking to the expectant mother and her father, and eliciting help from the hospital's ethics committee, the CNS called a meeting with the expectant mother's primary physician. The CNS discussed the ethical principles surrounding the patient's right to make this decision for herself and her child. The CNS utilized Rubin's[6] theory of maturation, which describes the taking in and taking hold process that occurs during pregnancy. The theory helped explain why the patient was not ready or able to make a decision about adoption at that point in her pregnancy. This information led to collaborative discussion and resulted in mutual agreement to provide the education and support necessary to allow this young woman to make an informed decision on her own.

Nurse-to-nurse consultation is the greatest trust and compliment shared among nurses as practice partners. Nurses at Sioux Valley Hospital have learned to strengthen their practices through valuing and using the knowledge and expertise of others. Expertise holds limited worth unless it is shared.

From the historical perspective, consultation at Sioux Valley Hospital has changed and is continually in the process of change. When the differentiated practice model of nursing was first initiated, consultation followed a traditional horizontal and vertical pattern. Specifically, horizontal consultation occurred among nurses in similar roles, whereas vertical consultation occurred among nurses in different roles based on expertise. It is important to illustrate what was gleaned from these traditional patterns of consultation to convey why consultation can evolve into a model that is more empowering and collaborative.

The result of horizontal consulting was affirmation and validation for the consultee. Much of the consulting took place on the horizontal plane, with nurses in like roles consulting each other, and within confined boundaries, usually limited to nurses they knew. Horizontal consultation was used for eliciting assistance from someone specialized or from someone with special experience in specific topics.

Exhibit 6–2 Case Study: "I Wonder"

The phone had an inquiring ring that cold, cloudy October day, so that it was no surprise when the quiet, modulated voice said, "I'm the education consultant for the _____ Board of Nursing, and I'll be coming to Sioux Falls in about 2 weeks to do some work with the South Dakota Board of Nursing. I wonder if you have time to see me to talk about your Summer E program. The board tells me it's a well-documented model, and we're exploring the concept and related regulation in our state." (Sioux Valley Hospital's Summer E is a formal 10-week shared clinical enrichment program for senior nursing students enrolled in baccalaureate programs. The externs receive excellence in education, experience, and employment. The extern, under the direction of clinical resource instructors, works in a one-to-one relationship with an experienced and qualified registered staff nurse.)

On still another colder, ice-framed day, the same voice said via phone, "The roads are snow packed and travel not advised, but, please, could I have an overview of your program when I come next week?" Appointments were hastily changed, and it was with a true sense of sharing that materials were gathered and a clear, unbiased, factual documentation of the student enrichment program with special emphasis on board rules and regulations was prepared.

The appointment was kept and lasted nearly twice as long as scheduled, in part because of our mutual sharing and high interest. The educational consultant came with prepared questions, and our current printed materials gave factual responses. We took the prerogative to play "what if" games, and more possibilities and questions led to more challenges and fewer answers. It was a highly stimulating and fulfilling time of collegial interest and professional direction setting. Our formal encounter had given rise to the best inquiries, communication, and critical thinking and created an interest and proposed outcome bond. This information would be shared with the _____ Board for discussion before accepting inquiries from agencies wishing to offer clinical enrichment programs. It would again be reviewed if rules and regulations were to be amended to include regulation of such programs.

Many of the first units to have self-scheduling also consulted with other units. They helped these units by giving hints as to steps to do or not do in the process, what obstacles might occur, and how they worked these problems out. Through this consulting process, these units and nurses became more comfortable with the consulting process in both seeking resources and serving as a resource to others. This affirmation and validation among nurses and nursing units helped strengthen the professional and collegial nursing practice at Sioux Valley Hospital.

As nursing staff confidence in the consulting process increased, more nurses started consulting in the vertical plane. Here nurses were looking for expertise, specialized knowledge, and/or problem-solving abilities. The vertical consulting process helped the consultee become empowered via the mentoring and coaching offered by the consultant.

Exhibit 6–3 Case Study: A Change Is Imminent (Team Contractual Agreement)

A nearby medical/education facility requested assistance from Sioux Valley Hospital when it was unsuccessful in filling its director of nursing position. The management group at the facility was dedicated, conservative, and traditional in their thinking, working in an environment where nurses and nursing were considered a secondary function of the organization. Therefore, nursing practice had little support to be anything but secondary. Consultation was requested to manage the facility until a permanent director of nursing replacement could be found.

The invitation to work together in this process came as an acknowledgment of the expertise and trust from previous working relationships with Sioux Valley Hospital nursing administration. On a contractual basis, a nurse trimanagement system was used to facilitate change in the contract organization over a short time frame. This nurse management team consisted of advanced practitioners from education, supervision, and special projects. The team was responsible for assessing the nursing care delivery system, outlining a new direction for nursing, and implementing as much as was feasible in the uncertain but short time frame until a new director of nursing could be hired and mentored.

In addition to the trimanagement team, a Sioux Valley administrative nursing director served as a liaison to the facility's top management to demonstrate and mentor the group on management skills. This administrative nursing director facilitated the creation of the management proposal and contract, coordinated the trimanagement system, assisted with brainstorming and problem solving, and ultimately facilitated the hiring of a new and permanent director of nursing for the contract organization.

To manage the organization, the team assessed the depth and intensity of needs and developed an action plan to meet these needs. The assessment revealed that change would need to occur over the course of many years. Team-building programs, such as the Myers-Briggs instrument and focus groups, were utilized to gain insight into the present nursing team and to foster trust in the group.

Each member of the team contributed a unique talent or perspective to the change process. The nurse supervisor had the task of managing the nursing team. She spent 30 hours a week in the organization. Others on the team recognized her skill in seeing a vision for the organization, having strong interpersonal skills and a keen ability in building trusting relationships, and giving constant positive reinforcement to the staff undergoing the changes toward the new vision. The educator and the special projects director each spent approximately 5 to 10 hours a week at the facility, depending on the needs. The educator was responsible for implementing team-building programs and addressing team-building issues. The educator also counseled staff undergoing struggles related either to job performance or to personal issues and developed an education committee to address continuing education needs. The special projects team member addressed the staffing ratios, reimbursement issues related to wage and hour, and overall acuity issues of clients presently in the organization.

The team met weekly with the organizational management team to provide progress updates and to seek further understanding of the contract organization's

continues

Exhibit 6–3 continued

philosophy and culture. This communication was imperative for successful implementation. The team was present for 1 year, and many changes were implemented.

For this ambitious and talented group of four who responded as one, it was an extremely positive experience. Each of the four recognized the strengths of the others and could visualize how they all fit into this unusual picture. Team management can work, and it can be mutually satisfying and growth producing.

Presently, the consultation process is moving toward the practice partnership model, as described by Koerner and Bunkers.[7] In this model (Figure 6–2), each nurse is an equally valued and functioning practice partner regardless of role or responsibility. The model identifies the underlying philosophy necessary for consultation to occur on a professional level and addresses the way nurses execute the role of consultant. The seven capacities described by Koerner and Bunkers[7]— clarity, congruence, commitment, connectedness, communication, caring, and creativity—are inherent components of the relational, humanistic culture of nursing at Sioux Valley Hospital. These capacities promote validation, affirmation, and empowerment of the practice partners.

This evolutionary or transformative consultative process is still developing in the practice at Sioux Valley Hospital. This novice-to-expert development occurs with each individual involved in the consultation and within the organization as all practice partners learn from each other. The process of consultation deals with

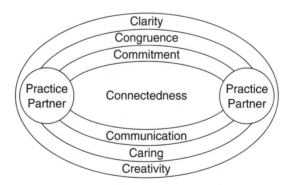

Figure 6–2 Practice partnership: The model. *Source:* Reprinted from Koerner, J.G. and Bunkers, S.S. The M-I-D-D-L-E-G-R-O-U-N-D: Part II, Developing Partnerships in Practice, *Nursing Connections,* Vol. 5, No. 3, p. 55, with permission of Nursing Connections, © 1992.

relationships and promotes empowerment through sharing of expertise. Nursing at Sioux Valley Hospital is still in its infancy on the continuum from the traditional model to the practice partnership model of consultation. Throughout the hospital, nursing consultation is in many places on the continuum from the merely horizontal/ vertical consultation model to practice partnership relationships or, in essence, on the novice-to-expert continuum of consultation.

> *Our relationships can be the fastest and the most*
> *powerful route to the deepest truth, if we know*
> *how to use them.*
>
> SHAKTI GAWAIN

Throughout the changes in the environment, the mutual valuing of each individual nurse as a professional with inherent knowledge, rights, and responsibilities led to questioning and consulting on a peer-to-peer level. As each nurse's self-esteem grew, he or she became ready to question and consult on a vertical plane as well as on the familiar horizontal plane. Thus the introduction of the advanced practice nurse into the practice environment was a natural event. Valuing had become inherent. Nursing then needed to enlarge its team and open its boundaries with the goal of creating a seamless environment for nursing practice. Furthermore, consultation outside the basic realm of nursing was duly enhanced.

The next generation of consultation will be interdisciplinary. This evolution is occurring at Sioux Valley Hospital with the inception of interdisciplinary team practices such as geriatric assessment, nutrition support, and pain management. The interdisciplinary focus will continue as it becomes the foundation of two new patient-focused care units at Sioux Valley Hospital (see Chapter 5 for a discussion of patient-focused care).

> *If we are to achieve a richer culture, rich in*
> *contrasting values, we must recognize the whole*
> *gamut of human potentialities, and so weave a less*
> *arbitrary social fabric, one in which each diverse*
> *human gift will find a fitting place.*
>
> MARGARET MEAD

Health care is demanding more interdisciplinary consultation on the client's behalf. It may be easier as nurses to consult within our own profession, however, because of common language and philosophy. Goal and role conflicts may hinder the effectiveness of the interdisciplinary process. Shared values as well as common understanding of operationalization of those values are important in interdisciplinary consultation. Trust and security in one's own profession, valuing of other professions, continued refueling, and a professional support system can play a major role in productive interdisciplinary consultation.

This transformation of the consultative process could not have evolved had there not been some team building by design. Two team-building strategies were used. One was an Ecology of Excellence philosophy. This philosophy addresses the champion, architect, mentor, and worksmith roles; commitment to first party communication (see Chapter 3) and other ecocentric behaviors (see Chapters 7 and 8 for more discussion about Ecology of Excellence and shared governance); and use of the Myers-Briggs Personality Type Inventory. The second team-building strategy was the implementation of shared governance and the differentiated practice model of nursing. These team-building strategies have strengthened the professionalism of nursing at Sioux Valley Hospital and have had a great effect on the continuing evolution of consultation.

Team building has helped build trust, promoted valuing and acknowledgment of all practice partners, created mutual acceptance, and enhanced recognition of the strengths and unique contributions each person has to offer to the practice. Instead of zooming in on our differences, as has happened historically, team members focus on valuing all practice partners, which has led to professional and personal empowerment.

> *If you have knowledge, let others light their candles at it.*
>
> MARGARET FULLER

THE ART OF SHOWING

The snapshot is fuzzy at best. The legs of one nurse are missing, and the other nurse is minus half her head. How and when does this candid shot come into focus? Can the image of both nurses be captured completely, and are the missing areas important for the message? Does this distorted, blurred exposure have relevance to the client, the nurses, or the delivery system? Perhaps of greatest concern, where is the client?

Nurses have long recognized that professional collegiality is founded on trust. The advanced practice nurse-care provider relationship affords extraordinary examples of mutual acceptance and positive exchanges, both of which are elements of trust. The advanced practice nurse concept, which embraces the tenets of mentoring, supporting, and sharing, has become a hallmark of the profession. Contemporary nursing attempts to define, crystallize, and implant this role within a staff and culture of many nursing units; thus the print comes slowly into focus. As advanced practice nurses begin to explore their role in relationship to other nurses, they soon find that their expertise is validated only as they acknowledge and enhance the strengths of their colleagues. This valued collaboration, which begins the consultation process, can be initiated by a simple question, a passing remark, an

"I wonder" or a formal "What do you think?" Bennis[8] tells us that truth begins with questions, and soon this exchange between the staff nurse and advanced practice nurse moves to sharing and eases into consultation. In the search to meet patient care accountability, the associate or primary nurse is offered expertise through the advanced practice nurse's explorative questions, new resources and correlations, and vivid past experiences, all through a casual remark or inquiry. This process is demonstrated in Exhibit 6–4.

> *Always the beautiful answer who asks a more*
> *beautiful question.*
>
> E. E. CUMMINGS

CONSULTATION AND EMPOWERMENT

Just as the question initiates the process of collaboration, true empowerment recognizes the creative potential and inherent worth of the peer. In Exhibit 6–5 the nurses engaging in the exchange affect the client care outcomes but also enhance the role of both consultee and consultant. As this mutual acceptance is viewed and the nature of empowerment is more closely examined, it becomes apparent that the nemesis of this quiet, powerful quality has taken life from the foundation of the hospital's delivery system. Hotter tells us that "true empowerment is driven by philosophy rather than by technique."[9(p11)] As the Department of Nursing's philosophy is reviewed, it is obvious that the photographer has correctly placed the film because "nurses are responsible for achieving quality outcomes for the profession,

---

Exhibit 6–4 Case Study: The Value of Consulting

The pulmonary/renal unit was asked by the postanesthesia care unit to consult on the implementation of the primary nurse role. The primary nurses and nurse manager from the pulmonary unit talked with the nurses on the postanesthesia care unit about how the role had been implemented on the pulmonary unit, the obstacles they had run into, and ideas as to how the postanesthesia care unit might utilize the primary nurse role. Many creative ideas were generated, and both groups contributed much to the discussion. Both units gained insight from each other, and both were positive about the results of this relationship between what seemed to be vastly different nursing units. The consultant unit (pulmonary) nurses went into the consultation wondering about the value that their ideas and experiences would have to the postanesthesia care unit nurses. The pulmonary nurses came out of the relationship with good feelings about what they had to contribute to others and felt valued as a result of the consultation process.

Exhibit 6–5 Case Study: Consultation through a Casual Remark

It was a normally busy day on the surgical unit as the CNS opened a medical record. She was greeted by one of the primary nurses, who was describing her full day of patient interviews and discharge planning. Across the unit came the loud voice of a patient sounding agitated and belligerent. The primary nurse looked at the CNS and said, "Now there's a patient for you!" They discussed the patient's history and exchanged possible reasons for his behavior. The primary nurse noted that the elderly patient was oriented and that his behavior was appropriate before surgery. Now on his second postoperative day he was exhibiting obvious signs of delirium. The primary nurse assessed his laboratory values as normal, and his pain medications had been carefully selected, taking into account his advanced age. The CNS reviewed the medical record and agreed that none of the documented data pointed to a cause for the delirium. She asked the primary nurse for permission to interview the patient. The primary nurse encouraged her to do so.

The CNS spent nearly a half hour interviewing the patient and his wife. She learned that the patient had had surgery 7 years ago for prostate problems. During his postoperative recovery at home, he had experienced difficulty sleeping. His physician had prescribed a sleeping pill that was effective in allowing him to sleep through the night. Over the past 7 years he had continued to take the sleeping pill almost every night. His wife stated that sometimes he woke up during the night and took another sleeping pill. The surgeon who was caring for the patient on this current hospital stay was not aware of the sleeping pill usage.

The CNS left the room and reported her findings to the primary nurse. They both understood the implications of abruptly discontinuing a sleeping medication and recognized those symptoms in this patient. The CNS consulted a pharmacist to suggest methods for safely weaning the patient from this medication. The recommendations of the CNS and pharmacist were documented in the medical record and shared with the surgeon by the primary nurse. Within 24 hours, appropriate interventions assisted the patient back to his preoperative mental status.

the client, and the organization" and because nurses "are entitled to practice as partners in a collegial and collaborative environment that promotes competency, commitment, and empowerment."[10] Certainly nurses in every role see their practice as the embodiment of this philosophy. The stated philosophy also serves as the channel through which their patient care responsibilities and therapeutic interventions meet the established professional standards.

Empowerment accompanies the fulfillment of role aspirations within such an environment and is neither separated nor divided from practice (or care) but rather blends and matches in planned congruence. The nurses in the original snapshot take on new dimensions and clarity as the camera is held steadily on a balanced tripod.

Advanced practice nurses have planned well for collaboration with nursing staff. A reflective posture is assumed if colleagues' questions seek only gentle affirmation, but resources are rallied if the inquiry is for facts. Problem solving requires sustaining input and critiquing broad options until the interdependence of seeking brings mutual direction and feasible outcomes. This realization of more similarities than differences in thoughts and possibilities among colleagues establishes interdependence as a strength. Nurses' mutual humanity forms a fundamental framework for the establishment of a relationship where role modeling and role internalization may occur.[11] It would be anticipated that, based on respect for their expertise and trust in their abilities, a mutual interdependence may grow and a synergistic relationship develop. As Hotter states, "Synergy is a situation in which members feed off the combined *strengths* (rather than weaknesses) and energy of others. This sense of synergy is often described as the 'chemistry just feels right.' While individual weaknesses may be recognized, they are often minimized or accommodated, rather than used as peer ammunition."[9(p14)] Synergy, as Hotter believes, is the highest form of interdependence.

Interdependence is sought and frequently mandated not only for nurse-to-nurse consultation but also for nurses consulting with other professionals as they seek to bring their expertise to the entire health care team. "The nurse must clearly be parallel in status, equal in function, and respected for the nurse's unique contributions in the delivery of health care." [12(p434)] What better way to foster interdependence than first through consultee to consultant and then by incorporating the nursing perspective within the interdisciplinary team?

The work of knowledge building, image building, and team building is ongoing at Sioux Valley Hospital. The process of knowing is being nurtured, as is the art of showing others the benefits of using the consultative process. A wide-angle approach to team building is now pulling in professionals from pharmacy, physical therapy, dietary, and other departments throughout the hospital. Empowerment has been demonstrated, interdisciplinary colleagues are serving the client, and professional standards are achieved. The picture now includes the missing legs and the entire head. The fuzziness has been replaced by a distinct outline. The would-be snapshot has become a living color photograph, all due to those who truly wanted to be in the picture.

*It is our attitude at the beginning of a difficult
undertaking which more than anything else will
determine its successful outcome.*
WILLIAM JAMES

THE EVOLUTION OF SUCCESSFUL CONSULTATION

The consultation process has been described as involving the phases of referral, assessment, planning, implementation, and evaluation. In reality, these phases remain fluid as a dynamic process between and within all phases.[13] Certainly no less important than the fluidity is the informality. A critical factor in the number and frequency of referrals is visibility. An advanced practice nurse educator at Sioux Valley Hospital reports that her time spent on the nursing units with a nurse resident has a secondary benefit. Not only is she able to mentor the nurse resident, but she always receives many informal consultations from the nursing staff while she is on the unit. The staff question her about upcoming workshops, development of educational standards, or opportunities for preceptoring. A CNS who works in collaborative practice with a group of cardiovascular surgeons spends most of her day on the patient care units assessing clients. Her visibility on the units has allowed the nursing staff to access her easily for consultations.

The assessment phase is the critical step in the consultation process. It is during this phase that the strengths and limitations of both the consultant and the consultee are identified and the nature of the problem or need for the consultant is defined.[13] It is imperative that this assessment process occurs in a time-efficient manner. One-to-one communication with the consultee is essential to involve him or her as a partner in the consultation process and to access necessary data. A good consultant has the ability to render down reams of information about one client or clinical situation to the key or striking issues, defined by Burgess[14] as salient factors. It is this ability that truly brings the art into the science of problem solving through consultation.

The planning and implementation phases of the consultation require effective communication among all persons or organizations involved. Koerner and Bunkers assert that "communication needs to be a continuous interchange of thoughts, opinion, and feelings through commonly understood symbols."[7(p56)] These symbols may be detailed nursing diagnoses and care plans when consulted by the primary nurse or brief descriptions of physical assessment data when communicating to a physician. Flexibility comes into the picture again as symbols and language that are best understood by the consultee are used. Timely and appropriate feedback to the consultee is essential. This effort, if made effectively, will increase referrals.

Evaluation is listed as the final phase of consultation, but in reality it is an ongoing process that can be accomplished in an informal way. In an arena where health care dollars must be spent wisely, the consumer or consultee must be assured of quality and effective service. The consultation process is not exempt from monitoring, which ascertains the effectiveness of the consultation. Evaluation is an opportunity for the consultee to determine whether needs were met and for the consultant to identify strengths and weaknesses of the process as well as whether and how goal outcomes were achieved. Personal growth as a consultant cannot occur without insightful evaluation of consultation.

For evaluation to be effective, objectives must be defined clearly before intervention. One must have a clear vision of what is to be accomplished and how one will determine effectiveness. Perhaps the mission of the consultation will be obvious with a clear path to achievement. Evaluation may be objective and relatively easy to determine. Many cases involving patient care, however, are not so easily focused. This may necessitate more subjective evaluation and may involve shades of gray as opposed to a crisp, bright picture. The consultant may need to determine whether to question the consultee about effectiveness, to look at the outcome, or perhaps to look instead at process and interactive aspects of the consultation when gauging evaluation of the consultation.

Three areas identified by Lippitt and Lippitt[15] for focusing effort in evaluation are the client/consultant relationship, consulting/training events, and progress toward specific goals. The latter two may be the focus of evaluations more often than the relationship. The relationship, however, is the area for true empowerment of the consultee. According to Barron,[16] valued relationships based on trust develop as the consultation process evolves. These may develop because of the complexity of the situation and probably because of the skill of the consultant. It is sometimes said that effective advanced practice nurses should work to put themselves out of a job. In other words, one should seek to empower the consultee in making critical judgments as well as in having the confidence to carry through with these judgments. This may be threatening to some consultants. To the most empowered and creative consultant, however, who continues to refill the pot, it may only mean that many more opportunities for consultation are generated.

Evaluation is an important tool that helps ensure quality in consultation. If effectiveness is not evaluated, an essential aspect of the process may be missed or opportunities for growth bypassed.

In the past, nurses have not consciously participated in consultation.[13] A learning curve exists in the utilization of clinical consultation by nursing staff. At Sioux Valley Hospital, this learning curve was shortened in some cases by informal marketing and educational programs on how to utilize the consultation process. This was necessary not only for the nursing staff making the potential referrals but also for advanced practitioners new to the consultant role.

The concept of nurse-to-nurse consultation seems ideal. Why, then, did Sioux Valley Hospital's advanced nursing practice experience a low number of referrals initially? One of several explanations, as discussed by Law et al,[17] may be applicable. Although nursing consultation appears to have many benefits, it also has some perceived risks. Nurses may be hesitant to request a consultation because they feel that this may indicate a personal weakness or incompetency. Some nurses may respond defensively or with feelings of guilt if someone suggests that they ask for help. Others may perceive a loss of control over the situation when a consultant becomes involved. Feelings of anger may surface in interactions with another nurse who has greater clinical or educational experience. These reactions can be avoided if nurses are educated in the process of consultation and understand that consultation is a two-way street in which knowledge is shared and gained by both persons. A final risk is accountability. Just as the nurse has the option of consulting, he or she also has the option of rejecting the recommendations of the consultant. The decision to accept or reject the recommendations is one to which the nurse must remain accountable.[17]

By definition, the role of consultant could easily be viewed as a power position because the consultant, who has special knowledge or skills, is called on to help the consultee with a specific need or problem. The consultee may be perceived as being in a dependent position and the consultant as being in charge or in power. This is a dangerous view of an interaction that should actually be viewed more as a balanced and mutual partnership.

Chisholm[18] suggests that for one to be powerful there must be a receptive audience that will value what one has to offer, trust one's judgment, and allow itself to be influenced. Therefore, who has the power, the consultant or the consultee? Chisholm asserts that the power of consultation lies not with any one person but rather within the interaction and the relationship. She believes that power in consultation is in the between space. It is in that between space that mutual respect exists.

Advanced practice nurses provide consultative services by interacting with nurses functioning in many different roles. The success of differentiated practice is in the valuing of each other's contributions to nursing practice irrespective of job title, role, or function. This same valuing needs to be present in consultations. Successful consultations are those in which a balance of power exists between the two involved parties. There is a collaboration and trust that guard against the misuse of power.

THEORY-BASED CONSULTATION

Benner asserts that "theory is a powerful tool for explaining and predicting. It shapes questions and allows the systematic examination of a series of events."[19(p2)] When advanced practice nurses consult, they do so from a unique viewpoint. That uniqueness is the ability to assess, discuss, or problem solve issues from a theoretical framework. Calkin[20] explains that expert nurses, defined as those with years of experience, guide their nursing practice through a sharp intuition that has been honed through the years. They possess a vast source of knowledge but are unsure of how they know. They just know. Advanced practice nurses, by virtue of their experience and expertise, also have intuition, but because of their advanced educational background they are able to label. This means that they can describe a phenomenon and relate it in a common language, correlating it with other concepts.

> *What concerns me is not the way things are, but*
> *rather the way people think things are.*
>
> EPICTETUS

In the consultation process, theoretical models can help reframe the situation. When a situation is viewed from an original paradigm of usual practice, creativity can be stifled. When it is reframed or viewed from a paradigm shift, new possibilities arise.

The case study in Exhibit 6–6 shows that using a theoretical model helped a nurse reframe a situation into one that supported the patient in making decisions about his health care that were consistent with his life goals. Basically, the advanced practice nurse only asked these essential questions: "What are your goals?" and "How can I help you get there?" Fawcett looks at theories or models in this way: Conceptual models "inform and transform nursing practice by informing and transforming the ways in which practice is experienced and understood."[21(p224)] They serve as guiding lights that illuminate the path to desired outcomes in patients, in practice, and in health care settings. The nutrition CNS referred to in Exhibit 6–6 uses Parse's[22] theory frequently in her practice. Advanced practice nurses at Sioux Valley Hospital use a variety of theories or guiding lights in their daily work. Some theories can work as a telephoto lens to aid in understanding the details of a patient care situation, and others are wide-angle lenses helping the nurse capture the broadest view possible of a patient care situation.

> *[A person's] mind stretched to a new idea never*
> *goes back to its original dimensions.*
> OLIVER WENDELL HOLMES, JR

During the consultation process the nurse consultant may share information with the nurse consultee about the theory he or she is using. Nursing theorist Margaret Newman has visited Sioux Valley Hospital as a consultant and has offered the nursing staff first-hand information about how to utilize theory to guide nursing practice. The use of theory in nursing can increase professionalism, give a coherence of purpose, and enhance communication.[23]

Exhibit 6–6 Case Study: Creativity through Reframing

An elderly, cachectic man was approached multiple times by the nursing and medical staff to allow a feeding tube insertion. The patient repeatedly refused. A nutrition support CNS was consulted. Utilizing Parse's[22] framework, the nurse explored this patient's life goals, hopes, dreams, current life situation, and important aspects of day-to-day life with him and his wife. Discomfort due to pressure on bony prominences, lack of energy, and frustration with nursing and medical staff constantly urging him to eat were identified. The CNS explored options with him. The patient chose to try a small, soft feeding tube that would allow nutrition to be delivered directly, thereby diminishing frustration and the urgency to eat. This would help restore damaged tissue, thus decreasing bony prominence pain. The added nutrition would also increase his energy level, enabling him to focus on other life goals. The patient and his wife expressed gratitude for these new options.

Health care is demanding more interdisciplinary consultation on the client's behalf. It may be easier for nurses to consult within the nursing profession because of common language and philosophy. To facilitate interdisciplinary relationships, however, Ingram[23] and Stevens[24] caution that nursing theory development should use a language that may enhance communication among nurses as well as other disciplines rather than create a separate language. This common language is an integral part of nursing's future collaboration with other disciplines. Shared values as well as common understanding of operationalization of those values are important in interdisciplinary consultation. Trust and security in one's own profession as well as continued refueling and a professional support system can play a major role in productive interdisciplinary consultation.

OVERCOMING AMBIGUITY

Just as the camera lens can become foggy so that images are difficult to visualize, so might the image of the consultant become unclear. Many roles, especially when they are in the process of development, lend themselves to ambiguity. In contrast to the more well-defined roles of the associate nurse and the advanced practice nurse in education and management, the developing new roles of primary nurse, clinical care coordinator, and CNS initially tended to be ambiguous.

Role ambiguity can expose itself in what Arena and Page[25] name the imposter phenomenon. Although Arena and Page address ambiguity in the CNS role, many nurses may be functioning in a role that is not well defined by the institution, the administration, or the nurse. Because the role of advanced practice nurse, especially one in the CNS role, lends itself to varied interpretations that in turn can lead to role ambiguity, the rest of this section focuses primarily on the CNS role.

The sense of imposter, especially for the novice CNS or an individual filling a newly created or ambiguous position, is not uncommon. How can one give advice to others when one is uncertain of one's own ability? The act of being consulted, however, can increase feelings of usefulness by virtue of the fact that someone wants advice.

Common sources of role ambiguity for the CNS, as described by Loudermilk,[26] include inadequate socialization to the role, conflicting role expectations of administrators and staff, inconsistent job descriptions, multiple accountabilities, and inconsistency of placement within the bureaucratic framework of employment. Because many of these sources of role ambiguity have been experienced by the CNSs at Sioux Valley Hospital, some potential solutions are now suggested. Although these references relate to the CNS role, it is assumed that these solutions apply to other roles.

Inadequate Socialization

In addition to inadequate socialization to the role, the CNS may experience social isolation by virtue of the uniqueness of the role.[27] This isolation may leave the advanced practitioner with an inadequate support system. An essential element for the consultant to be successful, especially in an environment of ambiguity, is networking or developing a formal peer support system. A formal peer support group can serve as a means of networking by providing access to valuable information, can result in increased productivity, and ultimately can benefit client care in terms of referrals, problem solving, and interinstitutional visibility.[27] The peer group may be the rich source of new ideas and knowledge and may be the empowering strategy that minimizes isolation and promotes self-esteem.[28] This networking can enhance self-esteem and provide a reference base for assistance, support, and information, which are all important to the consultant. It is an empowering strategy that ensures goal attainment and career mobility.[28] Maintaining a networking system helps ensure that as pictures are developed the practitioner will be included in the photo. Perceptions of frustration often surface when the consultant is absent from the team photo because his or her expertise has not been requested. It is additionally disheartening not to be included in the team photo even when one's expertise was utilized. Thus diligent networking as a consultant will increase the probability that one's assistance is remembered and requested in the future.

At Sioux Valley Hospital, a CNS group was formed to meet these socialization and isolation issues. Initially, the CNSs met as a shared governance council. Later, this group met with advanced practice nurses in education and management to develop a job description and competencies for all advanced practice nurses. Presently, the CNS group meets weekly. These meetings have provided a form of support for members, enhanced peer networking, and helped new CNSs understand potential role issues.

Conflicting Role Expectations

Loudermilk[26] suggests that educating colleagues about the specific activities of one's role is essential. Seizing opportunities to discuss concerns expressed by administrators and staff about the functions or responsibilities of the role is necessary. It is important to address these expectations as soon as one enters the advanced practice role. Successful role implementation and recognition of advanced practice nurses' contributions are maximized with communication linkages and administrative support.[29] Nursing management support for the role of the CNS in an institution is essential. A collaborative relationship between nurse managers and CNSs is imperative. It is then the collective responsibility of nursing management and the CNS to communicate effectively the purpose of the CNS to patients, nursing staff, medical staff, other departments, and hospital administration. A Sioux Valley Hospital CNS who was the first CNS in the medical-surgical division chose to introduce herself to the nursing staff via a letter to all nurses along with a needs assessment. The introductory letter assisted in communicating the hospital's expectations of her new role, and the needs assessment questionnaire targeted issues for which the nursing staff might need consultation and education. The letter decreased some of the ambiguity associated with the new CNS position, and the needs assessment proved to be beneficial in identifying educational topics and patient care issues that were then addressed through the consultation process.

Inconsistent Job Description

The suggested solution to an inconsistent job description is negotiation of the CNS role.[26] A time-limited contract to define expectations, to assign accountability, and to measure effectiveness of performance may help clarify role expectations. At Sioux Valley Hospital, the development of a job description and the use of written goals for each year, or in some cases each quarter, have assisted the CNS in focusing time and energy on patient/unit needs. The peer review/credentialing process (refer to Chapter 4) has also been advantageous. It has given a common language and consistency to the method by which all nurses are evaluated and has provided a formalized opportunity to network and share ideas.

Multiple Accountabilities

The CNS has multiple accountabilities to staff (nurses and other team members), to patients, to the employing agency, and to financial reimbursers. Loudermilk[26] suggests that the solution to this problem is to share monthly and annual summaries of effective role responsibilities that demonstrate improved patient outcomes, improved staff education and practice, and cost savings to reimbursers. Sharing this information helps strengthen and lend support to the role functions and cost effectiveness of the CNS.

As demonstrated by a hospice CNS with multiple accountabilities to the oncology patient, the hospital, the physician, and the reimbursers, a significant cost savings was recognized and shared mutually by all involved. This was done through the CNS facilitating critical thinking among the hospice staff on a variety of issues and possibilities related to hospice care. The CNS encouraged the staff to reframe the way in which quality care was delivered in the home environment. This cost savings was achieved through a change in the delivery system and in the use of durable medical equipment. The staff were able to recognize the benefits of the team's efforts by the cost savings shown, by continued client satisfaction as evidenced by positive patient satisfaction surveys, and by quality assurance studies. In addition, by utilizing her consultation skills to build relationships with reimbursers and physicians, the CNS shared information about the cost savings of the hospice program and thus ultimately increased the utilization of hospice services.

Inconsistent Position

When addressing the issue of inconsistent position within the bureaucratic framework, Loudermilk[26] suggests that the ideal organizational role of the CNS combines both staff and administrative responsibilities. Ultimately, however, the CNS must be allowed to move across traditional organizational lines. Loudermilk reminds us that "role definition and function should be dynamic rather than static" and that "autonomy, self-governance, flexibility, and creativity are values that should be upheld by the CNS."[26(p11)] It is these values that allow the process of consultation to occur in our progressively seamless environment. This evolved at Sioux Valley Hospital over a period of 2 to 3 years. Several factors have contributed to this evolution. One was the development of a job description that has been shared with staff. In addition, the CNS's visibility and demonstration of expertise have promoted referrals of complex patients, ultimately creating a case management system. This referral and case management process has evolved to the point that the CNS manages complex patients from prehospitalization to postdischarge and across multiple units and settings.

Role ambiguity can be devastating to any position and must be addressed if success is to be achieved. These fixes are intended to be examples that might aid others in ambiguous roles.

THE TRANSFORMATION OF CONSULTATION TO COLLABORATION

In summary, the continuing goal of consultation should be to empower the consultee with new knowledge and resources and to increase confidence in the consultee's own unique nursing practice. As Chisholm describes, "empowering others to do their job more effectively, efficiently, and expertly requires the nurse consultant to respect the expertise inherent in the consultee and to use this knowledge in reaching solutions, fostering courses of action, and effecting change."[18(p57)] We concur with Rogers and Trimnell[13] when they describe the overriding goal of consultation as helping the consultee develop knowledge, skill, or confidence to deal more effectively with immediate and subsequent situations. Empowerment is the desired outcome of consultation. Empowered nurses—that is, those who are confident in their practice role—are more likely to consult the advanced practice nurse as a practice partner. Empowerment of nurses through consultative interactions and other methods is an important strategy for nursing's transformation.[9]

The work of knowledge building, image building, and team building is ongoing at Sioux Valley Hospital. The process of knowing is being nurtured, as is the art of showing others the benefits of using the consultative process. A wide-angle approach to team building is now including professionals from pharmacy, physical therapy, dietary, and other departments throughout the hospital. Empowerment has been demonstrated, interdisciplinary colleagues are serving the client, and professional standards are achieved.

At Sioux Valley Hospital, the creation of an Integrated Care model for nursing accompanied by the philosophy of shared governance has brought those involved to a higher level of understanding and valuing of each other as individuals and as practitioners. An environment of openness to seek help from each other in a variety of directions has been created. No longer is the nursing practice looking at vertical and horizontal patterns of consultation but rather at a transformation into a complex matrix of intradisciplinary and interdisciplinary collaboration as practice partners. This is a transformation by design.

REFERENCES

1. Oda DS. Consultation: an expectation of leadership. *Nurs Leadership.* 1982;5(1):137–139.
2. Rutherford DE. Consultation: a review and analysis of the literature. *J Prof Nurs.* 1988;4:339–344.
3. Nicolai C, Pitts-Wilhelm P. Weighting role competencies based on job role. Paper presented at the meeting of the Nursing Career Pathway Project; September 11, 1989; Sioux Falls, SD.
4. del Bueno DJ, Weeks L, Brown-Stewart P. Clinical assessment centers: a cost-effective alternative for competency development. *Nurs Econ.* 1987;5:21–26.
5. Koerner JG, Bunkers SS. Transformational leadership: the power of symbol. *Nurs Admin Q.* 1992;17(1):1–9.
6. Rubin R. Maternal tasks. In: *Maternal Identity and the Maternal Experience.* New York, NY: Springer; 1984:52–69.
7. Koerner JG, Bunkers SS. M-I-D-D-L-E-G-R-O-U-N-D: part II, developing partnerships in practice. *Nurs Connect.* 1992;5(3):53–59.
8. Bennis W. *Why Leaders Can't Lead.* San Francisco, Calif: Jossey-Bass; 1990.
9. Hotter AN. The clinical nurse specialist and empowerment: say goodbye to the fairy godmother. *Nurs Admin Q.* 1992;16(3):11–15.
10. Sioux Valley Hospital Department of Nursing. *Sioux Valley Hospital Department of Nursing Philosophy.* Sioux Falls, SD: Sioux Valley Hospital; February 1990.
11. Curtin L, Flaherty MJ. The nurse-nurse relationship. In: *Nursing Ethics: Theories and Pragmatics.* Bowie, Md: Brady; 1982:125–135.
12. Porter-O'Grady T. Nursing governance in a transitional era. In: Chaska NL, ed. *The Nursing Profession: Turning Points.* St. Louis, Mo: Mosby; 1990:432–439.

13. Rogers M, Trimnell J. Maximizing the use of the clinical nurse specialist as consultant. *Nurs Admin Q*. 1987;12(1):53–58.

14. Burgess C. Think tank discussion: case management, managed care, salient factors, centers of excellence. Presented at consultation visit to Sioux Valley Hospital; November 19, 1991; Sioux Falls, SD.

15. Lippitt G, Lippitt R. *The Consulting Process in Action*. 2nd ed. San Diego, Calif: University Associates; 1986.

16. Barron A. The CNS as consultant. In: Hamric AB, Spross JA, eds. *The Clinical Nurse Specialist in Theory and Practice*. Orlando, Fla: Grune & Stratton; 1983:91–113.

17. Law MSG, Smith MO, Igoe SN, Caplin MS. Nurses helping nurses. *Imprint*. 1989;36(2):65–69.

18. Chisholm M. Use and abuse of power. *Clin Nurse Spec*. 1991;5:57.

19. Benner P. *From Novice to Expert: Excellence and Power in Clinical Nursing Practice*. Menlo Park, Calif: Addison-Wesley; 1984.

20. Calkin JD. A model for advanced nursing practice. *J Nurs Admin*.1984;14(1):24–30.

21. Fawcett J. Conceptual models and nursing practice: the reciprocal relationship. *J Adv Nurs*. 1992;17:224–228.

22. Parse RR. Human becoming: Parse's theory of nursing. *Nurs Sci Q*. 1992;5:35–42.

23. Ingram R. Why does nursing need theory? *J Adv Nurs*. 1991;16:350–353.

24. Stevens B. *Nursing Theory: Analysis, Application, Evaluation*. 2nd ed. Boston, Mass: Little, Brown; 1984.

25. Arena DM, Page NE. The imposter phenomenon in the clinical nurse specialist role. *IMAGE*. 1992; 24:121–125.

26. Loudermilk L. Role ambiguity and the clinical nurse specialist. *Nurs Connect*. 1990;3(1):3–11.

27. Gilliland K, Tosch P, Hussey L, Hines C, Lane L, Loftis PA, et al. Specialty nursing council: a peer support group for nurses in independent roles. *Clin Nurse Spec*. 1990;4:38–42.

28. Fain JA, Viau P. Networking: a strategy for strengthening the role of the clinical nurse specialist. *Clin Nurse Spec*. 1989;3:29–31.

29. Hamric AB, Spross JA. *The Clinical Nurse Specialist in Theory and Practice*. 2nd ed. Philadelphia, Pa: Saunders; 1989.

30. Avery M, Auvine B, Streibel B, Weiss L. *Building United Judgment: A Handbook for Consensus Decision Making*. Madison, Wis: Center for Conflict Resolution; 1981.

31. Goleman D, Kaufman P, Ray M. *The Creative Spirit*. New York, NY: Penguin; 1992.

EXERCISE 6–1: CONSULTATION EXERCISES

1. What are the losses and gains to the consultant and the consultee in the interaction described in Exhibit 6–5 (consultation through a casual remark)? Who or what holds the power in this interaction?

2. Take an inventory of the consultative resources in your work, school, or home environment. First, list each person's name, his or her special skill or talent, and how that person can be contacted. Second, discuss how to promote the utilization of these persons as consultants.

3. Imagine you are out for a walk on a beautiful June afternoon. As you pass by a church, you are stopped by a woman who identifies herself as the mother of the bride and asks you to take photographs of her daughter's wedding. Unfortunately, she only has six exposures left on her film. As the photographic consultant, how would you decide which people and activities to capture on film? How does this exercise relate to your role as consultant?

4. Human Pretzels (for a group of six to eight people):[30] Have the group stand in a circle. Instruct each person to reach across the circle with both hands (not crossed) and to grasp hands with two different people. Then, without letting go, try to untangle. The goal is, if you are lucky, to find yourselves in a reassembed circle with everyone holding hands with the person next to him or her. Spend about 10 to 15 minutes trying to untangle.

   Now have an outsider (not a part of the group holding hands) assist the group in the problem solving for another 5 to 10 minutes.

   Compare and contrast the perception and outcome of the two different perspectives (with and without the outsider assisting with problem solving). Discuss how this exercise relates to consultation and your role as a consultant.

5. I Am a Camera (do this with another colleague or friend):[31] Determine which person will be the camera and which the photographer. Assume that there are 12 to 24 frames on this role of film.

   If you play the camera, assume that your eyes are the camera lens and that your right shoulder is the shutter button. Trust that the photographer knows what he or she is doing. Your eyes are to be shut until the photographer takes a photograph by tapping you on the right shoulder. At that instant your eyes should open and close quickly, just as the shutter of a camera does, and record the image in view (in your memory). All you have to do is see what is there in front of you without any preconceived notions about each of the pictures you take. Your task is to record every detail of the picture perfectly with no distortion.

   If you play the photographer, stand behind the camera. Your role is to walk the camera around, guiding him or her by the shoulders and positioning him or her so that different scenes will be in his or her line of vision. The photographer then takes a picture by depressing the shutter button (tapping the right shoulder) of the camera.

How is this experience an example of reframing offered by a consultant? See Exhibit 6–6, the case study of creativity through reframing. Discuss the similarities and differences between this exercise and consultation. The rapid series of recorded impressions gives the camera the experience of seeing without perception being filtered through expectations. Seeing without any predetermined concepts is important. Reducing your preconceptions when you face a new problem is a vital element in a creative process such as consulting.

7 Community

Connie K. Schmidt, Diana Berkland, and Doreen S. Miller

Community . . . is the being no longer side by side
but with *one another.*

MARTIN BUBER

The community of nurses at Sioux Valley Hospital has been united through the evolution of a professional practice. Challenge and change are frequently the focal points in bringing individuals together. This chapter describes the challenges and changes that influenced the evolution of a professional nursing practice.

The evolution of a new community of professional nurses has been promoted by interdependent processes. Refer to Exhibit 7–1 for a review of the characteristics of a profession. The processes that have most affected the community are the implementation of differentiated practice and the development of shared governance. Through differentiation of practice, distinct professional practice roles were developed for the community of nurses. The roles of primary nurse, associate nurse, and clinical care coordinator were identified and implemented. The process of developing a shared governance model at Sioux Valley Hospital aided the evolution of the professional practice.

Shared governance is defined as a professional nursing governance model that provides autonomy and establishes accountability for practice-related decision making of individual practitioners. Shared governance is an accountability-based governance system for professional workers and represents a transition from the traditional industrial model. With the industrial model, the worker might be asked to provide input, but lacks autonomy and authority for decision making (Porter-O'Grady, T. Personal communication, February 1, 1990).

Three types of shared governance models have been identified by Porter-O'Grady:[1] councilor, congressional, and administrative models. The councilor

214

Exhibit 7–1 Characteristics of a Profession

---

1. A profession uses a well-defined and organized body of knowledge that operates on a conceptual and intellectual level.
2. A profession constantly enlarges the body of knowledge it uses and improves its education process through use of scientific methods.
3. A profession educates its practitioners in institutions of higher education.
4. A profession applies its body of knowledge to practices that are vital to human and social welfare.
5. A profession functions autonomously, formulates its own professional policy, and controls its own professional activity.
6. A profession attracts individuals with intellectual and personal qualities that support the ideals of the profession, who serve the profession above personal gain and identify their professional activity as a lifetime work.
7. A profession strives to provide its practitioners with compensation through social and legal sanction, continuous growth, and economic security.

Source: Adapted from Bixler, G.K. and Bixler, R.H., The Professional Status of Nursing, *American Journal of Nursing,* Vol. 43, No. 9, pp. 730-735, American Journal of Nursing Company, © 1943.

---

model was implemented at Sioux Valley Hospital. It utilizes councils to structure the governance of staff and management. Delineation of clinical and management accountabilities is critical. By specifically defining areas of accountability, authority, autonomy, and control will exist in the organization.[1]

Five councils are utilized with Porter-O'Grady's model. The practice council is accountable for the work of the profession. The quality assurance council is accountable for the quality of the work and the competence of the profession. The education/research council is accountable for the generation of new knowledge. The management council is accountable for the management of resources. A fifth council is composed of the chairs of each of the other councils and is accountable for coordinating and integrating the work of the councils and addressing issues that affect every council.[1] The formation of these councils had a profound effect on the development of a community of professional nurses at Sioux Valley Hospital.

Before the introduction of shared governance, nurses at Sioux Valley Hospital had formed microcommunities (nursing units), minicommunities (nursing divisions), and a macrocommunity (the nursing department) (Figure 7–1). The shared governance process facilitated the restructuring of community to be defined as the professional nursing practice. Barriers, known and unknown, began to break down as nurses worked together to make decisions for the entire (macro) community rather than just for the micro- or minicommunity in which they practiced.

They cannot see the forest for the trees!
CHRISTOPH MARTIN WIELAND

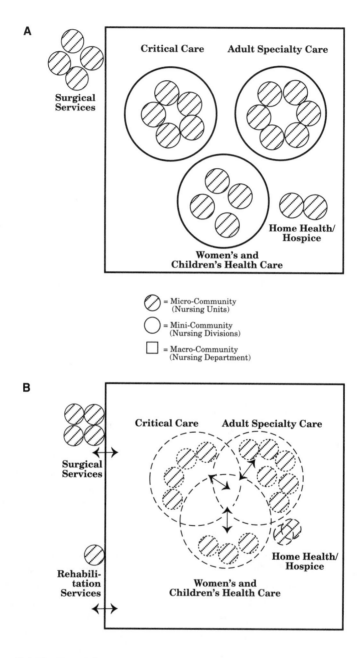

Figure 7–1 The Sioux Valley Hospital nursing community. (**A**) Before shared governance (1989). (**B**) After shared governance/practice consolidation. Note: Rehabilitation services department was newly developed in April 1990.

With the common goal of quality and cost-efficient patient care, the professional nurses came together as one community. The work of the community and of the organization was focused on the patient. Therefore, to support the work of the nurse at the bedside, shared governance and differentiated practice were implemented. In describing the process by which a professional nursing practice evolved, systems theory and change theory are used as a framework.

SYSTEMS THEORY

Systems theory describes how an organization processes information, energy, or matter to affect an outcome. Organizations are complex systems with boundaries and interrelated parts through which energy, matter, and information flow in the form of inputs, throughputs, outputs, and feedback. Refer to Exhibit 7–2 for definitions of these concepts.

Within each system are subsystems. The professional nursing practice at Sioux Valley Hospital is an ever changing subsystem within an ever changing system, the organization. Ultimately, the organization exists in the ever changing larger system of health care. Therefore, as each system and subsystem evolves, the effect of change is far reaching.

> *The real . . . community is when its members have*
> *a common relation to the centre overriding all*
> *other relations.*
>
> Martin Buber

Ideally, all the systems and subsystems of health care interact toward a common goal: quality and cost-efficient patient care. In spite of ongoing change, the system and subsystems are always striving to maintain equilibrium or balance. In theory,

---

Exhibit 7–2 Concepts of Systems Theory

Input: Any information, energy, or matter entering a system from the external environment.

Throughput: The process through which information, energy, or matter is transformed.

Output: Any information, energy, or matter leaving the system to the external environment.

Feedback: Output that becomes input to the system; usually used to evaluate how the system is functioning.

this state of equilibrium may be stationary, a fixed point to which the system returns after a disturbance. This state of equilibrium can also be dynamic: Equilibrium may be found at a new point after the disturbance. The entire system responds to external disturbance in one of three ways: refusing to acknowledge the disturbance, taking action to restore equilibrium, or accommodating to a new equilibrium.

The flow of information in a system has been described in the literature. Buckley[2] suggests that all systems belong to a hierarchy of systems. Those at upper levels within a hierarchy of systems presumably have more information available to them. Also, a small amount of information, energy, or matter at high levels triggers a large amount of activity at other levels, creating more energy (Figure 7–2). If this is accurate, it follows that subsystems and individuals at lower levels of the hierarchy receive less information, energy, and matter. Also, the information available at lower levels will ultimately have a lesser effect on the entire system than information at higher levels.

Organizations can be described as either being open or closed systems. Those organizations that attempt to exert strong control over the subsystems and external environment are relatively closed. Conversely, those that do not use control in this way are relatively open. Some fall to the middle ground by attempting to exert a reasonable degree of control over both internal subsystems and the external environment to maximize efficiency.

Figure 7–3 depicts systems theory applied to the community of professional nurses at Sioux Valley Hospital. The processes of differentiating practice and implementing shared governance are the throughput, along with the unique and therapeutic relationship between nurse and patient. As these factors evolved, the output emerged: a professional nursing practice and empowered, knowledgeable patients. It is important to examine closely the impact of input, internal factors, and external factors on the system (throughput).

INPUT

Input is defined as any information, energy, or matter entering a system from the external environment. The inputs that have been identified include nurses' educational backgrounds, nurses' values, patients, and consultants. The educational background of the nursing community can be considered part of the input to the system. Sioux Valley Hospital offered a diploma nursing program until 1986. As a result, many of these graduates practice at Sioux Valley Hospital. The hospital also attracts nurses from two baccalaureate degree programs and three associate degree programs that are located within 70 miles. The values of the nurses who practice at Sioux Valley Hospital are another input (see Chapter 2). The nursing population is quite homogeneous. The vast majority are white women who originated in the Midwest. The strong work ethic associated with this region is prevalent. Patients are probably the most important input;

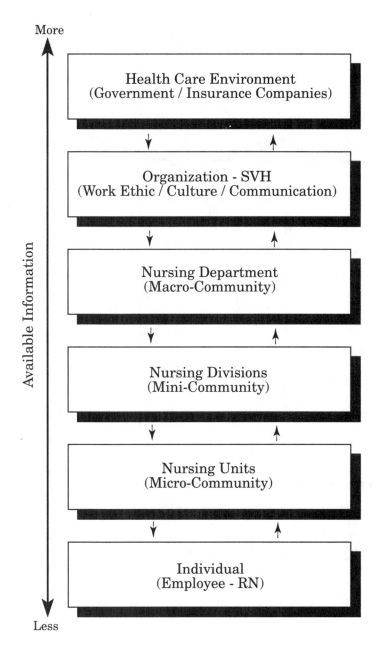

More

Available Information

Less

Health Care Environment
(Government / Insurance Companies)

Organization - SVH
(Work Ethic / Culture / Communication)

Nursing Department
(Macro-Community)

Nursing Divisions
(Mini-Community)

Nursing Units
(Micro-Community)

Individual
(Employee - RN)

Figure 7–2 Organizational systems hierarchy before shared governance. *Source:* Adapted from *Role Theory Perspectives for Health Professionals,* 2nd ed. by M. Hardy and M. Conway, p. 113, with permission of Appleton & Lange, and M. Conway, © 1988.

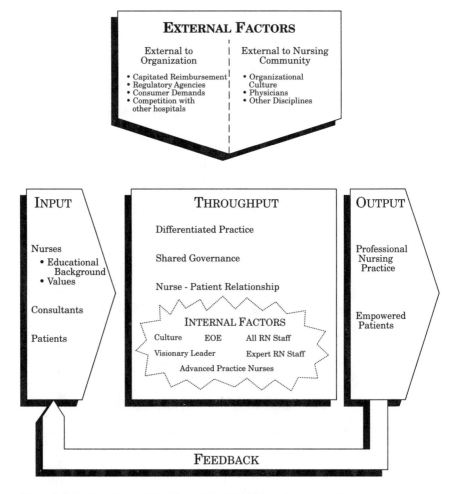

Figure 7–3 Systems theory and the Sioux Valley Hospital nursing community.

after all, patients are the focus of nursing. Patients are admitted to hospitals for nursing care. Thus one cannot exist without the other.

> *Nothing happens unless first a dream.*
> CARL SANDBURG

Two key consultants also enhanced the evolution of a professional nursing practice by the ideas and information they shared. They were also important inputs (see Appendix 1-A for a list of key events at Sioux Valley Hospital). The community was exposed to the visionary thinking of Dr Peggy Primm in 1987. Several nursing units (microcommunities) participated in a demonstration project for differentiated practice. The community brought this experience and exposure into the processes on which they embarked. Dr Tim Porter-O'Grady was invited as a consultant in 1989 to expand further the thinking of the community. He shared his expertise on developing a shared governance model. These consultants, as well as others, served as inputs to the system.

> *VISION is the Art of seeing Things invisible.*
> JONATHAN SWIFT

The educational backgrounds of the nurses, the nurses' values, the patients, and the consultants all provided input for the processes of implementing differentiated practice and developing shared governance with the community of nurses.

Internal Factors

Internal factors are factors preexisting within a system or subsystem that affect the process that is taking place. The internal factors that affected the implementation of differentiated practice and shared governance and the nurse-patient relationship included a visionary leader, the nursing culture, an all-registered nurse staff, an expert staff, and advanced practitioners. In addition, the entire organization, including the Department of Nursing, had been introduced to the concept of empowerment through a philosophy called Ecology of Excellence.

The nursing practice at Sioux Valley Hospital has a visionary vice president of patient services. This position carries legitimate authority. This vice president also carries a large degree of personal charismatic authority. When these two types of authority combine, a leader has sapiential authority. This enables him or her to gain support for decisions from those who are needed to implement a plan. It is truly these visionary capabilities that stimulated the community of Sioux Valley Hospital to seek the outputs of a professional nursing practice and empowered patients. The vice president's vision included empowerment of the nurses who worked as administrators and managers as well as of those nurses touching the patient at the bedside. This vision and ability to facilitate empowerment of others were internal factors in this process.

> *We are what and where we are because we have*
> *first imagined it.*
> DONALD CURTIS

The process was also internally affected by the advanced practice nurses in the community. During the past 5 years, a number of nurses have completed graduate degrees. The number of nurses in advanced practice roles has increased significantly as the nursing community has developed (see Chapter 10). With the implementation of differentiated practice and shared governance, the nurse managers, nurse educators, and clinical nurse specialists (CNSs) worked together to carry out the visionary plan and to empower the nurse at the bedside.

In 1986, nursing administration was faced with the reality of increasing patient acuities, and cost consciousness was imposed by the prospective payment system. Patients were needing care that required a different set of nursing skills. The decision was made that by January 1990 all nurses in the Sioux Valley Hospital nursing department would be registered nurses. Licensed practical nurses (LPNs) were given the opportunity to continue their education to the registered nurse level. Sioux Valley Hospital offered financial assistance through a tuition reimbursement program and loans to those returning to school. In addition, through collaboration with a nearby university, classes for an associate degree program were offered at the hospital. The majority of nurses pursued their education, with 56% entering the registered nurse role by January 1990. Those who chose not to seek registered nurse licensure were assisted in finding new positions/roles within the hospital system or in other organizations. Within the hospital, LPNs are utilized in quality assurance, medical record or business office positions or in nursing assistant, health unit coordinator, or monitor, obstetric, or surgical technician roles. Only 8% of the LPNs left the organization. By 1991, most units had implemented differentiated practice. When the implementation of shared governance occurred in 1990, all nurses in the community were registered nurses. They were also expert and experienced nurses. The turnover (attrition) rate was 6.2% in 1989.

The culture of the nursing community was another internal factor. Some nurses had embraced the concepts of teamwork and empowerment. These seeds of support were scattered throughout the organization and had been planted by the Ecology of Excellence philosophy. This philosophy emphasizes the value of diversity and capitalizes on this diversity by forming teams. Individuals, through self-assessment, can identify their strengths. Four types of team members are identified: champion, architect, work engineer, and worksmith.

The champion is the person who has the idea but may be unable to operationalize it. The architect has the ability to take an idea and develop a plan for its implementation. This plan may be too idealistic, however, so that the work engineer's strength lies in making the plan realistic and workable. The worksmith is the person whose strength is implementation of the plan. Thus all types of individuals are needed to have a highly functioning and productive team.

This philosophy, along with knowledge of the Myers-Briggs Type Indicator, has been useful in practice. For example, one of the authors consults on a regular basis with a colleague who has different strengths in problem solving and strategizing. Acknowledgment of diversity is acceptable in the organization and is frequently verbalized. Refer to Chapters 2 and 8, respectively, for more information regarding culture and Ecology of Excellence.

External Factors

External factors are factors preexisting outside a system or subsystem that affect the process that is taking place. In describing a system, one needs to consider environments with shared boundaries. For example, one environment is the community of nurses. This environment shares a boundary with the organizational environment. The organization in turn shares a boundary with the global health care environment (Figure 7–4). These environments and boundaries are important to recognize. Nurses as a community are truly a subsystem within a system, the organization. The organization is a subsystem within our local, state, and national health care system. Whatever happens in the larger system has tremendous potential for affecting its subsystems, and vice versa.

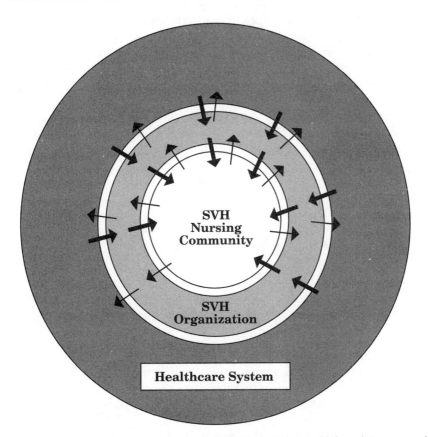

Figure 7–4 Boundaries in an open system. Arrows depict the exchange of information, matter, and energy across boundaries and between systems and subsystems. Whenever this exchange occurs, the potential for change exists.

With the evolution of a professional nursing practice, the boundary between the Sioux Valley Hospital nursing community and the Sioux Valley Hospital organization became open and fluid. The impact of this is discussed at the end of this chapter with the implementation of liaison committees.

The factors external to the nursing department but internal to the organization were identified as organizational culture, physicians, and other disciplines. The most influential factor external to the community of nurses was the organizational culture. The style of management of the organization had been traditional, with decisions occurring in upper and middle management positions as opposed to the employee or worker level. The concept of a shared governance model had never been considered outside the community of nurses. The organizational valuing of high quality and cost effectiveness permeates the nursing community also. The activities of physicians and other disciplines affect nursing, and vice versa, because all are practicing within the same health care system.

Factors external to the organization that had a potential effect on these processes at the time were capitated reimbursement systems, regulatory agencies (eg, the Joint Commission for Accreditation of Healthcare Organizations and Medicare), consumer demands, and competition with other hospitals. The first two were driving organizational decision making toward evaluation of financial aspects of delivering care to patients. Consumers have an increasing level of awareness regarding controlling the costs of health care. The consumer is also demanding an ever increasing level of quality of health care. These factors affected decision making of both the organization and the community of nurses.

Throughput and Feedback

Throughput, or the process through which information, energy, or matter is transformed, is described using change theory as a framework (see below). Feedback, or the evaluation of how effectively a system is processing, is discussed later in this chapter.

CHANGE THEORY

A basic understanding of change theory is also beneficial when one is examining the community as it relates to implementing differentiated practice and shared governance. Change theory has its beginnings in the work of Lewin.[3] In Lewin's theory, change is a three-step process involving the phases of unfreezing, moving (change), and refreezing.

Unfreezing involves the creation of motivation to change.[3] The individual becomes aware of the need for change. This stage is a cognitive one, in which the individual is exposed to the idea that perhaps there is a better way of accomplishing a goal. The second phase involves the actual change or moving. The process of change is planned in detail and then initiated. Lewin believes that in this phase a cognitive redefinition of what used to be must occur on the part of the individual, along with new responses to old stimuli. This is a period of disequilibrium. Lewin's third phase of change is refreezing. The new changes are integrated, and stabilization occurs. The cognitive process is an incorporation of the idea into the client's value system. As the value is internalized, it is reflected in the individual's behavior. The change is perpetuated because, as it becomes internalized by a critical mass of individuals, it becomes part of the value system (culture) in which the system operates.[3]

Another component of Lewin's theory about change includes the idea that there are forces that work either to facilitate or to impede the change process.[3] Driving forces are those that facilitate change, and restraining forces are those that impede change. It is beneficial to identify both driving and restraining forces in the planning stages of the change process. The change agent can then capitalize on those forces that can drive the process forward while avoiding or diffusing the forces that could potentially impede the process of change.

Lewin's theory of change can be applied to the community of nurses at Sioux Valley Hospital. In this experience, the client was defined as the macrocommunity of nurses, and the change agent was the vice president of patient services. Nurse managers, nurse educators, CNSs, and some staff nurses acted as driving forces, as did the consultants and the characteristics of the registered nurse staff discussed earlier. Restraining forces were identified as the organizational culture and some nursing staff members.

When one is embarking on a major change, it is important to remember that initially only a small minority of the individuals affected will actually support the change. This group will be the driving force. On the other hand, there will be a small minority that will be opposed to the change. This group will be the restraining force. The majority of individuals will not have a firm opinion. The key to successful change is to unfreeze and move the undecided majority toward embracing the change. By doing so, a critical mass of individuals will evolve. As the critical mass internalizes the change, behaviors will change, and subsequently the culture of the subsystem will be affected.

The three-step process described by Lewin can be thought of as the throughput in systems theory. Remember, throughput is the process through which information, energy, or matter is transformed (Figure 7–5).

Unfreezing

During this phase, the ideas of differentiated practice and shared governance were introduced to the leaders of the community. Consultants were used by the visionary leader to describe the concepts and to support the leaders. It was during

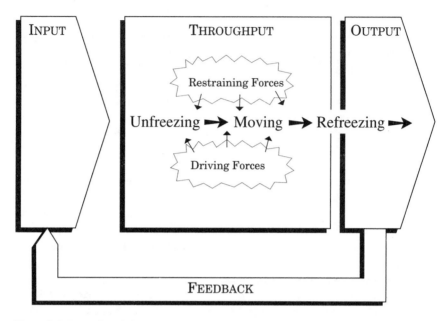

Figure 7–5 Integration of change theory with systems theory.

this time that the nursing leaders became aware of the need to change the care delivery system and the manner of governing the practice. A course on change was offered to nurse managers.[4] The differentiated practice demonstration project and open forum discussions about shared governance with staff and consultants, nursing leaders, and the visionary leader increased the cognitive awareness on the part of the entire nursing community regarding care delivery and the governance system.

The use of committees aided the implementation of shared governance. Before 1990 several committees had been established, each having a clearly identified objective. Through this format, participation of staff nurses in decision making was enhanced. Initially the majority of members of these committees were nurse managers, and the chair was usually a nursing administrator. Over a period of approximately 5 years, the committee composition shifted. Nursing staff were both members and chairs of these committees. This opportunity for participation provided staff nurses with mentors for professional growth. Staff nurses were able to acquire skills such as facilitating meetings, coordinating activities, and public speaking as well as to establish relationships with nurses from other micro- and macrocommunities.

Moving

A development council was organized to plan the implementation process for shared governance. This council was composed of individuals selected by their peers in the preexisting committees. During the year of its existence, this council was accountable for establishing the structure for the model. The various councils of shared governance were established in a well-planned order of events. The four councils described earlier were established: practice, education/research, quality assurance, and management. The term *nursing congress* was later prefixed to these councils to differentiate them from the unit-based councils. With a shift in the organization to continuous quality improvement, the Nursing Congress Quality Assurance Council is now referred to as the Nursing Congress Quality Improvement Council. The fifth council was named the Nursing Executive Council. The Nursing Executive Council is composed of the chairs of each of the nursing congress councils, four nursing executives, the vice president of patient services, and the administrative director of surgical services. This council coordinates and integrates councilor activities and addresses issues that affect every council.

In addition, a sixth council was temporarily established, contrary to the advice of a consultant. This council was the Advanced Practice Council. When it was established, the role of advanced clinical practice was not well defined at Sioux Valley Hospital. The major accountability of this group was to establish a role description for this practice. After this was accomplished the group disbanded, and representation was included on the four nursing congress councils.

Initially the nursing congress councils were each composed of 10 members representing diverse perspectives. In time these groups expanded to 25 to 30 members and included a member from each nursing unit. Sampson and Marthas[5] advocate 7 to 10 members as the ideal group size. This was acknowledged, but the benefits of enhanced communication and increased participation with more members were believed to override this recommendation. This change is a reflection of the culture of the nursing community.

Some of the earliest activities of each of the councils were participation in a group analysis and establishment of group norms, councilor accountabilities, and a councilor charter. The group analysis was completed by an advanced practice nurse certified in the administration of the Myers-Briggs Type Indicator. Suggestions were offered to optimize the group's process. Examples of norms, accountabilities, and a charter are included in Exhibits 3–3 and 3–4, in Appendix 3-A, and in Exhibits 7–3 and 7–4.

With the establishment of the nursing congress councils, unit-based council development began. Each nursing unit (microcommunity) established a practice, education, quality improvement, and management council. The unit-based councilor accountabilities coincided with the respective nursing congress councilor accountabilities.

Exhibit 7–3 Shared Governance Nursing Congress Education Council Accountabilities and Descriptor Statements

---

The Nursing Congress Education Council will be accountable for:

1. establishing standards of practice for educational activities (establish standards and guidelines for educational programs within and outside Sioux Valley Hospital, such as assessment of educational needs, evaluation tools, continuing education units, and patient education materials)
2. ensuring that systems are available for meeting educational standards (ensure that resources are available to meet the standards)
3. monitoring and evaluating outcomes that indicate whether educational standards are being met (reports on a regular basis from unit education councils)
4. providing leadership and direction for unit-based educational activities (help unit-based education councils develop their council structure, etc.)
5. implementing and communicating council activities (representatives from this council are responsible for reporting at unit-based councils)
6. developing and nurturing an environment for nursing research (value nursing research and communicate this throughout the department of nursing)
7. providing resources to enhance/assist individuals to achieve personal and professional goals and potentials (nursing center activities)
8. developing a mechanism for nursing practice communication (mechanism to communicate nursing practice activities, such as *Nursing Speaks* or another newsletter)

Source: Courtesy of Sioux Valley Hospital, Sioux Falls, South Dakota.

Some units, because of their size, chose to combine one or more councils. For example, the dialysis unit, which has 13 nurses, combined its practice and management councils and its education and quality improvement councils. Membership on the unit councils was left to the individual units to decide. Some units, because of their unique culture, chose to include other staff members such as technicians, health unit coordinators, and nursing assistants. One unit also has physicians included as councilor members.

The nursing congress councils address clinical issues that affect the entire nursing practice and are a mechanism for dissemination of information. The unit-based councils address issues that affect their specific unit. Collaboration among a small number of units may occur if an issue is limited to their unique practices. The work of the councils, especially the nursing congress councils, is accomplished in ad hoc committees. These committees have a well-defined purpose and a short-term existence.

The implementation of differentiated practice took place in the microcommunities. The steps toward change were planned in detail but differed from community to community. The change process time frames varied among communities. Some nursing units implemented the principles within a few months; others took more

Exhibit 7–4 Shared Governance Nursing Congress Practice Council Charter

---

Membership: Composed of one member per practicing unit, one nursing administrator, and one CNS. Each council member will also be a practicing unit practice council member.

Term of membership: 2 years.

Frequency of meetings: First Monday from 1300 to 1500 hours in Meeting Room B.

Chair: A clinically oriented Nursing Congress Practice Council member selected by the council for a term of 1 year, at which time the chair-elect will become chair. Elections will be held in May.

Purpose: The Nursing Congress Practice Council's purpose will be to address issues related to nursing practice and to provide for the determination of standards against which practice, nursing judgments, and activities may be measured.

Subcommittees: Nursing chart forms and procedures.

Source: Courtesy of Sioux Valley Hospital, Sioux Falls, South Dakota.

---

than 2 years to actualize fully the differentiated roles. The common language has served as a uniting force among nurses in the community. Microcommunities that were viewed as different have identified the commonalities in their nursing practices.

Refreezing

Once the shared governance councils were established and the system proved efficient, the nursing staff integrated the new methods of communication, decision making, and evaluation into their definition of community. Representation on the various councils changed as terms of service expired. The process moved smoothly and without much resistance. The entire community of nurses had reached a similar level of integration and stabilization in approximately the same time frame. The organization soon recognized the new structure and communication system. A subsystem in the organization had changed. As the boundaries between nursing and other departments became more open and fluid, interactions and communication patterns changed.

Refreezing is more difficult to describe in the differentiated practice process. Because time frames and levels of acceptance and resistance varied, the entire community did not reach stabilization and integration at the same time. The differences in application of the principles kept some microcommunities in the moving phase longer than others. This also served to keep macrocommunities separate, according to their level of development. All nursing units (microcommunities) are now functioning within the Integrated Care delivery system; this is uniting the community of nurses and producing a truly professional nursing practice.

Although a degree of refreezing has been reached in reference to the processes of differentiated practice and shared governance, the community is in a perpetual state of unfreezing and moving in other processes. For example, the implementation of Integrated Clinical Pathways has required unfreezing and moving of the community's medical record documentation process and has affected the differentiated practice nursing roles. Integrated Clinical Pathways have become tools to further the development of the professional nursing practice, to expand the community of nurses, and to promote collaboration with other disciplines. Pathways were developed to coordinate the care of the patient from admission through discharge. The process of developing Clinical Pathways required the expertise of many nurses. This is best displayed through an example.

The Integrated Clinical Pathway for caring for a patient undergoing a cardiac catheterization included input from nurses in the Sioux Valley Hospital community (ie, cardiac recovery unit, cardiology nursing unit, and CNSs), as well as from nurses outside the macrocommunity as previously defined. These nurses included those working in the cardiac catheterization laboratory, physician offices, and cardiac rehabilitation. See Chapter 5 for more discussion about Integrated Clinical Pathways. Thus the community has been expanded to include all professional nurses who touch the patient.

Therefore, some of the subsystems of the broader system of differentiated practice have reached refreezing, then have been required to unfreeze and move. The community has adopted the motto: "Change is the norm, stability is suspect," as unfreezing, moving, and refreezing continue.

OUTPUT

Output is defined as any information, energy, or matter leaving the system for the external environment. The vision includes as output the development of a professional nursing practice and empowerment of patients. Each of these outputs can be described in more detail.

With the evolution of the professional nursing practice, all nurses experienced an increased accountability through the application of authority, autonomy, and control. The nursing practice cannot truly be held accountable until individuals are empowered to be autonomous, the practice is given the authority to make decisions regarding clinical practice, and the practice is given control of its governance. This process took place in varying degrees depending upon individual growth and the cultures inherent in each microcommunity. For example, the process of peer review has evolved with the nurse manager no longer completing the annual evaluation. The accountability for credentialing the staff and peer review is now within the purview of the staff (see Chapter 4).

Another benefit of the increased accountability has been the opportunity for staff to self-schedule their hours; all nursing units currently self-schedule. This has increased their control of their practice. This accountability has also been a growth opportunity as nurses have acquired negotiation skills and a budgetary awareness.

The process of communication has been enhanced because there are now greater numbers of people involved and hence better informed staff. Being informed is a personal choice. Several avenues for obtaining information are available. Each unit council reports its activities regularly at the nursing congress council meetings. Because of the efficiency of councils, some units no longer hold unit meetings. Some of those units have created newsletters for their staff. A summary of nursing congress council activities is published in a monthly newsletter. This publication is distributed to the nursing units and is also mailed to the unscheduled part-time staff to keep them informed.

The members of the various councils are another source of information. Staff nurses know who represents their views. The representatives to the councils are expected to share information and to seek input on issues being addressed. The nursing congress council representatives are also members of the corresponding unit council. Meeting agendas and minutes are available for both the unit and nursing congress councils.

The flow of information has changed. In the past all information regarding other nursing units, other departments, and even the organization at large was funneled through the unit directors. Now with so many more people involved and having access to information, the flow of communication has been enhanced and expedited.

The role of the unit director, formerly referred to as the head nurse, has changed drastically. The key function of this role is to facilitate the operation of the unit. This involves coaching, mentoring, and ensuring that adequate resources are available. The role of a nurse manager within a shared governance structure can be compared to a helicopter. When things are operating smoothly, the manager, like a helicopter, hovers quietly above, observing the big picture of what is happening. When problems arise, the helicopter descends. In other words, the manager then coaches, facilitates, or mentors staff to resolve the problem. Once the problem or issue is resolved, the helicopter once again ascends. Each unit director has unique leadership qualities and, like everyone else, may vary in his or her stage of professional development. One unit director recently stated that she could not even imagine going back to the previous method of management.

Staff now have an established mechanism for identifying inefficiencies and suggesting alternatives. This has become especially important in the present health care environment. An example is the implementation of unit-based cardiopulmonary resuscitation recertification. Formerly this had been provided by the staff development department.

The team approach to patient care has been enhanced as a result of shared governance and the crumbling of the invisible walls between the various communities. With the implementation of shared governance and differentiated practice, working relationships between micro- and minicommunities were enhanced. Because of the opportunity to acquaint people and to work together on councilor issues, bonds between micro- and minicommunities evolved. No longer does the person on the phone have just a name. This continues to strengthen the macrocommunity overall and supports a team approach to care. This same phenomenon is now occurring between nursing and other departments.

Through the process of developing a professional nursing practice, the culture of the macrocommunity began to embrace authority, autonomy, control, and, therefore, accountability. As individual nurses adopted the behaviors inherent in these concepts, those people in contact with them, including patients, other nurses, and support staff, experienced a transfer of empowerment.

The output of empowered patients is still developing. The nurse–patient relationship (throughput) is the process by which this can be achieved. By empowering patients, it is believed that quality of care and customer satisfaction will be enhanced. This goal is central to fulfilling the mission of the community and the organization. A driving force for patient empowerment is the consumer himself or herself. Today's health care consumers are cost conscious and demand more information regarding their care, options available, and cost. To empower patients requires a shift in thinking and values of the health care team and the organization. Two units are being redesigned and will have patient-focused care as their philosophy. Care will be provided from an interdisciplinary approach with some decentralization of services. This process will enhance patient empowerment.

Empowerment of patients is evidenced by a plan of care mutually determined by the patient, nurse, physician, and other members of the health care team. Upon admission, patients are informed of their rights as well as their responsibilities as patients. Integrated Clinical Pathways also inform patients of the expected course of recovery, equipping them with the information they need to ask appropriate questions about their recovery. A goal of the case management model being developed is to empower the patient further as an ongoing participant in the life care plan (see Chapter 5 for more discussion about the case management model).

FEEDBACK

The feedback system, or evaluation of the process, was especially apparent in the developmental phases and during implementation of shared governance and differentiated practice. The feedback obtained as a result of evaluation indicated a need for change or modification.

During the developmental phase of shared governance, many changes were made as a result of feedback. The most drastic was the expansion of councilor membership. Feedback regarding the differentiated practice process in the developmental phase was at the microcommunity level. The changes that resulted from this evaluation process affected only the microcommunities. Some of these communities became diverse as a result of the feedback process. For example, some microcommunities initially implemented the primary nurse role as a direct caregiver and integrative role; others implemented this role primarily as an integrative role. Feedback in the later phases of the evolution of shared governance brought less change to the entire community. Feedback in the later phases of development of differentiated practice greatly affected the macrocommunity. The microcommunities eventually evolved to a care delivery system where the primary nurse is foremost in an integrative role. The community was able to accept role expectations for all nurses that could be implemented in any setting.

Evaluation is ongoing. Since the development and implementation of shared governance and differentiated practice, many subsequent changes have occurred as a result of feedback obtained.

THE FUTURE

The future holds bright horizons for the community of professional nurses at Sioux Valley Hospital. The growth and development of a professional practice are ongoing, and the shared governance structure may go through the change process once again. Through feedback, the community has become aware of the need to redesign the council structure. It became apparent that the work of the nursing congress councils focuses on the clinical practices of the associate, primary, and clinical care coordinator roles. Although they are interrelated, the practice issues of CNSs, educators, and managers are not being addressed.

This new awareness represents the unfreezing step in the change process. As a result, the CNSs have developed a group practice, complete with councils (practice, management, quality improvement, and education) similar to those of each nursing unit. The chair of each CNS council is a representative to the related nursing congress council. Advanced practitioners in education and management have also created councils within their practice. These additions to the council structure have prompted the community to reevaluate the entire governance system.

The refinement of roles also has prompted a reevaluation. As the barriers between micro- and minicommunities began to break down, nurses practicing in the roles of associate nurse, primary nurse, and clinical care coordinator began to identify issues common to the role, not necessarily those common to the micro- or minicommunity. Ad hoc committees of nurses in one role were formed to evaluate specific topics. The need for a councilor structure that promotes collaboration among nurses within a role was obvious.

As the current shared governance structure was fully operationalized, some inefficiencies surfaced. One example relates to the Nursing Congress Practice and Management Councils. The Nursing Congress Practice Council has the accountability for making decisions regarding clinical practice. Because of the impact that these decisions have, however, fiscal implications are present. The Nursing Congress Management Council has the accountability for providing adequate resources to support clinical practice. Thus the clinical practice issues ended up needing the approval of the management group to be operationalized. This has delayed implementation of decisions and has contributed to frustration. The new model of shared governance that has been proposed addresses the issues that have been discussed. Implementation of the new model is anticipated in the near future.

This community of professional nurses exists within an organization and continues to interface with many other departments. The community has identified the benefits of collaboration with these departments. The formation of several interdepartmental liaison committees has created a forum for collaboration. For example, the Nursing/Pharmacy Liaison Committee addresses issues of importance to both professions. This group consists of representatives who are empowered to make recommendations. Within the nursing community, some issues must then be reviewed by the various and appropriate councils. Liaison committees have also been formed with the laboratory and the supply departments. The community has been further expanded through a liaison committee formed to address issues between nurses in the macrocommunity who care for cardiac patients and nurses who work in a large cardiology clinic. This process has served to improve communication and to assist with decision making.

In addition, several advanced practice nurses recently facilitated the development of an organization of clinic nurses. Monthly breakfast meetings are held to provide a forum for interaction between the Sioux Valley Hospital nursing community and the community of clinic nurses. Through collaboration with the community of nurses, other disciplines have been exposed to the evolution of the professional practice. Some of those outside nursing have become interested in the process of creating a shared governance model. Unfreezing is now occurring at the organizational level. A task force composed of administrators and various disciplines is discussing the development of an organizational shared governance model.

Differentiated practice is also experiencing unfreezing and moving. The need for a system of case management has been identified. Unfreezing has occurred, and the moving process of change has started. The model involves expanding the differentiated practice system and includes the use of Integrated Clinical Pathways. Associate nurses manage on each shift the care of patients who follow the Pathway. Primary nurses manage from admission to discharge the care of patients who deviate from the Pathway in a limited number of areas. CNSs are consulted to manage the care of patients who become outliers and are high users of resources. This management is on a continuum from preadmission through postdischarge. Detailed planning has occurred, and a demonstration project has started.

The implementation of Integrated Clinical Pathways has also caused changes. A new system of documentation is required for the Pathway to be efficient. The primary nurses and associate nurses have come together to design this system. Each role will need to integrate this tool for managing care and documentation within their definition of care delivery and the value system of the community. When this integration is accomplished, refreezing will have occurred.

CONCLUSION

The implementation of differentiated practice and shared governance has brought many challenges and much change. When nurses were faced with the challenges, it was helpful to be reminded of the vision or output being sought: a professional nursing practice and empowered patients. Because of the personality type of most nurses, this vision needed to be expressed in a more concrete manner. The vice president of patient services provided the vision. Nursing leaders in various roles then acted as change agents. The unification of the nurses at Sioux Valley Hospital as a community was an unanticipated output. Its impact has been tremendous, however, and has potentiated the successful implementation of differentiated practice and shared governance.

Change is never easy. By objectively identifying driving and restraining forces, strategies can be formulated to ensure success. The work of change is never finished. The health care system and subsystems and the mini-, micro-, and macrocommunities are constantly evolving. A change in one component affects all other components. Therefore, beware: A sense of completion may be unrealistic.

Is your practice ready for a major change? What is your vision? What outputs do you wish to achieve? An organizational assessment should be the first step you take. It will help you establish a baseline understanding of your organization. The authors recommend the tool developed by Reddencliff, Smith, and Ryan-Merritt.[6]

Change requires risk taking, but nothing ventured is nothing gained. In the Sioux Valley Hospital experience, risk taking resulted in the foundation of a community of nurses. The full impact has yet to be realized.

No endeavor that is worthwhile is simple in prospect; if
it is right, it will be simple in retrospect.

EDWARD TELLER

REFERENCES

1. Porter-O'Grady T. Shared governance and new organizational models. *Nurs Econ.* 1987;5:281–286.
2. Buckley W. *Sociology and Modern Systems Theory.* Englewood Cliffs, NJ: Prentice-Hall; 1967.
3. Lewin K. Group decision and social change. In: Maccoby E, ed. *Readings in Social Psychology.* 3rd ed. New York, NY: Holt, Rinehart & Winston; 1958:197–211.
4. Koerner JG, Bunkers SS. Change: a professional challenge. *Nurs Admin Q.* 1991;6(1):15–21.
5. Sampson EE, Marthas MM. *Group Process for the Health Professions.* 3rd ed. Albany, NY: Delmar; 1990.
6. Reddencliff M, Smith EL, Ryan-Merritt M. Organization analysis: tool for the clinical nurse specialist. *Clin Nurse Spec.* 1989;3:133–136.

EXERCISE 7-1: COMMUNITY-BUILDING EXERCISES

Rationale: This is an exercise to demonstrate the process of change as it relates to your group or organization. This process can facilitate the implementation of change, can challenge conventional thinking, and can promote brainstorming. Initially it is important to clarify what the goals are and to identify a common mission. A values clarification exercise can be helpful.

Exercise 1

1. Write down five things you value in your professional life.
2. Write down five things you value in your personal life.
3. Write down five key areas where you spend your time.
4. Discuss those things to which you devote enough time and those things to which you do not devote enough time.

If you really value something, it should be an area for which you make time. Otherwise it may be an ideal: something you value but do not make time for. This process should help each person define areas of personal and professional value.

Exercise 2

Before implementing change, it is important to assess the organization in various areas. The organizational flowchart does not give a complete picture of the complexity of an organizational system. The formal structure does not represent many essential informal structures in place in an organization. Reddencliff, Smith, and Ryan-Merritt[6] offer a fine example of an organizational analysis:

1. Discuss the formal and informal organizational system. Discuss the formal mission statement and its congruence with the organizational values (where the time is spent).
2. Identify and discuss the formal and informal power bases in the organization.
3. Discuss the change process (unfreezing, moving, and refreezing) as it relates to your group or system. Include the extent of involvement of nursing staff at the unit level (microcommunity). Become familiar with the leadership, formal and informal, at each level.
4. Describe the decision-making process at the various levels. Are the decisions made by consensus or command, and are the decisions made with all involved having access to the necessary information?

5. Identify and discuss the leadership styles of the formal and informal leaders.
6. Identify and discuss the communication network, formal and informal. Are openness and honesty values in the organization and various communities? Discuss also the clarity and distortions of organizational communication.

8 Corporate

Cindi Slack, Judith K. Crane, Vicki J. Tigner, and Richard M. Jones

> *If we don't change directions, we'll end up where we're headed.*
>
> CHINESE PROVERB

In most organizational structures, decision making contains three levels. At the top is the corporate level, composed primarily of the board of directors, the chief executive officer, and the vice presidents of various departments. These individuals as a group are responsible for the financial performance of the organization, the corporate image, and the community services the organization performs. In the middle is the business level, or those managers who generally translate the corporate mission into functional objectives. The third level is the operational or grassroots supervisors, who develop short-term objectives and implement the corporation's strategic plan. In hospitals, often it is the third-level people who directly manage the delivery of services to the patient but who feel least empowered. This was well documented when Sioux Valley Hospital performed an analysis of the strengths, weaknesses, opportunities, and threats (SWOT) that composed our business eco-system. This was facilitated through a consultative relationship with Dr Frank Steiner and Ecology of Excellence training. A few introductory definitions may help the reader understand the basic principles underlying Ecology of Excellence.

> A business environment will produce its own Ecology based on the relationship between the ECOsystem elements of the Employee * Customer * Organization. We believe it is this ECOsystem interdependence which establishes and/or sustains a business Ecology of Excellence required for success in today's marketplace. Business performance is directly linked to an Ecology of Excellence and these links are forged from the interaction of the key elements of the ECOsystem: Employee behavior produces Customer outcomes which impacts

238

the Organization. Successful results gained from these cause/effect relationships in the ECOsystem will produce an Ecology of Excellence teamed with a winning business performance.

In a successful business ECOsystem [see Figure 8–1], the expected behaviors, outcomes, and impacts can be defined. The definition characteristics of each can best be identified within a framework of three major components of an Organization. STRUCTURE is the policy, procedure and routine of daily business operations supported by standards of excellence which evaluate employee performance. CULTURE is the motivation of the workforce to achieve business success linked with an expectation of excellence seen as an employee attitude of service quality. PERFORMANCE is the realization by employees that independent and team contributions produce margin-based workforce incentives. These contributions promote excellence through continued innovation of product line to meet the changes in customer needs and challenges in market demands.

Structure: Business Operations/Standards of Excellence

There is a relationship between the mechanics of business operations, and the standards of excellence through which performance is measured. This structural relationship expects an employee to exhibit COMPETENCE, an inventory of skills and abilities with which a product or service is delivered to the customer to assure quality and continued customer SATISFACTION. This customer trend will realize MARGIN for the organization, the bottom line financial performance which produces the revenue to support employee incentives and the resources to deliver the highest quality product.

Culture: Business Motivation/Expectations of Excellence

In order to maintain a motivation for business success and set expectations of excellence, the employee must have a COMMITMENT to the philosophy and goals of the organization, and the internalized desire to achieve and succeed for the benefit of the customer, the organization and self. The customer demonstrates a LOYALTY to the product/service by selecting the organization as sole provider and establishes a pattern of return business. In turn, the public perception or business IMAGE becomes one of excellence based on the organization's high regard for customer satisfaction and employee contribution.

Performance: Business Incentives/Promotion of Excellence

The incentives of business which promote expectations of excellence target employee behavior to be one of EMPOWERMENT, the belief in self responsibility and actions of internal control.

The employee takes responsibility for influencing "best result" outcomes in the workplace delivering to the customer real VALUE for the dollar. Such employees recognize that their contribution helps to secure MARKET share for the organization which in turn produces revenue that makes incentives available to the workforce and reinvestment capital available to the business. An empowered work force will strengthen market share for the organization.

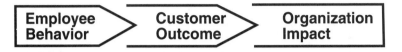

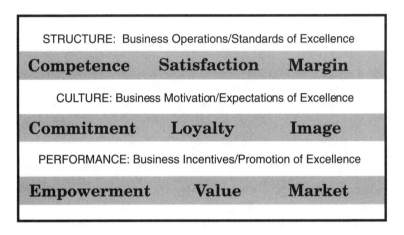

Balanced ECOsystem® = Competitive E.D.G.E.

Employees **D**elivering **G**rassroots **E**xcellence®

Figure 8–1 The business ECOsystem®. *Source:* Reprinted from *Ecology of Excellence®: A Balanced ECOsystem for Business Performance* by Educational Professional Services, p. 2, with permission of Frank Steiner, President, © 1987.

The ECOsystem employee behavior profile is one of competence, commitment and empowerment which delivers to the customer a sense of satisfaction, loyalty and value; the organization realizes the benefits of strong margin, a business image of quality and market dominance and expansion. These are the elements of the ECOsystem which deliver the competitive EDGE for the corporation and that E.D.G.E., we believe, is Employees Delivering Grassroots Excellence."[1(pp1-3)]

Through this assessment of the nursing department's strengths and weaknesses, it was identified that nurses at the third level of management and at the grassroots level at Sioux Valley Hospital felt a high degree of competence and commitment but that empowerment was ranked as the lowest value of the entire ecosystem.

These elements identified several of the basic premises of the culture of Sioux Valley Hospital. Culture refers first to content (shared understanding, artifacts, and behaviors), second to a group, and third to the relationship between the group and the content, a relationship of distinctiveness and specificity. Culture refers to the shared understanding peculiar to and specific to a group (Sioux Valley Hospital's culture is discussed in Chapter 2).

In *The Fifth Discipline,* Peter Senge wrote, "If any one idea about leadership has inspired organizations for thousands of years, it's the capacity to hold a shared picture of the future we seek to create. One is hard pressed to think of any organization that has sustained some measure of greatness in the absence of goals, values, and missions that become deeply shared throughout the organization. IBM had 'service'; Polaroid had instant photography; Ford had public transportation and Apple had computing power for the masses."[2(p9)] Sioux Valley Hospital had committed nurses who delivered highly competent clinical care. Senge continues, "Though radically different in content and kind, all these organizations managed to bind people together around a common identity and sense of destiny. . . . What has been lacking is a discipline for translating individual vision into shared vision—not a 'cookbook' but a set of principles and guiding practices."[2(p9)]

Steiner was invited to Sioux Valley Hospital in late 1987 to assist hospital employees in developing their shared vision through learning team-building principles and communication practices. In nursing the people who perform the management function often have been ill prepared to assume such a role. Bedside nurses must be as adept in the management process as those at the operational, business, and corporate levels. Empowerment may be a perceived value that indicates the grassroots view of their ability/authority to manage. Through the implementation of differentiated practice, Ecology of Excellence, and Myers-Briggs, by 1989, when the SWOT was repeated, empowerment's value had increased by 56%.

The process of empowering nurses began with the operational management level. Truly the corporate and business levels (with a few exceptions) of the organization were not vested in the project. The outcome of implementation, however, was a realization by the grassroots level that nurses at the bedside hold a position in a corporate structure and have accountability/authority defined by their roles.

CORPORATE CULTURE

This chapter seeks to create a mental image of the characteristics of the corporate culture at Sioux Valley Hospital. As the authors identified corporate culture features, the terms that prevailed included *old versus new health care structures, male versus female models,* and *linear versus systems models.* Other descriptors for these systems refer to how information is either closely held or shared, how communication is formally depicted through organizational charts, and how financial data and margin are either integrated into quality outcomes or independent variables.

Change was occurring rapidly in the external environment. It is recognized by the authors that in 1993 Sioux Valley Hospital's corporate culture was similar to what it was in 1987. The health care structure at Sioux Valley Hospital has been traditionally male dominated. On the corporate level there are 2 women: 1 of the 15 members of the Board of Directors who was appointed in 1986, and 1 who is the vice president of patient services. Traditional operational styles were male oriented in power, communication, hierarchy, and values and exhibited linear thought processing. Other descriptors are that they were systematic in knowing and following the rules and competitive within and among groups. The vice president of patient services recognized the difference between this operational style and the changing paradigm in management styles. Nursing, being composed primarily of women, had many skills essential in the changing paradigm of business. The word *paradigm* became a household word in the operational nursing management environment. Educational opportunities were offered to this level to enhance awareness of the phenomenal rate of change in the external environment. Some quotations from the readings distributed to the nursing management level may be helpful to exemplify the vision that was created for the culture.

Naisbitt and Aburdene, in *Reinventing the Corporation*, state, "Significant change occurs when there is a confluence of changing values and economic necessity."[3(p42)] As companies reinvent themselves, they need to find new structures and values. Those that learn from how women do things will have a start. Women can transform the workplace by expressing, not by giving up, their personal values. These values include:

- an attention to process instead of to the bottom line
- a willingness to look at how an action will affect other people instead of the "What's in it for me?" approach
- a concern for the wider needs of the community
- a predisposition to draw on personal, private-sphere experience when dealing with the public realm
- an appreciation of diversity
- an outsider's impatience with rituals and symbols of status that divide people who work together and so reinforce hierarchies

Both men and women pay heavily in trying to conform to a management style that reflects mostly masculine values. This style emphasizes rationality and solving technical tasks. In it, people's needs may get lost. Each gender must be taught and must integrate a blending of old and new or male and female. As Ferguson and Ferguson write:

Androgynous management embraces instrumental and expressive behavior, vicarious and direct achievement styles, collaboration and confrontation behavior, a proactive and reactive style and compliance and alliance producing skills.

Each sex may need to accentuate the behaviors of the other sex in order to be androgynous. Women need to discuss issues in a linear, systematic style as well as use intuition; to deal with power as well as emotion; to assert themselves and compete, where appropriate, as well as to foster collaboration. For men, of course, it is the reverse. Men need more than power and competitiveness in order to have a full repertoire of effective behavior. They need to learn to express and deal with emotions other than anger and frustration. They need to engage less in joking and jockeying to establish a position and more in sharing and nurturing to build a team. Thus, a synthesis is necessary, a blending of strong masculine and strong feminine characteristics."[4(p233)]

The new system of organizations created by Frances Hesselbein for the Girl Scouts is circular. Positions are represented by circles, which are then arranged in an expanding series of orbits. Hesselbein states that circles are important symbolically: "The circle is an organic image. . . . The circle is inclusive, but it allows for flow and movement. It doesn't box you in. As the circles extend outward there are more and more connections. So the galaxy gets more interwoven as it gets bigger."[5(p.40)] At Sioux Valley Hospital the nursing department's new organizational charts adapted this symbology of circles representing job roles and relationships to the client (Figure 8–2).

STRUCTURE

Much may be learned about an organization by looking at its reporting style. Traditional organizations have functioned through the authoritarian or linear structure. In the linear structure there is a definite upper and lower echelon. Decision making takes place at the administrative level and is handed down through the ranks. Rarely does this process involve input from the staff level, nor is there flow upward to affect the final outcomes.

This structure has a distinct reporting format and communication process. Sioux Valley Hospital's organizational chart (Figure 8–3) has the patients and Board of Directors at the top. The next level is the president followed by the vice presidents. Some of the vice presidents report directly to the president, and other vice presidents report to the executive vice president. The chart continues with the departments that report to the various vice presidents. An organizational chart is defined for each department and includes each level of employee within that area and the reporting process in place.

In the past, the nursing department chart had the vice president of patient services at the top and the clinical nursing directors of the three divisions next. The head

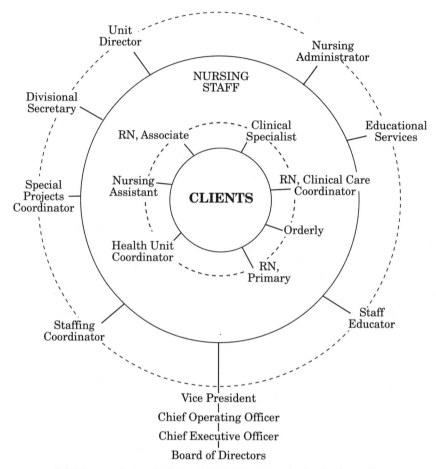

Solid lines reflect reporting relationships and accountability.
- - - - Dotted lines reflect communicating relationships and collaboration.

Figure 8–2 Sioux Valley Hospital Department of Nursing divisional chart. Courtesy of Sioux Valley Hospital, Sioux Falls, South Dakota.

nurse reported to the clinical nursing director with the specific staff roles following. In this structure there were many layers in place. The communication flow was up and down and rarely crossed to another department, except at the vice president level. This made communication slow and cumbersome. The message sometimes became altered or distorted by the time it reached its final destination. This process did not encourage prompt decision making or first party communication.

This flow of communication is best described by an example. When funds were needed for an expenditure, the requestor came face to face with the structure. The

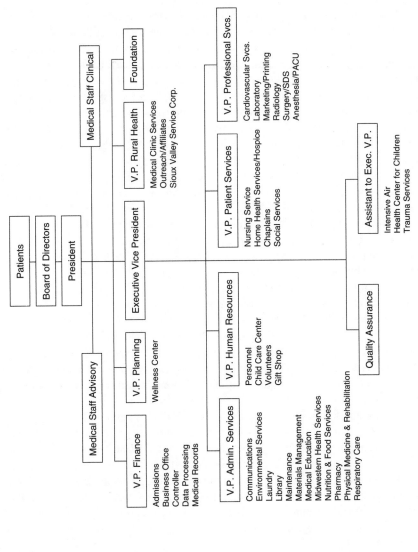

Figure 8–3 Sioux Valley Hospital organizational chart. Courtesy of Sioux Valley Hospital, Sioux Falls, South Dakota.

person in need met with his or her immediate supervisor and provided the necessary documentation. The request was then taken through the channels to the vice president. The vice president then went to the executive vice president. Depending on the dollar amount required, the next step was to secure approval of the president or the Board of Directors. The board met on a scheduled basis, so this request often was delayed because of the meeting schedule. Meanwhile, the need still existed.

The other concern in this system was who made the decisions. The decision may have been made by someone who did not have all the necessary information regarding the effect or outcome of the decision. In fact, a decision may actually have hindered another area from being able to perform its departmental functions related to lack of involvement in the decision. An example is the purchase of a payroll system that would affect every employee and department in the institution. If the decision were made by a select group without consulting all those who would be affected, it might be disastrous. The system might actually increase the workload of the managers responsible for the payroll of their employees. The system might not provide the necessary data needed to manage the payroll budget at the department level. Ferguson and Ferguson[4] call this a closed system. This type of system is self-contained and isolated from the larger environment of the institution. This can result in the organization becoming run down and even eventually dying.

According to Naisbitt and Aburdene, "yesterday's hierarchical structures do not work in the new information society."[3(p30)] Naisbitt and Aburdene also identify that cross-divisional teams work much better. This format integrates all who are involved with a specific service, who then work together as a team for the best outcome for all. This often brings together many departments that report to different managers and/or vice presidents. The process promotes buy-in to the outcome because the departments were involved in the development. This type of system is referred to as an open system.[4] The open system is receptive to a variety of inputs. The open system constantly imports energy; it does not run down. The open system adapts its design to the needs of the current situation. This structure involves in the process all those who will be affected by a decision.

This structure has begun to emerge at Sioux Valley Hospital. Examples of this process have become apparent through the nursing liaison committees. For example, as quality issues arose that involved the medical laboratory and nursing units, joint meetings were set up with representatives from the areas, who met to discuss specific topics. The problem solving involved all those affected by the issue and the resulting decision. The format was successful and was expanded to regular meetings with representatives from the nursing areas and medical laboratory personnel. An agenda was planned and circulated so that ideas could be generated before the meetings.

This committee laid the groundwork for future group meetings between nursing and radiology and between pharmacy and materials management. This process included a getting-acquainted time, where each group presented information about its department and gave specifics about the department functions to increase understanding. At the start of the process, the meetings were problem oriented. As the group matured the process became more future oriented, with strategic planning and problem prevention representing the primary agenda items of the committee. Quality and cost containment are now the focus of the committee's process. The meetings are held less often because of the enhanced communication that has resulted. Issues are more frequently addressed by the grassroots staff members who are involved in the issues as they occur, eliminating the need for frequent formal meetings.

The nursing department has changed its organizational chart to be consistent with the open system (see Figure 8-2). The new chart shows the patient at the center of the circle and all the nursing roles in a circle around the patient. The first circle around the patient is composed of those who are direct caregivers. This includes all registered nurses, nursing assistants, health unit coordinators, and orderlies. The next circle is the unit managers, nursing administration, educational staff, and staffing coordinators who support the caregivers. The department of nursing's conceptual framework describes the organizational chart as follows:

> The organizational chart for the nursing department was redesigned to reflect our new philosophy of shared governance. This innovative, organizational model placed the client at the center of the chart. The circular design reflected removal of hierarchy, depicting instead mutual valuing of all care delivery roles. Placement of administration at the bottom of the chart identified a role change of management from controlling, directing and supervising to one of facilitating, coordinating, integrating and supporting.[6(p6)]

The entire process of reporting and communicating has changed dramatically between the nursing and ancillary areas. There is flow back and forth at the frontline levels that encourages prompt problem solving. The formal hospital organizational structure remains unchanged.

In a linear system there are often tight reins on the financial components. Measurements usually relate to the bottom line. This can be detected by management of the budget, which looks at familiar concrete data such as patient days (which determine the number of care hours). Factors that influence the number of hours used, such as acuity and the blend of novice and experienced staff on a shift, are usually not considered relevant in such a system. The presence of the linear system's structure can be seen by decisions made that affect quality in ways that are not traditionally measured. For instance, a pharmacy computer system that does not communicate with computers present in any of the areas it serves creates additional work for all involved. Decisions are often made that will save money without realizing the effect of that decision on quality being realized. The decision to run a specific laboratory test once during the day to save expense for the laboratory may create a nightmare when those data are not available to physicians who are caring for patients.

The Work Engineering process, introduced by Steiner through the Ecology of Excellence philosophy, assisted the staff at Sioux Valley Hospital to look at economics while keeping the balance of quality. A Work Engineering technique that we found valuable to determine the extent of an issue was a pulse. This is an informal, quick method to investigate the need for further action regarding an issue or potential problem. To carry out this technique, a question about the issue should be asked of a group of staff. If the response indicates that many persons view it as a problem, a larger task force or work group can be implemented to identify further the extent of the problem and to address potential solutions. This technique is used to investigate the need for further action, rather than to solve or address solutions to problems (see Exercise 8–1 for further details). Work Engineering encourages a full examination of an issue, which includes having the correct people on the team to do the problem solving.

ACTION COUNCIL

The Sioux Valley Hospital Action Council was formed to address interdepartmental issues that could enhance the quality of work life and increase the business performance of the hospital. The intent was not to preempt the formal lines that already existed in the hospital but rather to serve as a clearinghouse for matters in the clinical areas of practice (grassroots decision making). The Action Council had members from each area of the hospital. Bylaws were developed to detail the structure of the council (see Appendix 8-A). Eligibility for membership was attendance at Ecology of Excellence classes. Staff members were elected by their coworkers to represent the department for a 2-year term. The Action Council was chaired by a staff member selected from the members of the council. A vice president served as an advisor to the chair and assisted with planning the agenda and facilitating the meeting.

One of the first issues brought to the Action Council came from executive management. The issue was the expense of worker's compensation benefits paid to employees who were injured during work. The council was asked to examine the issue and to make recommendations to executive management regarding a safety education program for staff. A task force that included Action Council members as well as representatives from the hospital safety committee and the employee health nurse was formed. After the data were evaluated, a proposal was made to and accepted by executive management. This proposal included evaluation of new employees who were at risk for a back or neck injury. The focus was employees with previous injury or placement in a work environment that put them at risk for an injury because of the type of work. A second proposal included a back to work program. This involved the evaluation of an injured employee by the physical medicine department and an exercise program directed at strengthening the employee. The goal was a reduction in lost work time due to an injury.

After the council had been meeting for 2 years, it became clear that the focus was changing. Many of the issues discussed related to employee benefits. Executive management utilized the council to gather information from employees. As a result, the Action Council has now become the Human Resource Advisory Committee. Membership on this committee continues to be by staff selecting peers with all departments represented. Terms are for 2 years with half the membership rotating each year. The chair continues to be selected from the members. Personnel policies and benefits are brought to the committee for input and recommendations. This committee has provided a forum for staff to receive information and to give feedback on issues that are important to them.

Work redesign, now an industry buzz word, surfaced at Sioux Valley Hospital during the time that the Action Council was formed. The nursing department viewed this as a possible solution for addressing the nursing shortage. In addition, some entry level positions in the institution could be expanded. Discussions were started interdepartmentally to evaluate the feasibility of housewide involvement in work redesign. When the project did not expand to involve other departments, the nursing department developed a demonstration of work redesign involving the nursing assistant role. Housewide work redesign is now being formally developed with the construction of two new patient care units. The project has support from executive management and multiple departments. The successful planning has been influenced by the flow of communication among the departments involved with the project. The fears and anxieties that exist with such a change are still present, but they are blended with trust.

COMMUNICATION

Trust and communication were integral to the success of this process at the corporate level. Communication tools were developed to facilitate more rational, direct, first party communication. Ecology of Excellence principles, which included first party communication and shifting of the masculine style toward androgyny, were the rationale for these tools. Interface agreements are one example of these tools. These agreements are described in Chapter 5, and examples can be found in Exhibits 8–1 to 8–3.

Recreating the vision of nursing at Sioux Valley Hospital required a change in communication styles and patterns. Naisbitt[7] has identified the next era as one of information. Past management literature discusses communication in terms of formal and informal information lines. The good manager must understand how information is transferred within his or her department and determine methods to control, manipulate, and investigate what information is moving through these communication channels. This information model works when information is viewed as a finite quantity that can be distributed. In our new model, information

Exhibit 8–1 Interface Agreement: Midwestern Health Services (MWHS, Teletrace) and Sioux Valley Hospital (Postcoronary Care Unit, PCCU)

Customers: Patient
           Cardiologist
           Sioux Valley Hospital postcoronary nurses

Quality requirement: The Teletrace patient and his or her family are assured of 24-hour coverage of pacemaker monitoring.

Needs:
1. To ensure that a registered nurse trained in Teletrace monitoring is on the PCCU to provide 24-hour coverage, to include:
   • 24-hour telephone monitoring
   • completion of calls
   • appropriate paperwork
   • patients who arrive on PCCU will be assisted to complete Teletrace transmission by PCCU nurse
2. To provide inservices to provide quality in Teletrace monitoring skills to staff nurses.

Interface action plan: PCCU staff will:
1. provide for charge nurse on unit with Teletrace rhythm interpretation skills to ensure 24-hour coverage
2. if off-hour calls are received, place tracing in white card from Teletrace file and complete appropriate off-hour forms
3. determine whether physician needs to be notified of off-hour call
4. be responsible to complete in-house transmission (use of transmitter and acoustic couplers)
5. provide time analysis to MWHS for reimbursement of time spent in interface
Monthly calls less than 6 minutes are free. For any call over 10 minutes, PCCU will be compensated for time.

MWHS Teletrace staff will:
1. forward calls to unit after hours
2. provide off-hour forms to PCCU
3. provide staff education as to use of transmitter, acoustic coupler, and Teletrace file every 6 months
4. provide for hours of intervention to be reimbursed to Sioux Valley Hospital for documentation as noted in 5 above
5. update card file on PCCU

Expectations:
1. Teletrace standards will be met on a 24-hour service.
2. Trained personnel will be available on unit 24 hours a day.
3. The nurses commit to each other that any variance will be handled via first party communication with copy of the variant tracing.
4. Referral to the PCCU quality assurance committees is to be reviewed on a monthly basis.
5. A 6-month report of corrective intervention will be prepared by PCCU quality assurance for MWHS quality assurance.

Courtesy of Sioux Valley Hospital, Sioux Falls, South Dakota.

Exhibit 8–2 Interface Agreement: Midwestern Health Services and Sioux Valley Hospital Pharmacy

---

Customers: All home infusion therapy patients

Quality requirement: Consistency in charging mechanisms

Needs: To develop accurate, fair charges from Sioux Valley Hospital pharmacy to Midwestern Health Services for emergency and after-hours pharmaceutical services.

Plan: Pharmacy will:
1. charge Midwestern Health Services for emergency and after-hours home infusion therapy utilizing the following formula: average wholesale price –10.5% + $4.75
2. bill Midwestern Health Services every 30 days for services provided:
   * These charges will be sent to Midwestern Health Services attention infusion therapy nurse.
   * Prepare no more than a 7-day supply of medication for any one client.

Midwestern Health Services will:
1. rely on the Sioux Valley Hospital Pharmacy Department to prepare home infusion therapy on an emergency/after-hours basis
2. continue to quality check pharmaceuticals prepared by the pharmacy and arrange for appropriate delivery to the client
3. provide 24-hour call with referral to consultants as needed
4. notify pharmacy regarding physician orders on new clients in an emergency or after hours

Both parties will review this agreement periodically. When costs of supplies, equipment, or services change, either party may modify the agreement at that time.

Courtesy of Sioux Valley Hospital, Sioux Falls, South Dakota.

---

is identified as a resource. The responsibility of management must be to identify what information is required by staff and to try supporting staff with information necessary for them to do their work. In the old model information is a control and power mechanism, whereas in the new model information is a tool used to empower staff to accomplish their own responsibilities.

It is easy to identify when the old or new system is in place. When the old norms are in force, persons are concerned with whom to include at a meeting and their need for the information presented at the meeting. There is a dependence on the use of formal organizational structural lines to transfer information. New information moves up the organizational chart, over to another department, and then back down that branch of the organization. When staff are empowered and use new systems of communication, there is no dependence on the organizational chart for decisions regarding who should have information. Rather, the decision is based on who may

Exhibit 8–3 Interface Agreement for Researchers Obtaining Records from Medical Records Department

---

1. Researchers will give the Medical Records Department a minimum of 2 days notice when patient records are requested. Requests will be written.
2. Researchers will request only those records that can be reviewed on the day requested. Researchers will make every effort to finish reviewing all charts on the day requested.
3. Researchers will obtain the patient records requested on the day and time specified.
4. The Medical Records Department will make every effort to have patient records requested by researchers available at the time requested. If a patient record is on a patient unit, the Medical Records Department can tell the researcher where the record can be reviewed.
5. If the researcher wishes to review the patient record outside the Medical Records Department, the researcher will inform the Medical Records Department where the record will be.
6. All patient records will be returned to the Medical Records Department by 1700 hours without exception.
7. If the researcher wishes to review records after 1700 hours, the researcher will do so in the Medical Records Department.

Courtesy of Sioux Valley Hospital, Sioux Falls, South Dakota.

---

be affected by the information or who should be included to make an effective decision.

Financial information is often closely guarded in a closed, controlled organization. In an organization that uses information in the new system, financial goals, targets, and productivity language are common at many levels. Several techniques were utilized at Sioux Valley Hospital to bring a change in thinking to the nursing staff regarding financial information. First, information about the relationship between patient days and productive hours was sent to each unit and placed on graphs. Trends of this information were then discussed at staff meetings to increase each staff member's understanding of the costs of the patient care provided.

One example of how information flow has changed comes from an unrelated project. A group of staff from many departments and levels of management and staff were discussing the problem of space in the cafeteria during lunch times. During one of their discussions, a staff member stated the perception that there would be more funds to allocate to a new cafeteria if the hospital had not put dollars into landscaping and adding trees to a new parking lot. There was considerable discussion that this perception was shared by many staff members. As a result, a hospitalwide communication was distributed that identified that when the city granted the permit for construction of the new parking lot it required the addition of trees and appropriate green space. Previously it would not have seemed necessary to share this information with staff.

The changing style of information management and communication affects the corporate culture. Eisler[8] identifies two basic organizational styles: dominator and partnership. The dominator model could be compared to the military and is organized by rank and control. The partnership model uses linking and networking, which stress relationship rather than control and power. Naisbitt and Aburdene[3] searched for examples of a new breed of manager, one whose top responsibility is creating a nourishing environment for personal growth. This shift from control to partnership can be identified as more women achieve management positions in the information society. Naisbitt and Aburdene[9] also have listed the six components of women's leadership as questioning, openness, ability to role model, emphasis on teaching, restructuring, and empowerment. With the new vision of professional practice, the nursing department at Sioux Valley Hospital has attempted to use partnering as a model for interaction with other departments. This was described earlier in relation to nursing liaison committees.

Improved communication patterns are not the only changes that occur with a professional model such as the current Sioux Valley Hospital model. How people organize to get work done is also affected. The formal organizational chart becomes less identifiable, and committees, task forces, or work groups are formed by identifying which persons have the input and know-how to get the job done. Peters and Waterman[10] identify this phenomenon as chunking, an action orientation that uses think tank style work groups. These work groups do not show up on the organizational charts, but they are integral to getting the work of the organization accomplished.

For Sioux Valley Hospital, this change in who should be involved in getting the work done can be charted by the development of a strategic planning process. The nursing department over the years had developed a planning process that included setting short-term and long-term goals at the unit and department level. In the early years of this process, the departmental goals were developed at a meeting of all nursing managers and nursing administrators. After this action, unit managers would involve their staff at unit meetings to develop goals specific to the unit. Currently the nursing departmental goals are determined at a day-long planning session, where representatives are present from all levels of nursing professionals: associate, primary, clinical care coordinators, nurse managers, clinical nurse specialists, nurse educators, and nursing administrators. Each group is responsible for contributing to the work, and all contributions are considered equally.

Within the corporation, the strategic planning process has also been altered. It has changed from a plan determined by the hospital administrators to a month-long process where each manager presents the issues, potential growth opportunities, and service changes for his or her department. These presentations are given to executive management and an advisory council of selected department mangers called the Management Advisory Council. Before making his or her presentation, each manager is directed to discuss and develop these presentations with input from staff in his or her department. Staff members and other managers are encouraged to attend the presentations. After all presentations have been made, the Management Advisory Council submits a summary of issues confronting the hospital and a list of proposed items prioritized for inclusion in the strategic plan.

Many forms of communication at Sioux Valley Hospital have changed. One change that is still in process is the development of communication tools known as Integrated Clinical Pathways (see Chapter 5). In the early 1980s, the Health Care Financing Administration (HCFA) instituted diagnosis-related groups (DRGs) as a means to facilitate hospital reimbursement. A crisis occurred, and Sioux Valley Hospital took measures to respond. First, it was believed by the nursing department that the underlying culture had to change. This culture is only now changing organizationally. Second, a system of control for the new culture had to be implemented. The system of control, the control of information or Clinical Pathways, is thought to be an answer to the control of spending and facilitation of patient care at the bedside.

CONTROLLING HEALTH CARE COSTS

Sioux Valley Hospital began to review the steps necessary to control the problem of rapidly escalating health care costs by managing patient care delivery through a process called Integrated Clinical Pathways. As McManis writes, "In 1990, hospital mergers, conversions and closures will accelerate, not only for administrative efficiency but also for clinical integration that in the long run will make healthcare delivery more effective and less costly."[11(p60)] Some futurists predict that managed care will become the preferred reimbursement method by the year 1995.

Efforts to control escalating health care costs have resulted in shorter hospital stays and an increased level of dependency of hospitalized patients who have needs for support after discharge. Who is in control at this crucial time? Too often, as Anthony and Young state, "the control structure is assumed to be identical to the organizational structure and, therefore, no additional thinking needs to be done. Also structure can be a rather complex problem, involving several dimensions. . . . Although controllability may be difficult to pinpoint, it is a fact that someone in an organization has control over each resource-related decision."[12(p233)] This premise holds true in the health care environment. Who the controller is in a community-based hospital environment is often the question. Most would agree that it is not the patient.

If control is defined "as the power, the authority, or the influence that one person has to direct the actions of others,"[13(p507)] then control may be said to be in the hands of the physician and nurse at the bedside because they direct the actions of the patient. At this time, and until physician reimbursement is directly linked to hospital reimbursement, administrators in a hospital environment exert control over physicians and nurses by monitoring, evaluating, and influencing their behavior to control direct costs.

As Bedford states, "For control to exist there must be something, an activity or a process to be controlled. . . . Control cannot be applied unless the way in which the variable components of the process are to be directed has been determined."[13(p508)] The HCFA has determined this for hospitals through the process of reimbursement for DRGs. The reimbursement is specified for a DRG and its average length of stay tied to a regionally adjusted fixed dollar amount. In the health care environment, then, cost minimization is the performance criterion.

When DRGs were first introduced, Sioux Valley Hospital executive management and nursing division management used control methods of informal and formal education of physicians to promote the concept of cost minimization. This was initially met with physician responses varying from acceptance to hostility. Although certain physician groups responded favorably and decreased the length of stay of their patients, some continued to practice without changing their behavior, and a few others seemingly rebelled and actually increased length of stay. The last two groups obviously recognized no adverse effects, and because some physicians were towing the line the hospital continued to realize financial success. The HCFA, however, continued to provide declining amounts of reimbursement for each DRG category. As a result, hospital administrators recognized that more significant control measures needed to be implemented.

Because staff nurses were not included in the initial educational process, a plan was developed to increase responsibility and accountability for nursing outcomes. This plan utilized many of the cultural diagnosis elements described by Deal and Kennedy.[14] One of these diagnostic techniques is to study the physical setting. A company that is proud of itself will reflect this pride in the cleanliness of its environment and in its overall structure. Another technique is to read printed literature about the company. Often an observer can track company statements over time to see how the corporate culture has evolved. Other diagnostic techniques include evaluating the guest relations program, observing how people spend their time, reviewing personnel policies, listening to stories, and interviewing employees. The interview process can be done via employee surveys such as a SWOT. The need for a change in paradigm was authenticated to the grassroots at Sioux Valley Hospital by the outside consultants who were brought in to facilitate our mourning and our education in the new way.

Nurses had a perception of little empowerment, as revealed by the SWOT conducted in 1987, and saw themselves as shift workers with little or no responsibility for the patient outcome or for the hospital outcome. Deal and Kennedy[14] specify the tips for managing change. Some of the ingredients for a successful change include a hero in charge of the process, recognition of external threats, mourning the old ways, training in the new ways, and bringing in outside consultants. Sioux Valley Hospital's heroine was the vice president of patient services, who led the nursing practice successfully through the change process. The awareness of the external threats of health care reform was a lived experience and was clarified by the consultants who were brought in to educate us about the new paradigm. Mourning was facilitated through a ritual of actually burying symbols of the old ways. From 1987 to 1992, Sioux Valley Hospital nurses have undergone a transformative process and now communicate via employee questionnaires that they feel empowered and have a definite role in shaping the outcome of both the patient and the hospital.

Although the process of education, Work Engineering, and financial awareness building was implemented and the last few days of patient stays in the hospital were eliminated by extensive nurse–physician collaboration, this was not enough. The hospital continued to experience increasing losses from the Medicare program, the highest user population, and from other insurers that were now implementing similar controls. It became apparent that the physician–nurse team must make the patient well in the most cost-effective manner, that is within a designated or appropriate length of stay, using appropriate resources. Therefore, it was imperative that this team examine what happened to a given case type on each day of hospitalization and plot out the course of hospitalization.

Using DRG 410 (chemotherapy administration) as an example, a Clinical Pathway was developed and tested through a retrospective study of 32 randomly selected patient charts. This was done by outlining the key incidents that must occur for the specific case type while simultaneously considering the time frames that need to be followed to meet length of stay parameters and to control resource utilization. Because in the initial phase of the study the purpose of the Clinical Pathway was informational, the variable of physician practice patterns had to be considered, and six Pathways that correlated with the number of physicians practicing differently were defined for DRG 410 to allow for further study. The six Clinical Pathways appear in Appendices 8-B to 8-G. DRG 410 has a defined length of stay of 2.6 days and a reimbursement of $1,477.99 at the time of this writing and for this facility.

Analysis of the data revealed that 21 of the 32 clients or 66% of the population met the criterion of control of costs as evidenced by actual costs falling below the $1,477.99 allowable reimbursement. This means that $31,037.79 of reimbursement was derived from these 21 cases, of which $17,454.92 represented expenses, for a gain of $13,582.87. Seven physicians' clients, all with an oncology specialty, were sampled (although seven physicians were included in the study, two of the physicians had practice patterns so similar that six Clinical Pathways were derived).

Eleven of the 32 patients (34%) exceeded allowable reimbursement. Total *charges* averaged $3,083.10 per case or a variance of $1,605.11 per case over reimbursement. The range of charges was $1,987.18 to $4,387.78. Total *costs* for the 11 cases not meeting Clinical Pathway criteria averaged $2,083.26 per case or a variance of $605.27 per case over reimbursement. This totaled $6,658.03 in actual losses to the hospital for these 11 cases (total costs – DRG 410 reimbursement × 11 cases).

A review of these data (Table 8–1) indicated that, given DRG 410, physician G's practice pattern caused a loss to the hospital of $414.40 for each of his total caseload (6 patients), physician E caused a loss to the hospital of $9.40 for each of his total caseload (8 patients), and physician C caused a loss to the hospital of $72.13 for each of his total caseload (6 patients). Interestingly, it was also noted that physicians G and E were practicing partners. Their other practice partner, however, was physician B (a physician who received many referrals from outlying areas according to his verbal report), who showed a gain for his total caseload (4 patients) of $362.15. In the final analysis, this physician produced profit for the hospital.

Much more information could be extracted from the 32 cases analyzed, but a larger sample would need to be reviewed. First of all, from this random sample one would assume that physicians A and D are practicing appropriately within the criteria set by the HCFA. This may indeed be true, but physician A treats only female reproductive organ carcinoma, and physician D had a sample limited to one patient. Randomization then must be specified as 30 charts on each physician randomly sampled from all cases over the age of 65 years. Also, to limit other confusion, a geographic boundary of the sample population must be set to provide for control of the distance patients must travel to undergo therapy. Distance may limit the physician's ability to order preadmission diagnostics in an effort to control in-hospital costs. Because chemotherapy may be administered for a variety of cancers at a variety of stages, an effort must be made to define the population sample further than by DRG. In other words, treatment for a relatively stable group of patients in the initial stages of chemotherapy may vary from that of a group of patients with advanced disease and debilitating comorbidities. Also, the 2-day chemotherapeutic practice of physician A may vary significantly from the chemotherapeutic regime for leukemia. Unfortunately, as of this writing the HCFA groups all these disease states into DRG 410. Also, in-depth analysis of this population of patients 65 years old and older should include specific age-related dosages of medications to determine whether further readmissions could be prevented by administering geriatric doses of dye or chemotherapeutic agents.

Once the study is redesigned and completed, the Integrated Clinical Pathway will be standardized to fit the population of patients in DRG 410. It will show the critical or key incidents that must occur in a predictable and timely fashion to facilitate an appropriate length of stay. The key incidents of an Integrated Clinical Pathway are discussed in Chapter 5. The Integrated Clinical Pathway is individualized to the patient by the primary nurse and physician at the time of admission to the hospital with consideration of comorbidities and socioeconomic factors. If changes are to be made from the standard, they are defined at this time. Any deviations from the standard Integrated Clinical Pathways are considered variances and are identified by cause and

Table 8–1 DRG 410: Chemotherapy Administration (Allowable Reimbursement, $1,477.99)

1	2	3	4	5	6	7	8	
Physician	Average Length of Stay	Number of Cases Meeting Criteria	Total Cost	Average Cost Above/Below per Case	Number of Cases Not Meeting Criteria	Total Cost	Average Cost Above/Below per Case	Profit/Loss for Total Cases*
A	2.0	3	$1,659.09	+$924.96	0	0	0	+$924.96
B	4.0	2	$1,965.59	+$495.20	2	$3,222.07	–$133.05	+$362.15
C	3.83	4	$3,575.40	+$584.14	2	$4,268.52	–$656.27	–$72.13
D	3.0	1	$814.89	+$663.10	0	0	0	+$663.10
E	4.75	5	$4,581.76	+$561.64	3	$6,147.10	–$571.04	–$9.40
F	3.0	3	$1,658.26	+$925.24	1	$2,287.02	–$809.03	+$116.21
G	4.33	3	$3,199.93	+$438.01	3	$6,991.21	–$852.41	–$414.40
Approximate totals		21	$17,454.92		11	$22,915.92		

*Column 5 minus column 8.

Courtesy of Sioux Valley Hospital, Sioux Falls, South Dakota.

rectified or justified. Integrated Clinical Pathways provide nurses and physicians with a tool for controlling and planning utilization of hospital services. As Etheridge writes, "Clinical pathways mark the track for clinicians in the health care relay. They visibly and clearly show key milestones on the course that must be achieved in order to have an appropriate length of stay. Time, resource utilization, and patient outcomes are the essential markers that demonstrate to clinicians when they are on course."[15(p4)]

Health care in the 1990s is faced with an environment that will require that it change not only the structure and the basic nature of its business but also its culture and philosophy. In the coming years, health care must capitalize on trends rather than hide from them. Managing patient care utilizing Clinical Pathways or information as a control mechanism is a strategy that will assist in rationalizing the health care delivery system by eliminating redundancies and excess spending at the patient's bedside under the collaboration of qualified personnel before outside forces step in and do it for us.

> *I find the great thing in this world is not so much where*
> *we stand, as in what direction we are moving: To reach*
> *the port of heaven, we must sail sometimes with the wind*
> *and sometimes against it—but we must sail, and not*
> *drift, nor lie at anchor.*
> OLIVER WENDELL HOLMES, SR

In this chapter, the authors have described the corporate culture of Sioux Valley Hospital and the manner in which the nursing department sought cultural change. The organization, as the authors have described it, remains male dominated in executive management with linear thinking in its approach to financial management. Certain changes have been effective in the shift to a new paradigm as described in this chapter, such as Integrated Clinical Pathways, work redesign, empowerment of the nurse at the bedside to facilitate clinical decision making, and enhanced interdepartmental communication. The most challenging of opportunities arises when nursing interfaces with the finance department. Sioux Valley Hospital is implementing an approach or process to integrate financial data into quality outcomes. This process will facilitate the awareness that margin is not an independent variable.

Until 1990, budgets and financial management were purely an administrative function. Budgets were calculated and negotiated at the administrative level and were handed down to the unit manager, who was allotted a specified number of full-time equivalents and directed to manage his or her nursing unit within budget guidelines and with allotted dollars. There was little or no input given by the unit manager in determining resource needs for the upcoming year. Worse yet, computer reports containing voluminous pages of numbers were periodically sent to the manager as a tool for monitoring and evaluating the impact and outcomes of ongoing decisions related to the budget. These reports provided little readily useful information unless the unit manager had the time to conduct extensive analysis.

Society has entered a health care era in which the buzz word is cost containment. Nursing managers and personnel have a heightened awareness of costs and are being held to a higher degree of accountability to perform within budget restrictions. Individuals at the point of care delivery are making decisions that have a great impact on use of human and supply resources and, therefore, dollars. Thus managers and individual employees must be given a mechanism for systematically sifting through the volumes of financial data in a way that provides insight as to the impact of day-to-day decisions on bottom line financial outcomes.

Staff at Sioux Valley Hospital had adapted well to the outcomes evaluation process used in the quality improvement program. It was believed that the same basic concepts and processes could be used to enhance staff awareness regarding fiscal matters and individual nurses' abilities to manage financial resources more effectively. The end result was the creation of a system where quality outcomes are balanced with fiscal outcomes via an ongoing monitoring and evaluation process (Figure 8–4). The program was initially called fiscal improvement. It was believed that the staff would more readily recognize the intent and process if a name similar to continuous quality improvement was adopted.

The Fiscal Improvement Planning and Development Committee, consisting of unit managers and representative clinical care coordinators, was established. The first meeting agenda consisted largely of education on financial management and dialogue related to the committee's purpose and make-up. Also, this committee identified the accountabilities for the Fiscal Improvement Council (Exhibit 8-4). Monthly meetings were held, and a charter for the committee was developed (see Chapter 7). The first task was to educate the committee members about current

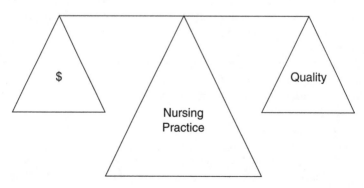

Figure 8–4 Quality and fiscal outcomes in balance.

Exhibit 8–4 Shared Governance Fiscal Improvement Council Accountabilities, 1993

---

1. To write and implement the fiscal improvement plan for nursing services provided at Sioux Valley Hospital.
2. To establish the fiscal improvement calendar for the nursing practice.*
3. To coordinate monitoring and evaluation activities using the 10-step methodology and to institute corrective action or refer to the appropriate council when such action is beyond the scope of this council.
4. To review and approve the indicators to be monitored by each practice.
5. To review and approve the composition of the fiscal improvement team.
6. To identify processes that are multidisciplinary in nature and interdepartmental teams that are formed.

*Nursing practice is broadly defined as the discipline of nursing at Sioux Valley Hospital regardless of the department in which the nursing practice is provided.

Courtesy of Sioux Valley Hospital, Sioux Falls, South Dakota.

---

hospital financial reports and management operations. Nursing management felt that everyone needed to know where Sioux Valley Hospital currently was before the process of determining where Sioux Valley Hospital wanted to be began. Committee members agreed upon a time frame for implementation of the fiscal improvement program (Exhibit 8–5).

Initial work leaned heavily toward developing consensus on a common language to be used within this program. There was consensus that the quality assurance process of continuously monitoring and evaluating outcomes would fit nicely with the goals of better cost containment. With minor revisions, all quality assurance forms were adapted to the program (see Appendices 8-H and 8-I).

A standard set of aspects of financial management and performance indicators, along with their respective thresholds, were identified. These are monitored and evaluated on a regular basis at the unit level. This is primarily a function of the management council of each nursing unit. The majority of members on the unit level management councils are clinical care coordinators, who are responsible for a large number of decisions affecting budget performance. See Appendix 8-J for a list of aspects of financial management and their performance indicators and thresholds.

The financial management monitoring and evaluation process is new. The first meetings began in the spring of 1992. Therefore, the committee is continuing to adapt the process and is facilitating its evolution into everyday operations. In the future, once staff become competent with the financial management process, the plan is to automate a number of the monitoring and evaluation functions. The ultimate goal is to provide monthly updates via computerized graphs so that trending can be communicated easily and quickly to all nursing personnel. Also, the committee plans to implement a computerized tool that has real-time impact. These computer generated "what if" programs will become the ultimate financial management decision-making tool within the organization.

Exhibit 8–5 Fiscal Improvement Committee Development Timeline

1. Conduct initial meeting and establish mission statement, purpose, and group guidelines. (May 1992)
2. Educate all members of committee about nursing budget pay period report. (June 1992)
   - Define concepts
   - Explain spreadsheet
   - Identify report auditing mechanisms
3. Develop a reporting deadline flowsheet and justification guidelines. (July 1992)
4. Start up maternal–child health and critical care divisions. (August 1992)
5. Set monitoring and evaluation targets for productivity and workload ratios. (August 1992)
6. Initiate a group reporting and sharing program. (September 1992)
7. Develop mechanisms for computerized trending and strategies for sharing this information with general nursing staff. (September 1992)
8. Educate Fiscal Improvement Committee members about nonpayroll expense concepts, calculations, monitoring, and evaluation (October 1992)
9. Educate Fiscal Improvement Committee members about income concepts, calculations, monitoring, and evaluation. (October 1992)
10. Begin education program on marketing concepts. (November 1992)
11. Develop specific unit marketing plans. (January 1993)

Courtesy of Sioux Valley Hospital, Sioux Falls, South Dakota.

The corporate environment at Sioux Valley Hospital continues to change, much as an amoeba writhing its way through fluid. More and more employees at every level of the organization are taking personal responsibility for the success of the organization. People want to make a commitment as long as they have the freedom and environment to do so. Sioux Valley Hospital nurses believe that it is not authority that produces results but rather the collective decision making that has been exemplified in this chapter.

REFERENCES

1. *Ecology of Excellence: A Balanced ECOsystem for Business Performance.* Educational Professional Services; 1987.
2. Senge PM. *The Fifth Discipline.* New York, NY: Doubleday/Currency; 1990.
3. Naisbitt J, Aburdene P. *Reinventing the Corporation.* New York, NY: Warner; 1985.
4. Ferguson SD, Ferguson S, eds. *Organizational Communication.* New Brunswick, NJ: Transaction; 1988.
5. Helgesen S. *The Female Advantage: Women's Ways of Leadership.* New York, NY: Doubleday/Currency; 1990.

6. Nursing Practice of Sioux Valley Hospital. *Sioux Valley Hospital Department of Nursing Conceptual Framework and Strategic Plan.* Sioux Falls, SD: Sioux Valley Hospital; 1990.

7. Naisbitt J. *Megatrends: Ten New Directions Transforming Our Lives.* New York, NY: Warner; 1982.

8. Eisler R. *The Chalice and the Blade: Our History, Our Future.* San Francisco, Calif: Harper & Row; 1988.

9. Naisbitt J, Aburdene P. *Megatrends for Women.* New York, NY: Villard; 1992.

10. Peters T, Waterman R. *In Search of Excellence: Lessons from America's Best Run Companies.* New York, NY: Warner; 1982.

11. McManis GL. Challenges of a new decade demand break with tradition. *Mod Healthcare.* 1990;20(1):60.

12. Anthony RN, Young DW. The control structure. In: *Management Control in Non-Profit Organizations.* New York, NY: Prentice-Hall; 1984:233–280.

13. Bedford NM. Managerial control. In: McGuire JW, ed. *Contemporary Management: Issues and Viewpoints.* New York, NY: Prentice-Hall; 1974:507–521.

14. Deal T, Kennedy A. *Corporate Cultures: The Rites and Rituals of Corporate Life.* Reading, Pa: Addison-Wesley; 1982.

15. Etheridge MLS. Definition, the center for nursing case management. *Collab Care Nurs Case Manag.* 1989;2(3):4.

EXERCISE 8-1: PULSE EXERCISE

Definition: This is a quick method to determine the scope of an issue, to determine the extent of a problem/concern, or to get feedback from the staff involved with an issue. The goal of a pulse is to provide one or two pieces of information, not to resolve the problem.

Steps:

1. Identify the group that is affected by the issue. This could be a staff or customer group.
2. List one or two questions specific to the problem or issue to be studied. A pulse question should take about 1 minute to answer. Make your questions specific. Examples:

Issue	*Pulse Question*
There are not sufficient supplies stored on the unit.	On this shift, did the shelf supply of intravenous tubing become depleted?
Patient lights are not being answered quickly.	What is the average time you have had to wait for a nurse to answer your patient call light?

3. Prepare a form to record responses to the question(s).
4. Identify a group of staff to ask the pulse question(s). Instruct the group to ask the questions as they are written.
5. Staff should perform the pulse during the same time period.
6. Summarize results.

Appendix 8-A
Sioux Valley Hospital Dakota EDGE
(Employees Delivering Grassroots Excellence)
Action Council Bylaws

PREAMBLE

The Action Council is a facilitating body established to enhance the quality of work life and business performance of the organization. The council will give guidance and recommendations on issues of Dakota EDGE and will serve as a clearinghouse for matters of the practice. It will not preempt the formal lines of responsibility, being legally bound by all operational policies and procedures of the parent organization.

NAME

The Action Council is the name given to the body of partners elected by their peers to represent their interests in the new business environment at Sioux Valley Hospital.

PURPOSE

1. To serve as a clearinghouse for the collection, categorization, and distribution of information pertinent to the business of Dakota EDGE.
2. To coordinate the general activities of the various enterprises that serve as parts of Dakota EDGE.
3. To coordinate the study by partners of ways to improve the cost effectiveness of venture operations.
4. To provide a systematic conduit for the exchange and resolution of issues between executive management and other partners.
5. To encourage the continuation of present intradepartmental and interdepartmental issue resolution by using the ECO process.

6. To advise partners by reviewing issues and referring to appropriate resources with monitoring of progress toward resolution.

MEMBERSHIP

1. Because the Action Council represents partners throughout the hospital, the membership will consist of elected partners from departments within areas of vice presidential responsibility and two ex officio members appointed by the executive vice president.
2. Representatives will be elected from the following vice presidential areas;
   - executive vice president—one (includes external operations and human resources)
   - administrative services—three
   - professional services—three
   - finance—two
   - patient services—four
   - ex officio members—two

   Each representative will have an elected alternate.
3. To be elected, representatives and alternates should have the following qualifications:
   - completed ECO training
   - active in activities in Dakota EDGE
   - Full- or part-time employee
4. Vice presidential areas that do not have qualified candidates will be left vacant until the next election.
5. Each representative and alternate shall serve a 1-year term and shall be elected either in the spring or fall, so that all members' terms shall overlap by 6 months to help ensure continuity of representation. Elections for these terms shall be in December and June of each year, with appointments to begin in January or July.
6. Responsibilities of representatives or alternates shall include:
   - attendance at all meetings of the council for the duration of their term using the following criteria:
     — in the event that an absence is necessary, the representative is responsible for arranging the alternate's attendance at that particular meeting
     — absences due to emergencies, illness, or planned vacation will be excused; representatives still need to arrange an alternate for missed meetings whenever possible

— two unexcused absences per 6 months are grounds for suspension from the council, in which case the department affected must elect a new representative to serve the remainder of the term involved

— any area not represented at a council meeting will be subject to any decisions made in its absence

- communication of council decisions to the area represented
- provision of feedback and awareness of council issues and how peer constituents view and/or might be affected by these
- assumption of their share of any subcommittee or task force responsibilities related to the work of the council
- advocacy and support of council decisions to all hospital staff

7. Each representative shall carry one vote on actions considered by the council. In the event that an alternate will need to be present, the alternate will assume all rights and responsibilities of the representative relating to voting procedure.

8. Each representative shall serve no longer than two full terms. He or she may be reelected to the council after a 6-month period away. Anyone elected to serve the remainder of another representative's term may be elected to serve one immediately successive term. (Exception: Any area where the number of eligible staff will not allow this criterion to be met will be exempt from the stipulation.)

   Terms as alternate will not affect one's possibility of becoming a representative.

9. Alternates have the responsibility to be aware of Action Council activities through communication with the representative.

OFFICERS AND RESPONSIBILITIES

1. Chair—shall be elected from among the council representatives for a 1-year term. The representative's position vacated by the chair shall be filled through election of another person from the affected department for the duration of the term involved. This election shall immediately follow the election of the chair so that the new representative can take office at the appropriate time. Elections for chair shall be in December to take office in January.

   Duties shall be as follows:

   - to chair all meetings of the council
   - to develop an agenda for distribution at least 1 week before regular meetings of the council
   - can appoint ad hoc committees as necessary

2. Vice chair—Shall be elected from among the council representatives for a 1-year term.

   Elections for vice chair shall be in December to take office in January.

   Duties shall be to chair meetings in the absence of the chair.

3. Secretary—Hospital administration shall appoint a support person for this position from outside the council membership.

   Duties shall be as follows:

   • to record, type, and distribute minutes to council members, alternates, each department, and administration within 1 week of the meeting date
   • to post a copy of the minutes in the Dakota EDGE venture room
   • to maintain attendance records, election dates, and absence information about all council members

4. Administrative/management representatives—Will serve as ex officio voting members of the council to provide advice and counsel from the administrative perspective and to lend support to the activities of the council when needed.

   • The administrative/management representatives will be appointed by the executive vice president to serve for 1 year on a rotating basis every 6 months. Appointment will be made in December and June of each year; terms will begin in January and July.
   • The administrative/management representatives shall have the following qualifications:
     — completed ECO training
     — active in Dakota EDGE activities
     — hold an administrative/management position

MEETINGS

1. Regular meetings of the council:

   • Frequency and times of regular council meetings shall be established or confirmed each year by a two-thirds vote of the members in January.
   • Any changes to the meeting schedule must be communicated by the chair to the council members.
   • The quorum necessary to conduct business of the council is a simple majority of all representatives.
   • Duration of regular meetings shall be limited to 1 hour.
   • Each regular meeting agenda shall include at least a review of the six items under "Purpose," above.

- All meetings will be open to all partners. Those who wish to address an issue on the agenda may participate in the discussion surrounding the issues by following *Robert's New Rules of Order.*

2. Special meetings of the council:
   - Special meetings of the council may be called by a two-thirds vote of all council members, by the chair, or by hospital administration.
   - At least 48 hours advance notice is required for special meetings of the council.

3. Parliamentary procedure:
   - The council shall follow procedural guidelines of the current edition of *Robert's New Rules of Order.*

STANDING OR SPECIAL COMMITTEES

1. The chair of the Action Council may appoint, from time to time, standing or special committees for the purposes compatible with the objectives of the Action Council. All committees so appointed shall have a majority of their membership composed of Ecology of Excellence members. The chair shall be a member of the Action Council.

2. Standing committees of the Action Council:
   - Issue Development Committee:
     — Membership includes three members of the Action Council appointed by the Action Council chair.
     — Membership includes chairs from each of the enterprises.
     — The Action Council chair will act as an ex officio member.
     — The chair of the Issue Development Committee will be one of the Action Council members.
     — The purpose of the Issue Development Committee is to set the format of the issue and to assist with development, refinement, and completion of the issue.
     — Issues must be completed in compliance with the Action Council bylaws. They will then be directed to the Action Council.
     — The Issue Development Committee will develop the format for executing the issue.
     — The Issue Development Committee will meet the second and fourth Wednesday of each month at 1500 hours in the Dakota EDGE venture room.

- Information Enterprise:
  — The objective of the Information Enterprise is to collect and disseminate facts and events associated with Dakota EDGE and the business activities of the organization.
  — The Information Enterprise meets the fourth Tuesday of each month at 1400 hours.
- People Enterprise:
  — The objective of the People Enterprise is to enhance the quality of work life through mentoring employees in the growth process and negotiating solutions based on balancing workforce needs and organizational resources.
  — The People Enterprise meets the second Thursday of each month at 1230 hours.

VOTING

1. On issues other than bylaws and meetings, actions may be accepted or rejected by a simple majority.
2. See "Amendments to the Bylaws," below, and "Meetings," above.

AMENDMENTS TO THE BYLAWS

Bylaws of the Action Council may be amended as follows:

1. by two-thirds vote of eligible voters present on amendments published at least thirty (30) days before the vote
2. by unanimous vote of eligible voters present of amendments considered without prior notice

ELECTION PROCESS FOR REPRESENTATIVES ON THE ACTION COUNCIL

1. The Action Council chair will select two partners to act as a nominating committee from each area defined in "Membership," item 2, above.
2. The nominating committee will prepare a ballot that contains open positions from each area as defined in "Membership," item 2, above.
3. Any staff member may place his or her name on the ballot for election.

4. The nominees should have the qualifications defined in "Membership," item 3, above.

5. The nominee must be willing to commit and serve in this position for 1 year and approve placement of his or her name on the ballot.

6. The nominating committee is responsible for the balloting process.

7. The election shall take place the first week of December and the first week of June.

8. The slate of nominees will be posted 2 weeks before the election:
   - Balloting will take place in each area via secret ballot, and ballots will be monitored by the nominating committee or a designated person.

9. All staff members will be entitled to one ballot.

10. A single majority of ballots cast will decide the election.

11. Campaigning is allowed.

12. In the event of a tie, another balloting will take place between the tying candidates.

OTHER

Institutional grievances, wage negotiations, hours, and terms or conditions of employment are not governed by the Action Council.

Courtesy of Sioux Valley Hospital, Sioux Falls, South Dakota.

Appendix 8-B
DRG 410: Chemotherapy Administration
Option 1

Date	Admit 1	Discharge 2	DRG LOS 2.6
TEACHING	-Reinforcement/new chemo tx -Emotional/family support -Side effects (stomatitis; nutrition, pain, constipation)		
DISCHARGE PLANNING	-Discuss/confirm home arrangements -Stress imp of post D/C lab work	Home	
NUTRITION	-Diet as tolerated -Offer foods of choice when desired; frequent small meals		
PHYSICAL ACTIVITY	-Up as tolerated -Encourage BRP -Up in chair for meals		

MEDS
IV
	-IV start-Carafate 1 gm AC
	-Begin chemo drip/-Decadron 4mg BID
	  IV push chemo meds-Zantac 150 HS
	-Treat side effects as occur: N/V
	-Monitor drip rate to insure appropriate D/C time;
	  consult Dr to increase rate as needed
		DC IV	

TESTS	-CBC, chem 1, O2 sat., UA, PT, PTT -CXR, nonfasting 12P, Tumor marker		
TREATMENT	-Daily weight -I/O-TED hose -Routine vital signs -Routine nsg assessment		
PRIORITY NURSING DIAGNOSIS	-Knowledge deficit -Coping -Pain -Inadequate nutrition -Constipation		

Courtesy of Sioux Valley Hospital, Sioux Falls, South Dakota.

Appendix 8-C
DRG 410: Chemotherapy Administration
Option 2

Date	Admit 1	Discharge 2	DRG LOS 2.6
TEACHING	-Reinforcement/new chemo tx -Emotional/family support -Side effects (stomatitis; nutrition, pain, constipation)		
DISCHARGE PLANNING	-Discuss/confirm home arrangements -Stress imp of post D/C lab work	Home	
NUTRITION	-Diet as tolerated -Offer foods of choice when desired; frequent small meals		
PHYSICAL ACTIVITY	-Up as tolerated -Encourage BRP -Up in chair for meals		

MEDS IV	-IV start
	-Begin chemo drip
	  IV push chemo meds
	-Treat side effects as occur: N/V
	-Monitor drip rate to insure appropriate D/C time;
	  consult Dr to increase rate as needed
		DC IV	

TESTS	-CBC, chem 1 -CXR, nonfasting 12P		
TREATMENT	-Daily weight -I/O -Routine vital signs -Routine nsg assessment		
PRIORITY NURSING DIAGNOSIS	-Knowledge deficit -Coping -Pain -Inadequate nutrition -Constipation		

Courtesy of Sioux Valley Hospital, Sioux Falls, South Dakota.

Appendix 8-D
DRG 410: Chemotherapy Administration Option 3

Date	Admit 1	Discharge 2	DRG LOS 2.6
TEACHING	-Reinforcement/new chemo tx -Emotional/family support -Side effects (stomatitis; nutrition, pain, constipation)		
DISCHARGE PLANNING	-Discuss/confirm home arrangements -Stress imp of post D/C lab work	Home	
NUTRITION	-Diet as tolerated -Offer foods of choice when desired; frequent small meals		
PHYSICAL ACTIVITY	-Up as tolerated -Encourage BRP -Up in chair for meals		

MEDS
IV
	-IV start
	-Begin chemo drip
	  IV push chemo meds
	-Treat side effects as occur: N/V
	-Monitor drip rate to insure appropriate D/C time;
	  consult Dr to increase rate as needed
		DC IV	

TESTS			
TREATMENT	-Daily weight -I/O -Routine vital signs -Routine nsg assessment		
PRIORITY NURSING DIAGNOSIS	-Knowledge deficit -Coping -Pain -Inadequate nutrition -Constipation		

Courtesy of Sioux Valley Hospital, Sioux Falls, South Dakota.

Appendix 8-E
DRG 410: Chemotherapy Administration
Option 4

	Admit 1	2	3	DRG LOS 2.6 Discharge 4
Date				
TEACHING	-Reinforcement/new chemo tx -Emotional/family support -Side effects (stomatitis; nutrition, pain, constipation)			
DISCHARGE PLANNING	-Discuss home arrangements		-Confirm home arrange; -Stress imp of post D/C lab work	Home
NUTRITION	-Diet as tolerated -Offer foods of choice when desired; frequent small meals			
PHYSICAL ACTIVITY	-Up as tolerated -Encourage BRP -Up in chair for meals			
MEDS IV	-IV start-Carafate 1 gm AC -Begin chemo drip/Decadron 4 mg BID IV push chemo meds- Zantac 150 mg HS -5000 u subq heparin BID -Pericolace BID, Mylanta 30cc BID -Sinequan 1 gm AC	Treat side effects as occur: N/V Monitor drip rate to insure approp D/C time; consult Dr to increase rate as needed		DCIV

| TESTS | -CBC, chem 1
-CXR, nonfasting 12P
-O2 sat, UA
-PT, PTT
-Tumor marker | BS | -Chem 1
-BS, PT | BS |

| TREATMENT | -Daily weight
-I/O-Ted hose
-Routine vital signs
-Routine nsg assessment |

| PRIORITY
NURSING
DIAGNOSIS | -Knowledge deficit
-Coping
-Pain
-Inadequate nutrition
-Constipation |

Courtesy of Sioux Valley Hospital, Sioux Falls, South Dakota.

Appendix 8-F
DRG 410: Chemotherapy Administration
Option 5

DRG LOS 2.6

Date	Admit 1	2	3	Discharge 4
TEACHING	-Reinforcement/new chemo tx -Emotional/family support -Side effects (stomatitis; nutrition, pain, constipation)			
DISCHARGE PLANNING	-Discuss home arrangements		-Confirm home arrange; -Stress imp of post D/C lab work	Home
NUTRITION	-Diet as tolerated -Offer foods of choice when desired; frequent small meals			
PHYSICAL ACTIVITY	-Up as tolerated -Encourage BRP -Up in chair for meals			
MEDS IV	-IV start -Begin chemo drip -IV push chemo meds	Treat side effects as occur: N/V Monitor drip rate to insure approp D/C time; consult Dr to increase rate as needed		DCIV
TESTS	-CBC, chem 1 -CXR, nonfasting 12P			

TREATMENT	-Daily weight
	-I/O
	-Routine vital signs
	-Routine nsg assessment
PRIORITY NURSING DIAGNOSIS	-Knowledge deficit
	-Coping
	-Pain
	-Inadequate nutrition
	-Constipation

Courtesy of Sioux Valley Hospital, Sioux Falls, South Dakota.

Appendix 8-G
DRG 410: Chemotherapy Administration Option 6

Date	Admit 1	2	3	DRG LOS 2.6 Discharge 4
TEACHING	-Reinforcement/new chemo tx -Emotional/family support -Side effects (stomatitis; nutrition, pain, constipation)			
DISCHARGE PLANNING	-Discuss home arrangements		-Confirm home arrange; -Stress imp of post D/C lab work	Home
NUTRITION	-Diet as tolerated -Offer foods of choice when desired; frequent small meals			
PHYSICAL ACTIVITY	-Up as tolerated -Encourage BRP -Up in chair for meals			
MEDS IV	-IV start -Begin chemo drip -IV push chemo meds	Treat side effects as occur: N/V Monitor drip rate to insure approp D/C time; consult Dr to increase rate as needed		DCIV
TESTS				

TREATMENT	-Daily weight
	-I/O
	-Routine vital signs
	-Routine nsg assessment
PRIORITY NURSING DIAGNOSIS	-Knowledge deficit
	-Coping
	-Pain
	-Inadequate nutrition
	-Constipation

Courtesy of Sioux Valley Hospital, Sioux Falls, South Dakota.

Appendix 8-H
Continuous Fiscal Improvement Report:
Ongoing Monitoring and Evaluation
Monitoring Tool

Department _____ Year ____	Aspect of Fiscal Management _____ Data Collection _____		
	Indicators	Thresh-old	Fre-quency

Follow-up
Improvement/Integration/Communication

Action

Evaluation

Problem Cause

System

Behavior

Knowledge

Courtesy of Sioux Valley Hospital, Sioux Falls, South Dakota.

Appendix 8-I
Continuous Fiscal Improvement:
Ongoing Monitoring and Evaluation Standards

Department _____

Date Submitted _____

Aspects of Fiscal Management	Indicators	Threshold	Data Collection

Evaluation	Problem Cause System Behavior Knowledge	Action	Follow-up Improvement/Integration/ Communication

Courtesy of Sioux Valley Hospital, Sioux Falls, South Dakota.

Appendix 8-J
Aspects of Financial Management

1. Volume
2. Workload
3. Expenses
4. Productivity
5. Human resource management

PERFORMANCE INDICATORS

1. Volume indicators
   - Patient days
   - Discharges
   - Admissions
   - Acuity
   - Transfers
2. Workload indicators
   - Acuity per patient days
   - Acuity per discharges
3. Expense indicators
   - Supply
     — Supply expense per patient day (SEPD)
     — Supply expense per discharge (SEDIS)
   - Payroll
     — Payroll expense per total hours (PETH)
     — Payroll expense per patient day (PEPD)
     — Payroll expense per discharge (PEDIS)
4. Productivity indicators
   - Total hours (TH)
   - Productive hours (PH)
   - Productive hours–indirect (PH-I)

- Total hours per patient day (THPD)
- Productive hours per patient day (PHPD)
- Productive hours per discharge (PHDIS)
- Productive hours–indirect per patient day (PH-IPD)
- Productive hours–indirect per discharge (PH-IDIS)
- Acuity points per productive hour–indirect (APPH-I)
5. Human resource indicators
   - Productive hours per total hours (PHPTH)
   - Productive hours–indirect per total hours (PH-IPTH)
   - Sick hours per total hours (SHTH)
   - Undertime per total hours (UTTH)
   - Convenience time per total hours (CTTH)
   - Convenience time ratio (CTR)
   - Meeting time per full-time equivalent (MTFTE)
   - FTEs
   - Vacancies
   - Vacancy rate
   - Orientation costs
   - Education costs
   - Length of stay (LOS)

THRESHOLDS

Volume Indicators

Patient days	$0.95 \times$ budget
Discharges	$0.95 \times$ year to date (YTD) – number of months
Admissions	$0.95 \times$ YTD – number of months
Acuity	None

Workload Indicators

$$\frac{\text{Acuity per patient day (YTD acuity – number of pay periods) } (26 - 12)}{\text{Patient days}} \times 0.95 \text{ or } 1.05$$

$$\frac{\text{Acuity per discharge (YTD acuity – number of pay periods) } (26 - 12)}{\text{Pay period}} \times 0.95 \text{ or } 1.05$$

Expense Indicators

SEPD	1.05
SEDIS	1.05
PETH	1.05
PEPD	1.05
PEDIS	1.05

FINANCIAL ACCOUNTABILITY THRESHOLD CALCULATION (PERFORM ANNUALLY IN MAY)

Indicators*	Threshold	Frequency
Volume indicators		
Patient days	(Current pay period budget) ± 10%	Pay period
Discharges	(Prev annual dis ÷ 12) ± 10%	Month
Admissions	(Prev annual adm ÷ 12) ± 10%	Month
Acuity	(Prev annual acuity ÷ 26) ± 10%	Pay period
Workload indicators		
Acuity per PD	(Prev annual total acuity) ± 3%	Pay period
	(Prev annual PD)	
Acuity per discharge	(Prev annual total acuity) ± 3%	Month
or admission	(Prev annual dis or adm)	
Expense indicators	±5% of previous annual ratio	Month
SEPD		
SEDIS		
PETH		
PEPD		
PEDIS		

*It is mandatory to trend all indicators on all units. Exception: Total acuity and admissions or discharges, not both.

Courtesy of Sioux Valley Hospital, Sioux Falls, South Dakota.

Volume Analysis Worksheet

INDICATOR _____

UNIT _____
FY _____

	JAN	FEB	MAR	APR	MAY	JUNE	JULY	AUG	SEPT	OCT	NOV	DEC	TOTAL
19__													
19__													
19__													
19__													
19__													
TOTAL													
AVE													
0.95%													

Courtesy of Sioux Valley Hospital, Sioux Falls, South Dakota.

Expense Analysis Worksheet

UNIT _____

MONTH _____

A. Patient days _____   F. SEPD (E ÷ A) _____

B. Total hours _____   G. SEDIS (E ÷ C) _____

C. Total discharges _____   H. PETH (D ÷ B) _____

D. Total payroll expense _____   I.   PEPD (D ÷ A) _____

E. Total supply expense _____   J. PEDIS (D ÷ C) _____

Courtesy of Sioux Valley Hospital, Sioux Falls, South Dakota.

9 Compensation

Eloise Baker, Shari Aman, Roxanne Dietz, and Doreen S. Miller

> *Life is a series of experiences, each one of which makes us bigger, even though some times it is hard to realize this.*
>
> HENRY FORD

Upon embarking on the process of developing a professional nursing practice through differentiated practice and establishing a shared governance system, the community of nurses at Sioux Valley Hospital was aware of some of the potential benefits it would receive. These benefits served as motivation for the nurses who were participating. The vision also included benefits for others in the organization. Potential benefits were identified for the physicians, the patients, the institution, and the community. Not everyone was aware of the vision or the process that was evolving. They were to be passive recipients of the benefits of a professional nursing practice.

Beneficiaries can be identified as anyone receiving benefits or anyone identified to receive proceeds or benefits. Compensation is defined as payment, remuneration, and counterbalance; to supply an equivalent; or to neutralize the effect of some action. Each group and individual received benefits, or compensation, in a different form. This chapter describes the beneficiaries and their compensations.

Employees usually see compensation as payment in the form of money or benefits in return for their time and efforts. Compensation also can be received in other forms. One can receive an emotional reward for engaging in an activity. Being granted a privilege of some kind can also be viewed as compensation, as can self-fulfillment, self-esteem, or anything seen as valuable to the recipient. Difficulty can arise when the beneficiary of compensation believes the reward is insufficient for the effort required or when the beneficiary does not value the compensation he or she will receive. When there is a lack of motivation to complete the activity being requested, the one who is offering the compensation must change either the requirements or the compensation to create motivation in the beneficiary.

Not all nurses and other organization members were aware of the vision of a professional nursing practice. Some of those who were aware did not value the vision. Therefore, there were various degrees of motivation to participate in the process. It was apparent from our experience that in the process of change, approximately 20% of individuals in our nursing practice valued the vision for change, 60% were indifferent, and 20% did not value the vision for change. It was imperative to create a critical mass of those who valued the vision by motivating the 60% who were indifferent regarding the vision. By addressing the nurses as beneficiaries who would be compensated for their efforts, this critical mass was established. The compensation that was identified took the form of authority, autonomy, and control or accountability for their professional practice. When this was achieved, the beneficiary was empowered.

SYSTEMS THEORY

Systems theory describes how an organization processes information, energy, or matter to effect an outcome. The system is always striving toward equilibrium. Organizations are complex systems with boundaries and interrelated parts through which energy, matter, and information flow in the form of input, throughput, output, and feedback. For a more detailed description of systems theory, refer to Figure 7–3.

Systems theory can be applied to the concept of compensation as it relates to the experience of differentiated practice and developing a shared governance system (Figure 9–1). In this situation the beneficiaries identified earlier are input to the system, as is the vision provided by the vice president of patient services. The vision is described in more detail later. The throughput, or the process, is threefold: implementing differentiated practice, developing a shared governance system, and establishing the nurse/patient/physician triad. The output is described globally as the empowerment that comes to all individuals as a result of the processes through the compensations received.

Internal factors are characteristics of the organization and the individuals involved that affect the process in some way, positively or negatively. In this situation, the culture of the organization, which had always been that of a traditional or authoritarian management style, was an internal factor. Communication and decision-making patterns were well established from the top administrators and flowed down the organizational hierarchy. Of the individuals identified as input, only the nurses were directly associated in the process of developing a shared governance system. In light of systems theory, ultimately all individuals in the organization were affected in some way as the system reestablished equilibrium.

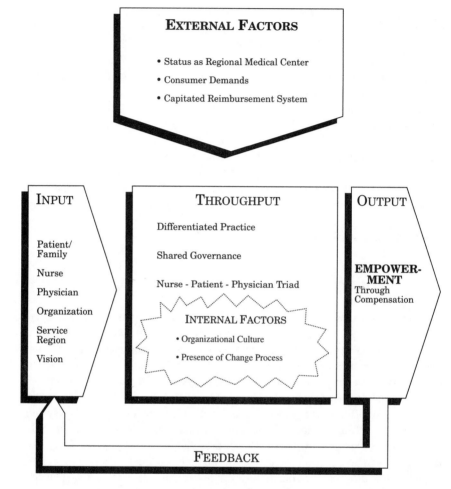

Figure 9–1 Systems theory applied to differentiated practice and the development of shared governance.

Another internal factor was the presence of the change process. Individuals and groups were at different stages of unfreezing, moving, and refreezing. This produced an environment displaying various levels of acceptance, motivation, and action. Inherent in this type of environment are differing views of adequate compensation. These factors must be considered when one is evaluating the system of empowerment through compensation.

External factors are characteristics of the environment in which the organization and individuals involved exist. The organization was viewed as a regional medical center serving portions of three states. It was seen as a progressive hospital and was expected to be on the cutting edge of service and treatment. The consumers utilizing the services were becoming more aware of their rights as consumers and of the need to control health care costs. The consumer was also demanding an ever increasing quality of health care, usually defined by technology. The organization was experiencing the effects of a capitated reimbursement system through the diagnosis-related group system and anticipated further restrictions from other payer sources. The health care environment was changing.

> *A vision without a task is a dream;*
> *A task without vision is drudgery;*
> *A vision and a task is the hope of the world.*
>   AUTHOR UNKNOWN

CREATING THE VISION

Differentiated practice is not only redefining tasks that are done by various people but also redefining the vision that guides these people. Creating vision is the process of determining an outcome, inspiring others, and creating a plan to implement change. Change may focus on different aspects of practice, such as quality patient care, patient satisfaction, or financial accountability. The vision is critical to the success of the change. Before deciding to take on a project such as this, the organization needs to decide on which aspect it is most crucial to focus.

Having vision serves different purposes. It gives a place to begin and allows people to discuss how they feel about patient care and practice issues. It also establishes where they would like to see change occur. Having a vision also serves to guide people through the process, gives direction to decision making, and provides strength when energy begins to dwindle. Eventually, the vision can also be used to actualize and measure progress and to create a sense of accomplishment.

The process of creating a vision is initiated by an individual or group, but it should include all who will be involved in the process. The ability to begin this process is strengthened by creating vision at the staff nurse level with support at the administrative level. Those who create the vision will ensure its success for this reason alone. Staff members are an integral part of forming a vision because the efforts of a critical mass are necessary to ensure success.

Once vision has been created, all must remain committed to it. This commitment is essential to maintain momentum throughout the process. Vision will change as time passes, so that in fact the vision is not as important as support and commitment. A motto in our change process was "Maintain the vision, but embrace the hybrid." We knew that as people adopted the vision it would be adopted based on unique aspects of practice on the various nursing units.

BENEFICIARIES: PATIENT AND FAMILY

Differentiation of practice significantly affects interaction among the nurse, patient, and family. Great potential exists to improve the delivery of care, which affects both quality of care and patient satisfaction. The outcome is compensation in the form of continuity of care, patient advocacy, participative care, nursing accountability, and cost containment for the patient and family.

Continuity of care is an issue that is significantly affected by length of stay and staffing patterns. Most patients see multiple nurses during their hospitalization. Patients are rarely assigned to the same nurse more than once. Lack of or poor communication and lack of follow-through with care planning may occur. Managing care can provide a greater sense of continuity, allowing the patient and family to feel that care is directed by a specific individual with whom they have the opportunity to develop a relationship and rapport (see Chapter 5).

Under a managed care system, patients and families experience care as organized and directed rather than as a hit-or-miss system that sometimes works and sometimes does not. The complexity of patient and family needs that are often identified and the number of individuals involved to meet these needs necessitate that one individual organize and direct activities. Before differentiated practice, patients and families occasionally fell through the cracks of the system because of lack of continuity and ambiguous role responsibilities. The role of the primary nurse was developed to address this issue. Continuity of care, patient advocacy, and care planning are integral pieces of the primary nurse role. This role clearly enhanced quality discharge planning, affecting long-term outcomes for both patient and family.

Because of the vision for differentiated practice, greater emphasis was placed on participative care. True participative care places the patient and family at the center of all activity and decision making, with most of the dialogue related to this occurring at the bedside. In addition to making participative care an expectation, the primary nurses were held accountable to ensure that patients and families were totally involved in all aspects of care. There was little doubt that doing this positively affected quality patient care and certainly patient and family satisfaction. There were multiple indicators and various ways that this was measured, such as increased discharge referrals, more interdisciplinary consultations, increased patient and nurse satisfaction, and improved care planning.

Patient perception of care and support by nursing staff was heightened by patient-centered care. Differentiated practice is designed to affect the way all staff relate to patients and families. It is often the subtle change in role responsibilities that begins to alter each nurse's beliefs and philosophy. Elevating the level of accountability affects patient outcomes and is the key to making a rewarding and satisfying role. The degree of a patient's perception of the change in quality of care depends on everyone adapting to a new set of norms and responsibilities. Patients who received care under this managed care system readily identified that they not only had received care but were cared about. It was possible to measure the patients' satisfaction under a managed care system.

One such study was conducted. Twenty-five patients from the postpartum unit completed a survey. They were asked to indicate whether they felt that primary nursing care improved their quality of care. One hundred percent of the patients believed that the quality of care was enhanced by primary nursing. Further data were collected utilizing patient questionnaires before and after implementation of differentiated practice, giving baseline data to use for future reference. These data also conveyed to staff that their efforts had made a difference.

From the nurse's perspective, a different level of accountability to both patient and family was actualized. Both groups had a greater level of accountability. Accountability relates to two key outcomes: quality of care and patient satisfaction. The primary nurse moved one step further and assumed greater accountability for groups as well as for individuals. These nurses looked beyond the individual patient assignment with a broader systems perspective. All who entered this role knew in advance that accountabilities as well as job responsibilities had enlarged. It was possible to identify whether these accountabilities were being met through anecdotal evidence, review of nursing documentation in the medical record, and performance appraisals.

Managed care also affected cost containment, primarily by decreasing patient length of stay. Discharge planning was not left until the day of discharge. The patient, family, and physician were aware of the plan well in advance. Integrated Clinical Pathways also aided in this process by serving as a map to guide expected and usual care and to define expected outcomes. It is important to note that decreasing length of stay can be accomplished successfully and without adversely affecting patient satisfaction if it is organized. Planning was enhanced by having a designated individual provide consistent guidance and direction, leading to an integrated and timely discharge. Managed care was achieved by involving the patient and physician in the discharge plan early in the hospitalization. Differentiated practice is one system that organizes care in such a fashion.

Our experience demonstrated that managed care can potentially decrease patient complications through the early identification of problems and timely intervention. The primary nurse can be instrumental in preventing duplication of services and delays in communication and can become a patient advocate. Outcomes, as mentioned above, should be monitored and evaluated. This monitoring and evaluation will provide direction as change occurs and affirmation to staff of the successes they have accomplished.

> *The mightiest works have been accomplished by*
> *[people] who have somehow kept their ability to*
> *dream great dreams.*
> WALTER RUSSELL BOWIE

BENEFICIARY: THE NURSE

The amount of compensation the nurse received in moving to this differentiated practice delivery system was directly proportional to the level of involvement undertaken. In the same way, the ability to realize the vision was a tremendously motivating factor toward achievement of goals only imagined previously.

For the nurses who became involved in the process of differentiated practice, there were rewards not envisioned at the onset. Nurses willing to take the risk viewed applying for the differentiated roles as a professional opportunity. The specific opportunities that became available were unknown early in the process, but once the nurse was involved they became evident.

In differentiating roles, nurses have the opportunity to choose which role will offer the most satisfaction. Although the responsibilities of the roles overlap slightly, each role has different and unique goals. The associate nurse plans and provides hands-on patient care on a shift-to-shift basis. The primary nurse manages and plans care for patients and families in the specific caseload while patients stay on the unit. The clinical care coordinator manages the unit environment on a shift-to-shift basis through human and material resource allocation and bed utilization. The clinical care coordinator also assists the associate nurse in providing quality care through crisis intervention and serves as a clinical resource. See the job descriptions in Appendices 4-A to 4-C.

As each role was developed, the individual nurse attained a greater level of autonomy. This autonomy became a benefit. Associate nurses acquired the autonomy to provide hands-on care in a manner that best met the patients' needs during that shift. In the primary nurse role, autonomy was realized through the ability to individualize the patient's plan of care throughout the episode of illness. The primary nurse had the opportunity to teach both patient and family, to encourage progress toward goals on a daily basis, and to serve as a consistent caregiver for the patient and family. Autonomy allowed nurses in this role to develop subspecialties focusing on a specific patient population. The primary nurse had become an expert clinical resource person in a chosen area of interest. Clinical care coordinators gained legitimate autonomy to assign nurses to patients in a manner that met the needs of both nurse and patient. The clinical care coordinator also had the autonomy to change patient assignments as the unit's environment changed.

Besides role-related autonomy, all nurses under a shared governance system gained the autonomy to influence change in their practice through the council structure. At Sioux Valley Hospital, nurses now collectively decide how they will practice within the guidelines of the profession and institution. Because of increased autonomy, nurses tend to value each role within the practice. It is expected in a shared governance system that one will honestly and openly voice one's ideas, opinions, and reactions regarding nursing practice to fellow nurses in a council setting that fosters trust and openness. Long-term answers are developed on issues that guide and impede professional practice.

One of the most rewarding benefits nurses received was emotional compensation through patient and family satisfaction. Nothing can make a nurse feel better about his or her contribution to the profession than a patient expressing thanks and appreciation for the care and concern received during the hospital stay. Patient expression of satisfaction is an immediate and direct reward for one's efforts, as opposed to delayed compensation such as money or peer recognition. Nurses were compensated also through physician satisfaction. Although physicians were passive players in the move to differentiated practice, their satisfaction was one of the goals identified in the vision.

Throughout the process of implementing differentiated practice, physicians were educated to the responsibilities of each nursing role. The physicians' trust and respect for nurses have evolved to a higher level since continuity of care has been enhanced. A collaborative practice between physicians and nurses is a result of having one nurse provide consistent, trended information to the physician on a day-to-day basis. The primary nurse is viewed as helpful for physicians' partners who are not as familiar with the patient's history. The primary nurse can relate the patient's history, response to treatment, and progress toward goals, preventing interruption in the flow of care or duplication of services.

Naturally, not all physicians bought into the concept of differentiated practice. The nurses focused their energy on enhancing the satisfaction of those physicians who realized the benefits of differentiated nursing practice. As the benefits were displayed, other physicians became aware of the positive impact of this process. Valuing each other's role is a major step toward a collaborative practice. Increased collaboration has been a major benefit to all the players affected by differentiated practice. Patients, families, nurses, physicians, and ancillary staff are compensated through improved communication and increased trust. The patient views himself or herself as important and cared about when all professionals involved in care take time to implement mutually determined goals. This level of collaboration ensures that all caregivers are informed and accountable for the actualization of goals.

Unit individualization of roles was one benefit of differentiated practice realized during the process. Although the general expectations and responsibilities of differentiated roles are the same housewide, the day-to-day practice of each role is operationalized differently from unit to unit. Because of vastly different patient populations, nurses were granted, and have utilized, autonomy to mold each role to meet their patients' needs. The main purpose of the primary role on all units is the same: managing care from admission through discharge. The methods of achieving that outcome vary, however. For example, work schedules may differ. Some primary nurses work 8-hour shifts on weekdays, whereas those in the adult intensive care unit provide 8-hour coverage 7 days per week. Other primary nurses believe that patients' needs are best met on their unit by working 12-hour shifts.

Although monetary compensation was offered to nurses who were willing to embark on this new practice, it was not a primary reason for them to take the challenge. Each unit had to work for 3 months toward its identified goals before being eligible for a monetary compensation. The wage structure now consists of three categories: the employee role, organizational operations, and the professional role. For a wage increase, the nurse must fulfill the employee role expectations. These expectations include obtaining the specified continuing education credits and cardiopulmonary resuscitation certification, meeting Joint Commission on Accreditation of Healthcare Organization's requirements, and following policies and procedures. The organizational operations include those incentives that maintain the organization on a 24-hour basis. Examples are pay differentials for the off-shifts and cross-training to another division. Within the professional role, the associate is a clinical I nurse and clinical care coordinators and primary nurses are clinical II nurses. The clinical II nurse has the accountability for meeting the goals and outcomes of the patients and for the practice. Master's-prepared nurses are at the clinical IV level and practice within their specialty. Previously described compensations have served as greater motivational factors than financial compensation.

Compensation in a differentiated nursing practice is bountiful and widely varied, but at Sioux Valley Hospital the nurses who received the greatest benefit from their new practice were those who committed themselves to the actualization of the vision. It was autonomy, authority, and control inherent in each role and the accountability for achieving identified goals that empowered the nurses involved. Empowerment was a motivating factor in this change process.

BENEFICIARY: THE PHYSICIAN

The physicians were one of the beneficiary groups who were passive recipients of compensation in the process of differentiating nursing roles. Although they were unaware of the vision responsible for motivating the change in practice, the transformation soon became apparent to them. The opportunity to work with nurses functioning in the same roles on a daily basis promoted continuity of care. Physicians were gradually oriented to the nursing roles and the purposes of each. As they became interested, physicians began to ask questions and became motivated to take part in the process. They benefitted from having the same primary nurses round with them every day. Both nurse and physician discussed patients' individual needs and the goals of the plan of care. True collaboration toward actualization of patient goals was manifest. The presence of the primary nurse on a daily basis fostered trust. Physicians were assured that information received was of high quality and comprehensive. This level of collaboration led to earlier intervention and prevention of potential patient complications. Time spent on patient rounds was often shortened because the needed patient information was readily available from a reliable, expert nurse. Physicians participated with the nursing staff to attain mutually determined goals of the plan of care in a timely fashion. With enhanced continuity of care, costs were decreased by avoidance of duplicated laboratory work and routine orders, prevention of complications because of early intervention, implementation of Integrated Clinical Pathways, and early discharge planning. Refined and organized discharge planning also saved physicians' time and effort. The most advantageous benefits from differentiated practice for physicians were quality, collaborative care, and increased patient satisfaction. Satisfied patients tended to have fewer complaints; thus physicians' work was more pleasant.

> *Whenever you see a successful business, someone*
> *once made a courageous decision.*
> PETER DRUCKER

BENEFICIARY: THE ORGANIZATION

Differentiated practice and shared governance must be actualized before the rewards can be measured. Therefore, it was essential for the organization to support the vision and the changes that took place as nursing professionalism evolved. The nursing practice had to acquire authority, autonomy, and control from supervisors and managers to succeed in the process of change. The institution became the beneficiary within the context of retention and recruitment of nurses; patient, family, and physician satisfaction (the customers); and cost containment as it related to continuity of care.

Recruitment of new nurses and retention of experienced professional nurses are important goals for any organization. The image of a nursing practice is viewed by those seeking employment as an important factor in accepting a position. Giving nurses the opportunity to become members of a professional nursing practice is a strategy that allows an organization to choose the most qualified and empowered nurses. The process of empowerment in a shared governance system leads to satisfaction that encourages nurses to remain within the organization.

The vision for a professional nursing practice at Sioux Valley Hospital included development of a well-defined orientation and nursing residency program. This program allowed nurses from all backgrounds to learn the process of shared governance nursing practice. The development of differentiated practice allowed the novice nurse to practice at a level appropriate to his or her experience. The flexibility to enhance a present role or to select another role positively affected professional development. Through the change process, nurses had the ability to make choices in career goals, participating in shaping a vision for their practice. Satisfaction within the work environment was a positive outcome for the organization because the nurse was an advocate for the organization and for the nursing practice.

Compensation to the organization can be measured by customer satisfaction, with the customers being defined as those individuals who utilize the services of the organization. Physicians have realized positive results through collaboration with nurses caring for patients in all roles. This collaboration has resulted in the facilitation of physicians' clinical practice. The physicians have become more loyal partners with the organization. Patients and families are now empowered to participate actively in the care being provided, enhancing the potential return of families for repeated hospitalizations. The organization is compensated as the physicians, patients, and families have become satisfied consumers of health care. A satisfied customer is an important marketing agent for the organization by sharing positive experiences with physicians, family members, and acquaintances.

Through the implementation of differentiated practice and shared governance, Sioux Valley Hospital has identified ways to utilize resources better. Establishing these processes did not come without costs. The initial costs included funding consultant fees. Existing education, orientation, and management time was focused on the demonstration project because no other funds were available. Pay differential funds were made available by streamlining the nursing organization with the elimination of assistant head nurses, clinicians, discharge planners, and supervisors. Nursing became a revenue center by charging for hours of nursing care. After implementation, the continuing costs of increased pay for nurses in clinical II roles, council time, and continuing education were vastly offset by Integrated Care savings. The organization has addressed the issue of decreased reimbursement in a capitated system with the use of Integrated Clinical Pathways, improved human and material resource utilization, and a case management system currently being developed for high users of health care resources (see Chapter 6 for more information about the case management system). The benefits of differentiated practice and shared governance outweigh the costs incurred to maintain this system.

After the implementation of differentiated practice and shared governance, the unit director also realized benefits. As the staff nurse attained authority, autonomy, and control, the director's role changed. The director became a mentor, coach, teacher, and advisor. Energy was focused on the professional development of the individual in the form of management and leadership skills. An example was the role of the nursing supervisor. As a result of this growth, the need for a nursing supervisor no longer existed. As the responsibilities of the clinical care coordinator increased, the need for the expertise of the supervisor decreased. This process began gradually in the maternal–child health division with the elimination of that supervisor. By 1991 the practice maintained one nursing supervisor with 24-hour coverage, and in 1993 the role was completely eliminated. The clinical care coordinators are now responsible for the daily management of the unit with the assistance of the unit director. It has been rewarding to recognize, challenge, and support this professional and personal growth.

BENEFICIARY: THE REGIONAL COMMUNITY

Sioux Valley Hospital serves a tri-state region, reaching into Iowa and Minnesota as well as the home state of South Dakota. The institution not only draws patients from that region but supplies outreach services to the communities in that area. The people who live in the service region are beneficiaries of the processes discussed.

Through differentiating practice and developing a shared governance system, the community of nurses began to address the needs of the patient on a continuum. Patient needs when returning home to the community are now recognized. This recognition has facilitated identifying the needs of the nurse caring for those patients. Previously established outreach educational programs have been expanded to encompass the needs of the patient and nurse. Examples of these programs are home uterine monitoring, fetal monitoring, and other high-technology services. Sioux Valley Hospital nurses are available to assist nurses in other institutions and communities to care for complex patients who previously would have been treated in the tertiary care setting. Learning experiences are offered on the Sioux Valley campus, including nurse fellowships in the areas of emergency department, perinatal nursing, and critical care nursing.

The community of nurses at Sioux Valley Hospital has begun the process of building partnerships with a local nursing home and some medical clinics to care better for patients in all stages on the care continuum. Partnerships such as this will allow broader application of programs already developed by multiple providers, further integrating client care. This process is serving to empower patients, physicians, and nurses in the entire service region.

As primary nurses developed their skill of anticipating patients' needs after discharge, community services experienced an increase in referrals. Within the first year of differentiated practice, the Visiting Nurses Association and other county health agencies experienced an increase in registered nurse visits as well as an increased need for supportive services such as homemakers and nursing assistants. One nursing unit, the postpartum/normal newborn nursery, had a significant increase in discharge referrals in a 12-month period. Exhibit 9–1 is an example of the change in referral patterns and compares referrals before (1987) and after (1988) differentiated practice. It is evident that not only the number but also the complexity increased. Social services, counseling services, and other organizations also experienced an increase in referrals.

In addition, the service region has experienced benefits from the development of a professional nursing practice through the relationships that individuals have developed with nurses over time. The region is learning about the different roles of a nurse (associate, primary, coordinator, and advanced practice) and the skills nurses have that make them unique as professionals. The image of a professional nurse is being developed and will continue to affect the service region.

Exhibit 9–1 Discharge Referrals before and after Implementation of Differentiated Practice

	January 1987		*January 1988*
1	Home Visit by Staff	9	Community Health/Visiting
1	Visiting Nurse Referral		Nurses Association
		4	Social Services
		1	Home Visit by Staff
		1	Dietitian
		1	Chaplain
		1	Mental Health Association
		1	Child Protection Services
			Numerous Calls and Visits by
		__	Clinician
Total 2		Total 18	

	February 1987		*February 1988*
3	Home Visits by Staff	4	Home Visits by Staff
5	Community Health/Visiting	10	Visiting Nurses Association
	Nurses Association	1	Threshold
		1	Red Cross
		1	Child Protection Services
		4	Social Services
		1	Pain Clinic
		8	Community Health Nurse
			Numerous Calls and Visits by
		__	Clinician
Total 8		Total 30	

	March 1987		*March 1988*
1	Visiting Nurses Association	11	Visiting Nurses Association
1	Child Protection Services	4	Community Health Nurse
4	Home Visits by Staff	3	WIC
		1	Home Visit by Staff
		1	Child Protection Services
		3	Dietitian
		1	High Risk Hearing Registry
		29	Social Services
			Numerious Calls and Visits by
		__	Clinician
Total 6		Total 53	
Grand Total		**Grand Total**	
16		**101**	

Courtesy of Postpartum/Normal Newborn Nursery, Sioux Valley Hospital, Sioux Falls, South Dakota.

Sioux Valley Hospital has emerged as the low-cost, high-quality provider of health care in the region.[1] The professional nursing practice has served to affect care in the region from both cost and quality perspectives. The community of nurses is developing a case management system that will further professionalize collaboration and partnerships. Providing high-quality care at a low cost is a strong commitment.

Table 9–1 demonstrates the fiscal impact that a clinical nurse specialist (CNS) can have on a patient population. The data were obtained after institution of a program in which the CNS manages postoperative cardiac surgical patients. The CNS is now responsible for ordering, in conjunction with the Clinical Pathway, laboratory tests, radiology studies, medications, intensive care unit transfers, and hospital discharges at the appropriate time intervals. It is an interdependent role with the surgeon, wherein the CNS acts as the primary care provider postoperatively. T-tests for significance of differences between "before" and "after" are shown in Table 9–1.

The length of stay has been considerably reduced by 2.02 days, primarily because there are no longer any nontherapeutic days that result when treatments and tests get ordered too late to be performed on the same day. These nontherapeutic days occur when the surgeon is operating all day and makes rounds during the evening hours. Because patient care is the primary role function, the CNS is able to round on all patients during daytime hours and to order necessary tests accordingly. The reduction in laboratory charges can be attributed to the CNS scrutinizing the results more closely and discontinuing serial tests when these are not indicated by the patient's clinical status.

The service region has also had opportunity to benefit from the institution's commitment to wellness. A comprehensive Wellness Center/Outpatient Rehabilitation Center is owned and operated by Sioux Valley Hospital. It serves outpatients in the region and offers memberships to individuals in the city of Sioux Falls and the surrounding area. Sioux Valley Hospital offers wellness and case management

---

Table 9–1 Effect of a Cardiac Surgery CNS after 3 Weeks

Variable	Before	After	Difference	Significance
Length of stay (days)	8.95	6.93	2.02	99.9%
Nursing care	$2038.56	$1597.19	$441.37	99.5%
Hematology	$306.43	$245.92	$60.51	99.6%
Chemistry	$1523.86	$1294.66	$229.20	93.2%
Room	$2482.45	$1917.93	$564.52	99.7%
Total charges	$7832.21	$6386.87	$1445.34	97.4%
	n = 31	n = 21		

Courtesy of K Karpiuk and DS Christenson, Sioux Valley Hospital, Sioux Falls, South Dakota.

services to the employees of area businesses. The CNSs are primary providers in this community model.

Redesign of professional nursing has offered compensation to the entire service region. High-quality, low-cost care provided in an empowering context has enhanced the roles, relationships, and outcomes for all involved in patient care.

REFERENCE

1. Gardner E. Study amends lore about CABG volume, cost. *Mod Health Care.* 1992;22(48):48–49.

EXERCISE 9-1: COMPENSATION EVALUATION

Choose one area of practice to be evaluated (eg, patient satisfaction, quality of care delivered, or fiscal awareness). Ask the group to answer the following questions related to the topic of interest.

1. What are the strengths?
2. What can be improved?
3. What are the benefits of change?
4. What are the barriers to change?

Identify the most important improvement to be made from the discussion.

Discussion questions:

1. How can differentiated practice assist in building strengths and improving areas of weakness?
2. How can a shared governance system assist in building strengths and improving areas of weakness?
3. Do the benefits of change outweigh the barriers to change?
4. How can the barriers be minimized to allow change to take place?

10 Celebration

Renee Schulz, Elizabeth Hindbjorgen, Carol McGinnis, E. J. Reid, and Georgia A. Stern

At our best we are passionate, not perfectionists.
At our best we are ourselves.
Let us be ourselves and enjoy each other.
WILLIAM L. COLEMAN

This final chapter on celebration is the culmination of much passion and enjoyment that was experienced in realizing the best that Sioux Valley Hospital nurses found in themselves. The dream of differentiated practice became a reality through the celebration of self and others. This celebration is only the beginning of the dreams that have yet to be fulfilled, cherished, and nurtured for a brighter tomorrow.

THE NEED TO CELEBRATE

Throughout history, the passage of great events has been marked with celebration. According to Webster, celebration is defined as follows: to perform publicly, to honor or observe (as in some special occasion or event), to praise, to sing the glories of, or to seize an occasion for being festive. Celebration itself is the art of celebrating. This chapter discusses the art of celebration as seen through the eyes of the celebrated. Throughout the Sioux Valley Hospital experience of implementing differentiated practice, celebrating became synonymous with the project itself.

To understand the need to celebrate, one has to understand the human spirit and what motivates each person to higher levels of performance. According to Maslow's hierarchy of needs, motivation stems from the desire to satisfy some need. If the need is strong enough, tension is created, and from that tension action results.[1] Maslow's hierarchy of needs, from the bottom up, recognizes five steps or levels of needs: basic or survival needs, safety and security needs, belongingness, ego status, and self-actualization.

To understand the Sioux Valley Hospital experience, one must realize at what level on Maslow's hierarchy of needs the project units were and what had to be accomplished for motivation to occur at the highest level of need or self-actualization. Those units that were involved in the demonstration project were, for the most part, at the belongingness level and were ready to move to higher levels. At the belongingness level individuals are less preoccupied with themselves and begin to form interpersonal relationships.[1] As this is accomplished and groups feel secure in the relationships that surround them, they are ready to move to ego status needs. Most of the units that undertook differentiated practice were secure in their interpersonal relationships at the unit level and were ready to forge ahead.

One unit that struggled initially had not fulfilled the belongingness need, and expecting the unit members to be at ego status level made their task more difficult. As identified by Maslow, a higher level need cannot be achieved until lower level needs are met. Had analysis of this unit been made earlier, the loss of time and the sense of disappointment may have been alleviated. More important, ego status is identified as the most difficult level to achieve because satisfaction at this level is dependent on the ability of others to respond to the individual or individuals.[1]

Maslow, in his studies, concluded that almost everyone comes into the world with the capacity to achieve self-actualization but that few do so because most become socially conditioned to the Jonah complex. The Jonah complex is based on a belief system of insignificance and feelings of unimportance and poor luck.[2] If an individual believes that he or she cannot make a difference, he or she will not make a difference. This has been identified in the literature as the theory of self-fulfilling prophecy.[3]

Other theorists agree. Rotter's[4] theory of locus of control asserts that individuals operating with an external locus of control believe that there is no such thing as personal control, autonomy, or freedom because stronger forces or powers make decisions. Because of the basic premise of "I am not worthy," recognition and awards are especially important to build the ego and to help the individual move to the self-actualization level. Hence the reason to celebrate. Celebration becomes a tool to nourish the ego so that individuals can focus on personal growth, become creative or use their creativity, take risks, seek autonomy, and develop the freedom to act.[1]

> *"Cause and Effect"*
> *Once, someone said something nice about me,*
> *And, all undeserved though I knew it to be,*
> *I treasured it there on my heart's deepest shelf,*
> *Till one day I quite surprised even myself*
> *By honestly making an effort to be*
> *That nice thing that somebody said about me!*
> HELEN LOWRIE MARSHALL

It was through celebration that stars were born. Whenever, wherever, and to whomever successes occurred (no matter how small), recognition was made. It became a growing experience for managers, staff, and physicians as each sought to receive the many accolades of praise and accomplishment that come with success. Success breeds success, and recognition truly feeds the human spirit to seek further success. Maslow would call this reaching self-actualization. It could be seen in many health care workers in each role involved in the project at Sioux Valley Hospital.

The key to success in celebrating is just that. Celebrating is a positive reinforcement of the successes attempted or attained. Because most nurses (70%) were sensing individuals, as defined by the Myers-Briggs Type Indicator, celebrating risk taking and progress toward a goal was imperative. Sensing as a preference style is seen in 70% of the US population. The data gathered at Sioux Valley Hospital were congruent with this. Individuals showing sensing as a preferred method of gathering data learn through experience and are applauded for their practicality and skill in using data from yesterday to understand today. Intuitive individuals (30%), on the other hand, understand the world through intuition and are lauded for their vision in seeing what is possible in the future and embracing the unknown. Therefore, intuitives may embrace change, whereas individuals whose preference is sensing will need greater encouragement to forge ahead into uncharted waters.

Differentiated practice was like untried waters with many unknown perils beneath the surface. Many were sure that just beneath that surface were sharks ready to tear them apart and spit them out in pieces. Celebrating the risk taking encouraged individuals to explore these uncharted waters because it was not just the finished product that was rewarded but also the attempts. No longer was *failure* a word to be feared. If anything, it became synonymous with success because recognition was given for the attempts made toward an unknown. The more attempts, the more recognition. Through these shared experiences of unknowns, the majority of nurses found themselves looking forward to the voyage toward the unknown. How could a person be wrong when no one else had charted the course before?

> *I desire that there may be as many different persons*
> *in the world as possible; but I would have each one*
> *be very careful to find out and pursue* his own *way.*
> Henry David Thoreau

Unforeseen was a commitment to the project that developed out of uniqueness or being different. Webster defines unique as existing as the only one or as the sole example, having no like or equal, standing alone in quality or being incomparable. Sioux Valley Hospital was unique even though it was a part of the Statewide Project. The hospital came to appreciate that distinction of being unique. Sometimes celebration can be as simple as identifying an individual or a group of individuals as unique in that no others are doing what that group is doing. The Sioux Valley Hospital experience caused nurses to walk taller, stand prouder, and develop a self-confidence not seen earlier. In being told they were unique, they became unique. Not only did nurses develop this sense of pride in being part of a unique system change, but patients and families embraced this new delivery system in the same manner.

Part of celebration is creating a different environment and a new belief system. The most effective way to change behavior is to put people into a new organizational context that imposes new roles, responsibilities, and relationships.[5] In the new roles created by differentiated practice, nurses were expected to choose the roles they would commit to fulfilling. Celebrating included the successful selection of role delineation. All roles were considered important to the success of the project. Therefore, all roles were celebrated.

As individuals sought recognition, communication became extensive, open, honest, and in some cases bold. As in the parable of the eagle and the chicken, lurking inside each individual (chicken) is an eagle just waiting to stretch forth its wings and fly.[6] In the parable, an eagle raised as a chicken refused to act as an eagle until a naturalist helped him realize his true potential. People born as eagles but raised as chickens sometimes need help to stretch forth their wings and fly. Eagles were emerging in every unit at Sioux Valley Hospital, and sometimes in stretching their wings and learning to fly another fledgling eagle's feathers were ruffled during the flight. As already identified, the key to success is rewarding all attempts and celebrating everyone's new wings. This can be one of the biggest challenges, yet it is absolutely necessary to nurture the ego status development of every individual.

As may be obvious, one key component of celebration is the recognition of project members that must come from management. This is especially important during the initiation and implementation phases of a project and is imperative to the success of the project. For managers to do this successfully, they also need to celebrate and be celebrated. Managers who are concerned about what might be perceived as a loss of status or role because of these newly born eagles (stars) will need to be celebrated as much as or more than their staff nurses. Managers will not be able to celebrate their units' successes if they feel any threat to their own survival. They will need to be nurtured and mentored by either peers or superiors into stretching their wings. It is imperative that managers see these new changes in their staff not as a threat but as an opportunity and a chance for them to expand their present role.

In the differentiated practice project, these managers were nurtured and supported to become facilitators of change and mentors to their staff. As staff nurses were rewarded for attempts, so were managers also rewarded for their ability to let go and allow these new eagles on their units to emerge. In the project units, these managers celebrated their newly found freedom because they no longer needed to serve as a surrogate parent to their staff. As nurses became eagles, they learned to solve their own problems.

It is important to understand that managers may have as much or more to overcome in this new paradigm than the staff. Mentoring and facilitating may not be skills they understand or have used previously. Recognition and reward are the fruits for ego status and the stepping stones to self-actualization. Managers and staff alike require these to move into higher levels of achievement.

With change may come power. Power does not have to mean the exertion of influence over others but rather can be seen as a process that involves actively working together toward a common goal. During this paradigm shift, it is important to celebrate the power and peace that are being achieved through the change. Peace is the means and the end and includes the process and the product. It means celebrating the praxis or thoughtful reflections that come from transforming the world. Nothing ever happens by just wishing it to occur. Transforming the world requires a careful and deliberate process and the time to achieve it. It means celebrating the empowerment that comes from acquiring new personal and/or professional strengths. It means celebrating the awareness that comes from the growing knowledge of self, others, and the world in which we live. It means celebrating the consensus that comes from active commitment to group solidarity and group integrity. It means celebrating the evolution of change and the transformation that is conscious and deliberate.[7] It means celebrate, celebrate, celebrate!

THE POWER OF CELEBRATION

> *Celebration is to be lived out*
> *not just read about.*
> *It is to be experienced*
> *not just explained.*
> *It will be known only to the degree*
> *with which we participate.*
>
> SCHNEIDER AND ORTEGEL

So how does one proceed with celebration? There is no party planning guide that has been developed to explain how to celebrate the death of a nursing delivery system and then the rebirth of a new practice, nor is it likely that one will be written that is applicable for all. Literature and history have been guides for how celebration has occurred in the past, however. Celebration is understood through its lived experience and the individuals or groups that live it. "Celebration happens in the hearts and the hands and voices of people."[8(p22)] How one celebrates can be as important as why one celebrates.

Ceremonies and rituals have been used throughout history as a form of celebration. They are a response to the human spirit's need to express a passion or emotion that perhaps is not allowed or encouraged at other times. Consider the number of civic, social, cultural, racial, and religious celebrations that are present in different societies. Such expressions are repeated according to some regular or irregular schedule, according to a need or an occasion.[8] Perhaps two of the most poignant examples of these are the ceremonies of births and deaths that are celebrated in various ways. Consider the number of celebrations or rituals that are observed by nursing. Who could forget the capping or pinning ceremony that new nurses celebrate as a rite of passage into the profession of nursing? Is not shift work ritualistic? Consider the delivery of nursing care: Has there not been a right time to give a bed bath? Is this not sometimes ritualistic?

In the Sioux Valley Hospital experience, burying the dead was celebrated with the death of the previous nursing care delivery system. An elaborate funeral at a funeral home occurred to allow a time and a place for grieving.[9] The grieving nurses were encouraged to bring their favorite nursing symbols of their past practice that represented something needing to have a final resting place. Funerals give honor to the departed and create memory for the living. For Sioux Valley nursing, it was important to honor old traditions and to celebrate them for the contributions they made to the nursing profession. It was also time, however, to bury old traditions and to create new traditions and new celebrations.

What can be shared about the Sioux Valley Hospital experience is the various manifestations of celebration that were used to move the nursing practice from the old to the new. These are the new rituals that express what is lived, and they inspire nurses to continue moving forward. A traditional form of celebration is sharing food and drink. In recognition of their new endeavor, the first units celebrated their new beginning by serving cake and coffee to unit staff and others in the institution. All were welcomed because this voyage would affect all the waters of Sioux Valley Hospital.

These events were not without other ceremony. Banners proclaimed the commencement of the project for each unit. Fliers were distributed throughout the hospital. Ribbon-cutting ceremonies were held, with physicians and executive management participating and adding their own fun. Photos were taken to commemorate the events. One physician lost half his necktie to a ribbon cutting and wore it with pride for the rest of the day, including during a speaking engagement away from the hospital. At one of these functions, another physician asked whether he would still be king. Another physician asked, "Who gave you nurses permission? Did this go to the medical staff?" It was an ambivalent time, and many staff, including physicians and nurses, were unsure of the future. Yet everyone believed it would never be the same. It was a time to celebrate! It *would* never be the same!

A common language of differentiated practice emerged. This can be compared to the liturgy of traditional religion that celebrates salvation. Liturgy brings to a group a common language and meaning. It forms tradition. In this instance, the liturgy of differentiated practice brought forth the words *primary nurse, associate nurse, clinical care coordinator, nursing diagnosis,* and *role development.* Common language adds unity to a practice and creates understanding.

Throughout history, groups have used symbols to represent visually that for which they stand. Be it a flag or a cross, a star or a crest, such symbols bring identity to a group. A special pin was developed for each project participant in the Statewide Project for Nursing and Nursing Education. Everyone was recognized for his or her efforts in forging through uncharted waters. The pin (Figure 10–1) served as a visual symbol of the practice, its scope, and its promise for the future.

A publication called *Nurses' Notes* was developed as a forum for celebrating nurse accomplishments and changes. As the project moved forward, other events were celebrated. An essay-writing contest entitled "I Took the Challenge" was held

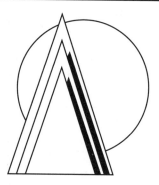

This logo, which represents differentiated practice in South Dakota, was designed by George and Diane Prisbe from Aberdeen, South Dakota. In developing the logo, the intent was to capture the major components of differentiated practice in a unique design.

The triangles represent the 3 types of nursing programs which prepare the graduate to write the N-CLEX RN licensing examination. The triangles also represent the 3 major components of nursing practice—direct care, communication, and leadership. The shaded areas between the triangles reflect the interaction of these components—patient teaching, delegation, and coordination. The circle in the background, like a rising sun, represents the entire scope of wholistic nursing practice, and provides promise for the future development of the profession.

Figure 10–1 South Dakota differentiated practice pin symbol. *Source:* Reprinted with permission from the South Dakota Council of Nursing Organizations.

to encourage nurses to share their differentiated practice experiences in written form. The winner received a gift certificate to a local restaurant and was recognized by having the winning essay published in *Nurses' Notes.*

Nurses' Week became established and celebrated during this time. It served as a vehicle for nurses to market themselves as professionals and then rewarded them for being professional. Since then, it has become a yearly celebration at Sioux Valley Hospital. It has evolved to include the Florence Nightingale Award, which is awarded to nurses for excellence at the bedside; the creation of the Ribbon of Life speaker for presentations of either historical or futuristic importance to nursing; the development of a unit poster or display related to the Nurses' Week national theme; the sending of balloon-o-grams; and drawings and raffles for gifts and prizes. In an early celebration, additional recognition was given to all nurses who were active on the various committees. These members each received certificates of appreciation and achievement.

One of the most popular events for acknowledging professional nursing has been the poster or display contest. Each year the poster or display contest creates a healthy competition among all nursing personnel to show off their area of work. The posters or displays are to reflect the area of work or the theme of Nurses' Week. Creativity is always considered. Judging is done by representatives from the Board of Directors, the hospital president or executive vice president, and other nonnursing department employees. Every contest entrant is celebrated as a winner because all displays receive either a blue, red, or white ribbon, but two traveling trophies are awarded to the best of the best. The challenge to be remembered is to celebrate and reward the attempts. Other awards that have been used to reward involvement have been professional nurse development books and magazine subscriptions.

EDUCATION AS CELEBRATION

> *Education is liberating!*
>
> PANKRATZ AND PANKRATZ

Celebrating education should be a primary consideration as an organization forges ahead into these uncharted waters. It is through education that new life can be created by unleashing that powerful organ called the mind. According to Litvak,[2] only 20% of the mind is used. Until education is valued and people understand what education can do for our changing world, it will not be valued to the extent it deserves. For most nursing organizations, no one would dispute the need for ongoing continuing education for nursing staff. Yet in periods of financial constraint (which now seem to be constant), the first place to look to limit dollars is in the amount or kind of education given to the employee. Remember the adage, "Pay now or pay later." It goes without saying that time and money spent well once are time and money that will not have to be respent when it is determined that costly mistakes resulted from lack of initial investment. Education is a motivating factor that gives a nurse the tools needed for growth and development in the practice. It is a motivation that cannot be bought but rather that comes from within. The gift of knowing is an investment that reaps benefits to be celebrated.

Investment in the mind is an investment in the future. There is no doubt that, without the money spent initially to implement the demonstration project, the outcome might have looked different at Sioux Valley Hospital. Dr Peggy Primm, the founder of differentiated practice, was brought into the organization as an expert on her model. It was her wisdom, insight, and expertise that gave the necessary direction to initiate the project. Although the nursing organization would have been able to proceed without her consultation, experts from outside the organization may be more strongly regarded than those who come from within the organization. In addition, there is a built-in safety mechanism for the management team in bringing in outside experts: Because they are not a part of the real organization, they can take the heat and say and do things that members of the organization cannot. The celebration of education at Sioux Valley Hospital came with this consultant and the others who were to follow. Major innovative changes can be enhanced by consultants who think, act, and react differently.

This inservicing time spent with Primm was mandatory to ensure that all players were hearing the same thing from the same expert. In the beginning, it looked not like a celebration of education but like a battleground of wits as tongues as sharp as swords fought for perceived safety. The constant attention to education, however, gradually changed the way people felt about change and life in general. In a 1987 nursing job satisfaction survey that was done at Sioux Valley Hospital, a secondary analysis of the demographic data revealed that only 48 of 357 registered nurses who returned the survey were enrolled in any formal educational program.[10] Since then, many nurses have pursued further education. In 1987, only 6 nursing personnel held a master's degree. As of June 1993, the number of master's prepared nurses had increased to 27; 1 nurse had earned a doctorate. Within 3 years another 18 nurses are expected to finish their master's degrees, and 2 others are expected to finish doctorates. Education has become a celebration of people's achievements and their acquisition of knowledge. It has been a hallmark and one of the driving forces that has helped Sioux Valley Hospital move more easily into the unknown. Knowledge gained can be power gained. Power gained can be change gained. That is celebration!

TIMING

There is a time when what you are creating and the environment you are creating it in come together.
GRACE HARTIGAN

In analyzing the celebration of Sioux Valley differentiated practice, it becomes important to understand the significance of time and timing. The use of paid time (discretionary), according to Pinchot,[11] is the most consequential and basic of corporate decisions that lead toward innovation. Pinchot contends that major corporations such as IBM, Tektronix, Ore-Ida, 3M, and DuPont permit people to spend up to 15% of their time exploring ideas. It is his belief that, without allowing employees paid time to explore and brainstorm, new ideas become only that: ideas. In the Sioux Valley Hospital experience, the eagles who emerged were the innovators. It was the time they spent in discussing how something would look and what might work that truly created the outcome that was realized and is still being realized. The use of discretionary time became a celebration to those who wanted to innovate and become part of groups that were doing just that.

Timing is the other aspect of when to implement change and celebration. There comes a period of time when it becomes advantageous to move ahead, a time to act or perform. Some of the great events of history have or have not occurred because of the timing. In some cases, it was as simple as being in the right or wrong place at the right or wrong time. Had Benjamin Franklin not been born when he was or lived when he did, perhaps there would have been no such thing as electricity or the Constitution. Had the seven *Challenger* astronauts, including the first teacher to go into space, not been chosen for that fateful flight in January 1986, that flight would have been just another space flight. Instead, to this day the event is forever remembered by the millions who watched in horror the explosion that ended seven people's lives. In these historical events, lives were forever changed.

So it was with nursing at Sioux Valley Hospital. It was not consciously planned to change the course of nursing to the extent that ultimately occurred. As identified throughout history, most events that are forever remembered were unplanned and unexpected. Because of timing, however, the events become a part of remembered history. Before differentiated practice, Sioux Valley Hospital nursing units/ divisions had little trust among themselves and were working in isolation. For Sioux Valley Hospital, the best timing came in the form of hiring a strong and capable leader who envisioned something different. That vision was the beginning of the process to change the way people were thinking and reacting. In addition, the time was right in health care as diagnosis-related groups and cost containment were forcing hospitals to consider the concept of working smarter, not harder. Finally, many nurse managers were believing that something different was imperative to their survival and the organization's survival. This perhaps was the biggest challenge and the biggest celebration, when 18 different managers became one unified manager group in its philosophy. When this group became viable and cohesive, it was the beginning of the celebration of change for Sioux Valley nursing.

REFLECTIONS

> *"The Song and the Echo"*
> *A song we sing. We cannot know*
> *How far the sound of it will go,*
> *How long its echo will be heard.*
> *We can but pray that every word,*
> *Each note in this, the song we sing,*
> *Will find its resting place and bring*
> *Some little measure of repose,*
> *Some strength, some happiness to those*
> *Who hear our song. If just one smiles*
> *To hear its echo down the miles,*
> *Then we should be content and know*
> *Our song was meant—God willed it so.*
>   HELEN LOWRIE MARSHALL

It has been approximately 6 years since the implementation of differentiated practice at Sioux Valley Hospital. Our song is presently being hummed in many circles of nursing practice across the United States. The words may not be there yet for all of nursing, but the melody is there. Once people feel the rhythm, the rest will come.

It has been asked by many organizations, How many people does it take to change anything? How long does it take for the change to become the accepted way of doing things? To answer the first, a quote from Steiner is appropriate: "If a plane is only five degrees different than the course thought on, over a period of time, that plane will be in an entirely different place than what was intended."[12] An organization does not need a majority of its individuals to be on the same path going the same direction. What is needed are those few individuals who remain committed to being five degrees off course. By maintaining the new heading, over a period of time a new destination is reached. That is celebration. It is when perseverance pays off and others have chosen the new direction. It is when that small minority wanting something different becomes the majority. That is celebration. There is no answer to how long it will take for a practice to change its style; every organization is different. Organizations can save themselves some pains by using the experts who have emerged in other practices. No one in this day of cost containment should reinvent any wheels. It in itself is a celebration when organizations learn to network comfortably and securely with each other without fear of reprisal or competition.

Would the participants of differentiated practice go back to earlier days? One needs only to look at some outcomes to determine an answer. As early as 1987, one of the most dramatic outcomes to be celebrated was the nursing report from the Joint Commission on Accreditation of Healthcare Organizations (Joint Commission). For the first time ever, the Joint Commission survey team had no suggestions or recommendations for the nursing department except that all nursing units needed to implement what the project units had begun. In 1990, the nurse surveyor commented that Sioux Valley Hospital should help the more rural, smaller hospitals meet the standards. "It should be your responsibility," was her statement.

In addition, the celebration of the Sioux Valley Hospital nursing practice has come in the form of the many visitors who have toured, visited, and consulted with the practice. Since 1988, more than 80 visitors from more than 35 facilities in the United States and two foreign countries have spent time at Sioux Valley Hospital to observe differentiated practice on the nursing units. With every visitor, the units had an opportunity to be celebrated as centers of excellence and innovation. Nurses who had never considered themselves anything but nurses were seen as the consultants to other nurses from other states. The more they shared, the more confident and self-assured they became. This has become evident in what the nurses have said and how they have said it.

Those who have gone on the road to make presentations or to consult have been all over America and to two foreign countries. These individuals have had an opportunity to see other nursing practices and to compare those practices with Sioux Valley Hospital's. That in itself has become a celebration because these nurses have found themselves visiting places they would not have had an opportunity to see otherwise. As they shared their thoughts and ideas, they also gleaned thoughts and ideas from colleagues in other places. A strong network has been established that continues to be celebrated.

In reality, nurses cannot go back to the old way, even if they wanted to. Once insight is gained and autonomy is practiced, there is never a way back. The physicians and nurses were correct in their belief that it would never be the same. The nurses at Sioux Valley Hospital have earned and gained decision-making power through hard work and professional development. It has been part of a complete overhaul of nursing. When differentiated practice (now called Integrated Care) was initiated, there was no way to know where it would lead except to know that it would lead to something different. It was a process. Process, according to Webster, is a systematic series of actions directed to some end; a specific, continuous action, operation, or series of changes; or a series of progressive and interdependent steps by which an end is attained. It may not have been totally systematic, because changes were made as necessary, but it was specific and continuous and required interdependent steps. It has become apparent in nursing that to move ahead it is not the finished product that is important but the process used to get there. When process is used successfully, the outcome is ensured.

There is no ending to this story because there is no finish; it is an ongoing saga. Integrated Care has been and is a process. The end has not been reached because the interdependent steps continue to change. It is evident, however, that the future will be filled with opportunities yet to be discovered and implemented. Celebration of Integrated Care continues. It is evident in the recognition of each nurse's accomplishments presented yearly in the form of a professional portfolio. It bursts forth in success stories from the bedside and in acts of human kindness and caring. It leaps out from nurses who have found a new way to work together as colleagues. It is seen in the creation of this book, which is a diary of an emerging practice. Finally it is seen in the practice itself, which has created a whole new generation of nurse advocates and health care reformists.

REFERENCES

1. Grazier PB. *Before It's Too Late: Employee Involvement . . . An Idea Whose Time Has Come.* Chadds Ford, Pa: Teambuilding; 1989.
2. Litvak SB. *Use Your Head: How to Develop the Other 80% of Your Brain.* New York, NY: Prentice-Hall; 1986.
3. Henshel RL. The boundary of the self-fulfilling prophecy and the dilemma of social prediction. *Br J Socio.* 1982;33:511–528.
4. Rotter JB. Generalized expectancies for internal versus external control of reinforcement. *Psychol Monogr.* 1966;80:1–28.
5. Beer M, Eisenstat RA, Spector B. Why change programs don't produce change. *Harvard Bus Rev.* 1990;68(6):158–166.
6. Chenevert M. *STAT: Special Techniques in Assertiveness Training.* 3rd ed. St Louis, Mo: Mosby; 1988.
7. Wheeler CE, Chinn P. *Peace and Power: A Handbook of Feminist Process.* 3rd ed. New York, NY: National League for Nursing Press; 1991.
8. Rivers CJ. *Celebration.* New York, NY: Herder & Herder; 1969.
9. Koerner JG, Bunkers SS. Transformational leadership: the power of symbol. *Nurs Admin Q.* 1992;17(1):1–9.
10. Schulz RG. *The Relationship of Registered Nurses' Demographic Characteristics to Their Perceived Autonomy.* Brookings, SD: South Dakota State University; 1992. Thesis.
11. Pinchot G III. *Intrapreneuring.* New York, NY: Harper & Row; 1985.
12. Steiner F. Speech at Harris Hospital Systems; August 1989; Fort Worth, Tex.

EXERCISE 10–1: CELEBRATE

Because knowing what to celebrate is probably as difficult as the actual celebrating, try this. Use the letters of the word *celebrate,* and ask group participants to name as many things to celebrate as they can using each letter. The idea here is to encourage a group-think about things that the members could celebrate in their unit or organization. There should be no wrong ways to use the letters. For example:

- **C**—create posters (colorful banners)
- **E**—enjoy the work that others have done through awards
- **L**—laminate cards with special sayings as an award or reward (long lists of stars)
- **E**—encourage group identification via a T-shirt, pin, cap, etc
- **B**—bring in food and drink for all to share (banquets to honor those involved)
- **R**—rave about accomplishments via notes, internal mail systems, etc (recognize achievements through certificates or rewards of time, money, or recognition)
- **A**—allow banners or balloons (acknowledging the stars)
- **T**—telling can itself be a reward (telling your story through consultations or book writing)
- **E**—entitlements and other symbolic gestures should be done

EXERCISE 10–2: CELEBRATION WORD SEARCH

Find the hidden words. All these words are kinds of celebrations that can be done to celebrate nursing or the nursing practice:

FOOD AND DRINK
BANNERS
POSTERS
CONTESTS
CERTIFICATES
DISPLAYS
SYMBOLS
SAYINGS
NURSE OF MONTH
NURSE OF YEAR
RECOGNITION
RIBBONS
TIME

```
R  I  B  O  T  L  F  C  O  N  T  S  G  P  D
A  C  E  R  T  Q  M  E  Y  S  R  U  N  O  I
D  Z  N  U  R  S  E  O  F  Y  E  A  R  S  H
R  I  B  X  R  F  M  C  O  N  T  E  S  T  S
D  O  S  S  L  O  B  M  Y  S  Q  K  N  E  Y
I  F  H  P  C  O  O  E  R  A  L  O  S  R  M
S  B  O  G  L  D  L  S  E  V  M  F  E  S  H
S  A  W  E  J  A  G  B  C  F  H  U  T  D  Z
I  N  H  B  R  N  Y  W  O  T  E  R  A  B  E
B  R  C  O  I  D  Z  E  G  C  E  J  C  M  S
M  Q  O  Y  G  D  S  S  N  O  B  B  I  R  P
A  E  A  K  Z  R  E  A  I  G  D  T  F  T  M
U  S  H  J  U  I  G  I  T  N  D  K  I  I  T
E  X  K  N  M  N  F  L  I  T  F  P  T  V  T
W  L  O  N  C  K  V  P  O  L  N  S  R  L  S
I  Y  O  Z  S  R  E  N  N  A  B  O  E  N  O
M  R  J  P  O  S  Y  A  S  V  D  E  C  A  P
```

List of Sources

p. ix   "If I can . . ." *Source:* Oliver Wendell Holmes, Sr.

p. xv   "It is good . . ." *Source:* Ursula K. LeGuin, *The Left Hand of Darkness* (New York: Ace Books, 1969), 220.

p. 1   "Drive thy Business . . ." *Source:* Benjamin Franklin, *Poor Richard: The Almanacks for the Years 1733–1758* (Introduction by Van Wyck Brooks, illustrations by Norman Rockwell) 1758 (New York: Bonanza Books, 1979), 279.

p. 2   "The history of . . ." *Source:* President Dwight D. Eisenhower, Address at the Hunt Armory in Pittsburgh, Pennsylvania on October 9, 1956. *Public Papers of the Presidents of the United States, Dwight D. Eisenhower, Containing the Public Messages, Speeches, and Statements of the President, January 1–December 31, 1956* (Washington, DC: Federal Register Division, National Archives and Record Service, 1958), 879.

p. 13   "Keep changing. When . . ." *Source:* Bruce Barton.

p. 16   "Saddle your dreams . . ." *Source:* Mary Webb, *Precious Bane* (New York: E.P. Dutton, 1926), 52.

p. 22   "Culture hides much . . ." *Source:* Edward T. Hall, *The Silent Language* (Garden City, NY: Anchor Press/Doubleday, 1973), 30.

p. 26   "It is not . . ." *Source:* Moliere.

p. 28   "The issue is . . ." *Source:* Bishop G. Bromley Oxnam, *On This Rock: An Appeal for Christian Unity* (New York: Harper and Brothers, 1951), 48.

p. 29   "The world hates . . ." *Source:* Charles F. Kettering

p. 30   "If you choose . . ." *Source:* Narcy Recker

p. 30   "In sharing the . . ." *Source:* Narcy Recker

p. 31   "A decision made . . ." *Source:* Narcy Recker

p. 31   "A clash of . . ." *Source:* Alfred North Whitehead, *Science and the Modern World* (New York: The Free Press, MacMillan Company, 1967), 186.

p. 33   "Culture is always . . ." *Source:* Friedrich Hertz.

p. 33   "Two may talk . . ." *Source:* Mary Hartwell Catherwood, "Marianson," *Mackinac and Other Lake Stories* (New York: Harper and Brothers, 1899), 6–7.

p. 34   "Put it before . . ." *Source:* Joseph Pulitzer.

p. 37   "Behold the turtle . . ." *Source:* James Bryant Conant

p. 46   "People are usually . . ." *Source:* Author unknown

p. 54   "Take time to . . ." *Source:* Napoleon Bonaparte

p. 58   "Many people in . . ." *Source:* George Peabody

p. 59   "There are no . . ." *Source:* Mary McCarthy, "The *Vita Activa*" in *On the Contrary* (New York: Farrar, Strauss and Cudahy, 1961), 155.

p. 59   "Self-expression must pass . . ." *Source:* Pearl S. Buck, "In Search of Readers," In Helen Hull, ed., *The Writer's Book* (New York: Barnes & Noble with Harper & Brothers, 1950), 2.

p. 63   "May we always . . ." *Source:* Facilitation Committee, Federation of Ohio River Cooperatives, as quoted by M. Avery, B. Auvine, B. Streibel, L. Weiss, *Building United Judgment: A Handbook for Consensus Decision Making* (Madison, Wisconsin: Center for Conflict Resolution, 1981), 26.

p. 69   "The strength, the . . ." *Source:* Muriel Rukeyser, "Nine Poems for the Unborn Child," VI Stanza 1, in *Waterlilly Fire: Poems 1935–1962* (New York: MacMillan, 1962), 139.

p. 71   "Other people . . . see" *Source:* President John F. Kennedy, Speech to Irish Parliament, Dublin, Ireland, June 28, 1963. "The Little Nations," *Let the Word Go Forth: The Speeches, Statements, and Writings of John F. Kennedy,* Theodore C. Sorensen, ed. (New York: Delacorte Press, 1988), 389.

p. 73   "Since the mind . . ." *Source:* Denis Waitley as quoted by John Roger and Peter McWilliams, *Life 101* (Los Angeles: Prelude Press, 1991), 234.

p. 78   "If a man . . ." *Source:* Barbara Proctor, advertising agency president

p. 80   "Never tell people . . ." *Source:* George S. Patton, Jr., *War As I Knew It* (Boston: Houghton Mifflin, 1947), 357.

p. 81   "Security . . . does not . . ." *Source:* Helen Keller, *Let Us Have Faith* (New York: Doubleday, Doran & Co., 1940), 51.

p. 81   "Making a choice . . ." *Source:* Edward Carpenter, "The Talk of the Town: Poet's Corner," *New Yorker,* January 6, 1986, 20.

p. 82   "Don't be afraid . . ." *Source:* David Lloyd George

p. 84   "No trumpets sound . . ." *Source:* Agnes De Mille, *Dance to the Piper* (Boston: Little, Brown & Co., Atlantic Monthy Press, 1952), 77.

p. 91   "We did not . . ." *Source:* Thornton Wilder, *The Eighth Day* (New York: Harper and Row, 1967), 107.

p. 129   "Seeing the same . . ." *Source:* Blaise Pascal, "The Apology and Translation" in *Pascal's Pensées* with an English Translation and Introduction, H.F. Stewart (New York: Pantheon, 1950), 203.

p. 131   "Cooperation is spelled . . ." *Source:* George M. Verity

p. 132   "Assets make things . . ." *Source:* Alfred Armand Montapert, *Inspiration and Motivation* (Englewood Cliffs, NJ: Prentice-Hall, 1982), 47.

p. 139   "Happiness lies . . . in . . ." *Source:* Franklin D. Roosevelt, First Inaugural Address, March 4, 1933, *Memorable Quotations of Franklin D. Roosevelt,* compiled by E. Taylor Parks and Lois F. Parks (New York: Thomas Y. Crowell Company, 1965), 258.

p. 158   "A thing that . . ." *Source:* John Miller.

p. 166   "Success is dependent . . ." *Source:* Sophocles, adapted from line 945 of *Electra.*

p. 188   "A single conversation . . ." *Source:* Henry Wadsworth Longfellow

p. 189   "All experience is . . ." *Source:* Henry Adams, *The Education of Henry Adams: An Autobiography* (New York: Houghton Mifflin Co., The Riverside Press, 1918), 87.

p. 192   "The greatest trust . . ." *Source:* Francis Bacon, *The Essays or Counsels, Civil and Moral, of Francis Ld. Verulam Viscount St. Albans* (Mt. Vernon, NY: Peter Pauper Press, n.d.), 81.

p. 197   "Our relationships can . . ." *Source:* Shakti Gawain, *Awakening* (San Raphael, CA: New World Library, 1991).

p. 197   "If we are . . ." *Source:* Margaret Mead, *Sex and Temperament in Three Primitive Societies* (New York: William Morrow & Co., 1963), 322.

p. 198   "If you have . . ." *Source:* Margaret Fuller

p. 199   "Always the beautiful . . ." *Source:* E.E. Cummings, *Complete Poems: 1913–1962; Introduction to New Poems [from Collected Poems]* (1938) (New York: Harcourt, Brace, Jovanovich, 1972), 462.

p. 201   "It is our . . ." *Source:* William James

p. 204   "What concerns me . . ." *Source:* Epictetus, as quoted by Roger von Oech, *A Whack on the Side of the Head: How to Unlock Your Mind for Innovation* (New York: Warner Books, 1983), 120.

p. 205   "(A person's) mind . . ." *Source:* Oliver Wendell Holmes, Jr.

p. 214   "Community . . . is the . . ." *Source:* Martin Buber, "Community" in *Between Man and Man,* translated by R.G. Smith (London: Kegan Paul, Trench, Trubner & Co., 1947), 31.

p. 215   "They cannot see . . ." *Source:* Christoph Martin Wieland, "Musarion," Canto II in *Musarion and Other Rococo Tales,* translated and introduction by Thomas C. Starnes (Columbia, SC: Camden House, 1991), 46.

p. 217   "The real . . . community . . ." *Source:* Martin Buber, "In the Midst of Crisis," *Paths in Utopia;* translated by R.F.C. Hull (Boston: Beacon Press, 1958), 135.

p. 220   "Nothing happens unless . . ." *Source:* Carl Sandburg, "Washington Monument by Night" from *Slabs of the Sunburnt West* (1922), *The Complete Poems of Carl Sandburg: Revised and Expanded Edition* (New York: Harcourt Brace Jovanovich, 1970), 282.

p. 221   "VISION is the . . ." *Source:* Jonathan Swift, "Thoughts on Various Subjects" in Vol. 4, *A Proposal for Correcting the English Tongue, Polite Conversation, etc.,* ed. by Herbert Davis and Louis Landa (Oxford, England: Basil Blackwell & Mott, 1957), 252.

p. 221   "We are what . . ." *Source:* Donald Curtis, as quoted by Anthony Robbins, *Awaken the Giant Within* (New York: Fireside, Simon & Schuster, 1991), 274.

p. 235   "No endeavor that . . ." *Source:* Edward Teller, *The Pursuit of Simplicity* (Malibu, CA: Pepperdine University Press, 1981), 152.

p. 238   "If we don't . . ." *Source:* Chinese proverb

p. 259   "I find the . . ." *Source:* Oliver Wendell Holmes, Sr., *The Autocrat of the Breakfast-Table* (New York: E.P. Dutton, 1906), 88.

p. 290   "Life is a . . ." *Source:* Henry Ford.

p. 293   "A vision without . . ." *Source:* Author unknown, quoted by Jacob M. Braud.

p. 295   "The mightiest works . . ." *Source:* Walter Russel Bowie, in "The Power of Imagination" Reader's Digest, August 1952, from *On Being Alive* (New York: Scribner's, 1952), 132.

p. 299   "Whenever you see . . ." *Source:* Peter Drucker.

p. 306   "At our best . . ." *Source:* William L. Coleman, "Forget the Stats," *Knit Together* (Minneapolis, MN: Bethany House Publishers, 1987), 118.

p. 307   "Once someone said . . ." *Source:* Helen Lowrie Marshall, "Cause and Effect," *Dare to be Happy* (Garden City, NY: Doubleday and Company, 1962), 41. Every effort has been made to contact the estate and heirs of Helen Lowrie Marshall, without success, to obtain copyright permission.

p. 308   "I desire that . . ." *Source:* Henry David Thoreau, "Walden: Or, Life in the Woods," *Walden and Other Writings of Henry David Thoreau* (New York: The Modern Library, Random House, 1950), 64.

p. 310   "Celebration is to . . ." *Source:* Kent Schneider and Sister Adelaide Ortegel, *Light: Language of Celebration* (Chicago: The Center for Contemporary Celebration, 1973), 14.

p. 313   "Education is liberating!" *Source:* L. Pankratz and D. Pankratz, "Nursing Autonomy and Patients' Rights: Development of a Nursing Attitude Scale," *Journal of Health and Social Behavior,* Vol. 15, No. 3, p. 211.

p. 314   "There is a . . ." *Source:* Grace Hartigan, as quoted by Cindy Nemser, *Art Talk: Conversations with 12 Women Artists* (New York: Charles Scribner's Sons, 1975), 171.

p. 316   "A song we . . ." *Source:* Helen Lowrie Marshall, "The Song and the Echo," *Dare to be Happy* (Garden City, NY: Doubleday and Company, 1962), 64. Every effort has been made to contact the estate and heirs of Helen Lowrie Marshall, without success, to obtain copyright permission.

Index

A

Abilene Paradox, 53–54
Accountability
See also Councils
  benefits of, 138, 231
  when consulting, 203–204
  defined, 132
  fiscal improvement council, *261*
  of nurses, 295
  process to achieve, 230
  in professional practice model, 13
Acuity, 44, 163–164
  increasing, 2, 6, *83*, 157
Admission assessment tool, *49*
  See also Database, Job descriptions and
  Job description standards
Adult specialty care services, 85, 157, 169, *216*
  See also Medical-surgical
Advanced practice nurse, 12, 13, 134, *140*, 221–222
  See also Clinical nurse specialist
  council, 207
  definition, 188
  educator, 188, 192, *195*, 202
American Academy of Nursing, 3
American Hospital Association (AHA), 136
American Nurses Association (ANA), 3, 12, *105*, *114–128*, 158–159
American Organization of Nurse Executives (AONE), 3, 136
Ants, 74–75, 131

Applicant evaluation, 86–*87*
Application for membership, 88–*89*
Assignment, 43, 44, 143, 144–145, *150*, 155
Associate nurse
  as consultant, 189
  job description, 84, *94–96*, 144
  role, 43–44, 85, 86, 132–134
  standards, *114–118*
Attrition rate, 138, 222
Augustana College, 82
Authority, 221
Autonomy, 13, *56*, 70
  as benefit, 296–297

B

Beneficiary
  community as, 301, 303–304
  defined, 290
  nurse as, 296–298
  organization as, 299–300
  patient as, 294–295
  physician as, 298–299
Benefits
  See also Empowerment
  of differentiated practice, 82–83
  financial, *140–142*
  of Integrated Care, 136–139
  of shared governance, 300
Blocking decision, 47, 60–*61*
Business, 2, 48
  competence, 15
  literature, 50

Note: Page numbers in italics indicate entries found in figures, tables, exhibits, or appendices.

C

Carpe diem, 71–72
Case associate, *49, 50*
Case management, *55, 140*, 209, 234
  See also Clinical nurse specialist
  Center for, *55*
  goal of, 232
Case manager, *49, 50*, 83, 135, *147–149*
Case study
  adult accident victim, *155–156*
  advocating for mother and unborn
    child, *193*
  change is imminent (team manage-
    ment), *195–196*
  Chin Lei, *151–153*
  consultation through casual remark, *200*
  corporate, *55*
  creativity through reframing, *205*
  I wonder, *194*
  Janet, *155–156*
  premature infant, *146–149*
  reducing costs in hospice, *140*
  Sam, *146–149*
  Staffing/Scheduling Committee, *56–57*
  transcultural perinatal nursing, *151–153*
  value of consulting, *199*
Celebrate, 16
  contest, 312
  funeral, 311
  how to, 310–313
  manager, 309–310, 315
  need to, 306, 307
  with pin, *312*
  with recognition, 308, 309–310, 312–
    313
  reward, 309
Celebration
  definition, 306
  education as, 313–314
  rituals, 310–311
  timing, 314–315
  visitors, 317
Change
  adapting to, 25, 28–29, 42
  agent, *98, 101, 105*, 225

  behavior, 225, 309
  choice and, 28–29, 73
  context and, 14
  course, 226
  culture and, 22, 34, 38, 39
  formula, 41
  as norm, 28, 41, 230
  principles, 14–16
  resistance to, 38, 229
  risk taking and, 235
  successful, 255–256
  theory, 224–230
  time to, 316
Charge nurse, 84, 132, 157
Chart audit, 45, *49, 50*
Chart monitoring and evaluation tool, 45
Charter, 227, *229*
Chemotherapy, DRG 410, 256–*258, 272–*
  280
Chin Lei, *151–153*
Choice, 22, 39
  change and, 73
  commitment to, 74
  fundamental, 77–78, *79*
  gender and, 78–79
  making decisions and, 30, 46–47
  outcome and, 73–74, 80
  pitfalls in making, 80–81
  point, 73, 75, 77
  power and, 70–71, 74, 76, 79, 81
  primary, 78, *79*
  process, 75, 80
  secondary, 78, *79*
  shared governance and, 70, 79
Circles, 27–28, 243–*244*, 247
Clinical care coordinator
  job description, 84, *100–102*
  role, 44, 85, 86–87, 132–134, 157
  standards, *124–128*
Clinical enrichment program, *111, 194*
Clinical I and II, *8–9*, 86, *111*, 138
Clinical nurse specialist (CNS), 28, *55*, 85,
  134–135, 167
  accountabilities, 208
  communication, *106*, 190–*191*
  as enabler, 190, 192

fiscal impact, *140–142, 303*
fluidity, 190
group practice, 233
isolation, 207
job description, *105–107*, 208
visibility, 202
Clinical Pathway. *See* Integrated Clinical
  Pathway
Collaboration, 13, *26*, 198–199, 200, 243
  definition, 130
  examples of, *147, 151, 155*
  of health care team, 130–131, 132, 133,
    134, 138, 209–210, 234, 297, 298,
    300
  tool, 162, 230
Collegiality, 131–132
Colon resection, DRGs 148, 149, *165, 166,
  182–184*
Committee
  composition, *56–57*, 226
  differentiated practice steering, 48, *49,
    50*, 82–83
  ethics, *193*
  fiscal improvement, 260, *262*
  human resources advisory, 249
  Integrated Care, *43–45, 51*, 135
  liaison, 234, 246–247
  nursing career pathway, 83–84
  nursing diagnosis, 159
  staffing/scheduling, *56–57, 66–68*
  unit selection, 86–87
Communication, 14, 15, 25, 31, 33–37, 42,
  44, 145
  See also Job descriptions and Job
    description standards
  board, 144–145, *150*
  common language for, 206, 208, 229,
    261
  consultation and, 190, *196*, 202, 205,
    208
  empowerment and, 130, 251
  first party, 36–37, 50–53, 249, *250*
  information and, 249, 251–253
  mechanisms, 29, *83*, 131, *228*
  multidisciplinary, 130, 207–208, 234
  patterns, 229, 291

process of, 231, 243–247
reframing of, 48, 50
as responsibility, *56*, 60
skills, *26, 27*, 53, 190
tool, 153, 158–166, 249–*252*
Community, 18, 215, *220*
  as beneficiary, 301, 303–304
  macro-, 215–*216*, 225
  micro-, 215–*216*
  mini-, 215–*216*
  relationships, 231–232
Compensation
  definition, 290–291
  differing packages, 3
  monetary, 8–9, 50, 83, *111–113*, 298
  systems theory and, 291
Competence, 25–28, 85, 135, 190–*191*
  See also Skills
  defined, *27*, 239–*240*
Compromise, 58, 80
Computer, 50, 168–169
Conference, multidisciplinary, *147, 151,
  152*
Conflict, 12, 13, 50, 61–62, 80, 84
Confrontation, 12–13, 37, 51–52
Consensus, 24, 31, 34, 41, 73, 82
  blocking, 47, 60–*61*
  definition, 46
  gender and, 79
  pitfalls, 61–63
  time required for, 54, *55, 57*, 62, 84
Consultant, *57*
  capacities of, 134
  educational, *194*
  peer support of, 207
  visibility, 202, 209
Consultation, 13, *90, 107*, 133–134, 222
  common language, 197, 204, 206, 208
  definition, 134, 189
  empowerment and, 199–201, 203
  horizontal, 193–194, 197
  interdisciplinary, 197, 206
  power and, 204
  practice partnership model and, *196–*
    197
  process, 201–204

strategy to provide, 144–145, 155
theory-based, 204–206
vertical, 193–194, 197
Continuity, *106*
defined, 129
as goal, 73, *83*
Context, 23, *27*
Coronary artery bypass, DRG 106, 163,
167–168
Corporate, *55*
culture, 241–242
decisions, 30, 246–247
structure, 243–246
Costs
controlling, *155–156, 166, 168,* 208–
209, 254–255, 260–261, 295
differentiated practice, 82–83, 300
shared governance, 300
Council, 88
See also Shared governance
accountabilities of, 215, 227, *228*
action, 248–249, *265–271*
advanced practice, 207, 227
charter, 227, *229*
development, 24, 227
education/research, 215, 227, *228*
fiscal improvement, 260–*261*
management, *57*, 215, 227
management advisory, 253–254
membership, 88, 227, *228, 229,* 231,
248, 249
nursing congress, 227, 231
nursing executive, 227
practice, 215, 227, *229*
purpose, *229*
quality assurance/improvement, 45, 88,
91, 140, 215, 227
size, 227
unit, 30, 227–228, 231
Creativity, 15, *26,* 33, 38, 75, *209*
consensus and, 47
in practice partnership model, *196*
through reframing, *205*
Credentialing, 28, 88, *91,* 208
Critical care services, 5, 85, 154–157, *216*
Critical thinking, 12, 13, 15, 25, *26, 27,*
208

See also Job descriptions and Job
description standards
Culture, 85, 89
change and, 22, 34, 38, 39, 225
corporate, 22, 23, 241–242
defined, 23, 241
formation of, 23–24
formula, 41
organizational, 23, 39, 41, 224
Sioux Valley Hospital, 6, 7, 84, 259
study, 24–*26, 35, 36,* 37, 38–39
understanding, 22, 38

D

Data collection tool, *49*
Database, 141, *146, 151,* 160, *180–181*
See also Job description standards
perinatal, 153, *176–179*
Dead Poet's Society, 71–72
Decision
See also Blocking
based on, 10, *26,* 224
made by, 30–31, 131, 251–252
power and, 46–47
Decision making, 13, 24
See also Consensus
empowered, 190–192
in integrative model, 2
process, 54
Decision points
career, 84–86, 299
organizational, 82–84
personal, 81–82
del Bueno, Dorothy, 27, 76, 190
Delegation, *44, 49, 50, 83,* 132–133, 169
See also Job descriptions and Job
description standards
Demographics
of Sioux Valley Hospital, 218
of South Dakota, 4
Demonstration project. *See* South Dakota
Statewide Project for Nursing and
Nursing Education
Devil's advocate, 59
Diagnosis-related groups, 254, 255
DRG 106, *167–168*

DRG 148, *165–166*
DRG 149, *182–184*
DRG 410, 256–*258, 272–280*
Dialogue, 34
Dialysis, 228
Differentiated practice
    See also South Dakota Statewide
        Project for Nursing and Nursing
        Education
    benefits, 10, 82–83, 136–139
    choice and, 70–71, 73–74
    common language, 311
    concept, 3, 14
    conceptual model, 190–*191*
    costs, 82–83, 300
    definition, 3, 10, 135
    history, 3
    implementation, 228
    Maslow and, 306–307, 308
    outcomes, 136–138, *155–156*, 190, *191*,
        239–240, 299–300
    pin, *312*
    process, 190–*191*
    reasons for, 10, 135
    recommendations, *83*
    structure, 190–*191, 240*
Director of ___ care services. *See* Unit
    director
Discharge planning, 12, *26, 43–44*, 137,
    147–149, 164
Diversity, 16, 18, 25, 32–33, 222
Documentation, 23, *43, 44, 49, 83*, 137, 163
    See also Job description standards, Inte-
        grated Clinical Pathway, and Tool
DRG. *See* Diagnosis-related groups
Dwarfism, *151–153*

E

Eagle, 76, 309, 315
Ecology of Excellence, 32, 38, 130, 221,
    222
    action council, 248–249, *265–271*
    culture, 239, *240*
    definitions, 238–*240*
    performance, 239, *240*
    pulse, 248, 264

structure, 239, *240*
    Work Engineering, 248
Ecosystem, 238–239, *240*
Employee role, *95–96, 98–99, 101–102*
Empowerment, 198
    consultation and, 209–210
    as goal, 73
    by manager, *103*
    motivator, 298, 299
    of patients, 167–168, 232
    of staff, *56*, 130, 139, 194, 239, *240*,
        291–292
    through team-building, 32
Environment
    boundaries and, 190–*191, 223*
    business, 32
    external, 3–5
    internal, 5–10
    seamless, 197, 209
    supportive, 38, 210
Evaluation tool. *See* Tools and Financial
    analysis
Exceptions, 163, *185–187*, 257, 259
Exercise
    celebrate, 319
    celebration, 320
    consultative inventory, 212
    education versus experience, 18
    financial analysis, 172–173
    for groups, 64–65
    human pretzels, 212
    I am a camera, 212–213
    individual values/choices, 93
    organizational, 93
    organizational analysis, 236–237
    photographic, 212
    pulse, 264
    SWOT, 305
    values clarification, 236
Extroversion, 32, 51

F

Facilitator, 58, 62
    focus group, 24–*25*
    manager as, 192, 231
Factioning, 61–62

Factoring Tool, 44, 86
Factors
  differentiating, 12
  external, 218, *220*, 223, *292–293*
  integrating, *11*
  internal, 218, *220–222*, *291–292*
Failure, 38, 47, 74, 308
Feedback, 14, *220*
  defined, *217*
  system, 232–233
  verbal, 34, 53
Financial
  analysis exercise, 172–173
  benefits, *140–142*
  integration, 259–260
  management, 261, *285–287*
Fiscal
  improvement standards, *283–284*
  outcomes, *140–142*, 208–209, *260*,
    303
Flexibility, *26*, 202, 209
Forces
  driving, 78, 225
  restraining, 225
Formula
  change, 41
  cultural identification, 41
  implementing Integrated Care, 172
  professional growth, 42
Fragmentation, 2–3, 7, 13, 157, 167, 170

G

Gender, choice and, 78–79, 90
Goals, *90*, 138
  choice and, 73–74, 77, 78, 299
  of group, 47, 55, 62
  patient, *43*, *44*, *49*, *94*, *97*, *116*, 131,
    133–134, *205*
Governance, 9, *90*, 192, 233
  See also Shared governance
Grief, 77, 89
Growth, professional, 34, 38, 53, 202, 226
Ground rules, 33, *43–45*, 51
Group
  focus, *24–26*, *35*, 41, *195*
  process, 47–48

H

Harvard Business School study, 12, 14
Head nurse. *See* Unit director
Healing Web, The, 15, 82
Health care
  changing, 1, 2–3, 29, 293
  continuum, 10, *11*, 13, 301
  Financing Administration (HCFA),
    254–255, 257
  goal of, 217
Hierarchy, *26*, 31, 218, *219*
Home health care, 134, *147–149*, 153–154,
  216
Hospice, *140–142*, 208–209, *216*

I

ICU, 154–157
Information, *217–220*, 231, 249, 251–253
Input, *217–221*, *291–292*
Integrated Care, 14, 33, 157
  See also Committee and Differentiated
    practice
  benefits of, 136–139
  defined, 135
  guidelines, *43–45*
  process, 139–158, 317
  transformative, 190–*191*, 210
Integrated Clinical Pathway, 159, 162–
  168, 234, 254
  See also Job descriptions and Job
    description standards
  documentation, 162, 230
  DRG 149, *182–184*
  DRG 410, 256–257, *272–280*
  exceptions to, 163, *185–187*, 257, 259
  task force, *52*, 162
Integration, 10, 12, 14, 130, 136, *149*, 157,
  226, 229, 246
  defined, 13
  of financial data, 259–260
Intensive care unit, 154–157
Interface agreement, 131, 249–*252*
Interpersonal relations, 12, *27*
  See also Communication
Interviews, 24, 44, 86–87
Introversion, 51

J

Janet, *155–156*
Job descriptions, *94–107*
Joint Commission on Accreditation of
    Healthcare Organizations (JCAHO),
    140, 159, 224, 316–317
Jonah complex, 307
Jung, Carl, 32

K

Kardexes, 159, 164

L

Labor and delivery, 150–*153*
Leadership, *103*
    See also Management
    transformational, 192
Learning, 32
    curve, 203
    life-long, 12, 13, 42, 154
    principles of adult, 28, 44, 192
    whole brain, 34–*36*
Length of stay, 129, *165*, *167*, 255, 257,
    258, 259, 295, *303*
    continuity and, *83*, 294
    goal to reduce, 73, 162, 165
Licensed practical nurses (LPN), 6, 7, *49*,
    50
    history, 3
    opportunity for, 222
    in South Dakota, 4–5
Lifeline, *148*
Literature, 41, 48–50, *55*
    used for making decision, 10
Locus of control theory, 307

M

MAIN, 4, 12, 14, 84
Managed care, *55*, *83*, 164, 166, 295
Management
    androgynous, 243
    responsibilities, 14, 31, 207–208
    styles, 30, 31, *56*, *57*

Manager. *See* Unit director
Maslow, Abraham, 306–307, 308
Maternal-child health, 5, 85, 139, 141–153
    See also Women's and children's health
    care services
Mediator, 58, 62, 63
Medical-surgical, 5, 85
    See also Adult specialty care services
Member
    application for, *89*
    full practice, 88, *91*
    provisional, 88, *91*
Mentor, 34, 37, *90*, *100*, *101*, 226
    See also Preceptor
    unit director as, 31, 192, 231, 300, 309
Midwest Alliance in Nursing, 4, 12, 14, 84
Midwestern Health Services, interface
    agreement, *250*, *251*
Moving, 225, *226*, 227–229, 230
My Fair Lady, 53
Mythology
    Aphrodite, 74–75
    Pandora, 72
    Psyche, 74–75
    Pygmalion, 53
Myers-Briggs Type Indicator, 32, 38, *195*,
    222, 227, 308

N

NANDA, *43*, 159
National Commission on Nursing
    Implementation Project (NCNIP), 3
Negotiables, 48, *50*
Negotiation, 13, 15, 34, 37, 133
    See also Job descriptions and Job
    description standards
Neonatal intensive care unit (NICU), 84,
    141, 143–153
Newman, Margaret, 15, 135, 205
Nightingale, Florence, 135, 313
Noise, 14, 75–76
Nonnegotiables, 48, *49*
Norms, 48–53, 54, *57*, 58, 62, 64
    Integrated Care committee, *51*
    Integrated Clinical Pathway task force,
        52

staffing/scheduling committee, *66–68*
Norms keeper, 58
North American Nursing Diagnosis
  Association, *43*, 159
Nurse
  as beneficiary, 296–298
  executives' responsibilities, 1, 2
  expert, 3, 28, *140*, 196–197, 204, 296, 299
  novice, 28, *140*, 164, 196–197
  students, 139, 164, *194*
Nurses Notes, 312–313
Nurses' week, 313
Nursing
  See also Job descriptions and Job
    description standards
  administrator, 85, 129, *195*
  care plan, *43*, *49*, *94*, *115*, 160
  common language, 197, 204, 208, 229
  conceptual framework, 247
  congress, 227, 231
  cost-effective care, 39, *106*, 135, 164
  divisions, 88
  diagnosis, *43*, *49*, *83*, 133, 138, 141,
    159–160
  orders, *43*, *44*, *49*, *50*, *83*, 159
  organizational chart, *6, 7, 9, 244*
  philosophy, 199–200
  plan of care summary, 160–*161*
  practice, 10–12, 15, *261*
  residency, 28, 85, 88, 299
  satisfaction, 138
  strategic planning, *104*, 253
  teams, *144–145*, *146*, *150*
Nursing Speaks, *52*, 228

O

Opportunity, 34, 39, 47, 85
  professional, 10, 138, 202, 226, 296,
    309
Organization
  as beneficiary, 299–300
  open, 246
Organizational
  chart, *6*, *244*, *245*, 247
  model, 2

structure, *7*, *9*, 243
styles, 253
Orientation, 44, 135, 164
  See also Performance Based Develop-
    ment System and Residency
  feminine, 79
  to group, 47
  time, *191*
Orientee, 32, 44
Output, *217–218*, *220*, 230–232, *291–292*

P

Pandora, 72
Paradigm, 75, 76, 89
  changing, 15, 242, 255–256
  shift, 164, 169, 204–205, 259, 310
Paradox, 32, 39
Partners, business, 32
Partnership, *101*, 130
  multidisciplinary, 134
  practice, 193, *196–197*, 210
Patient
  as beneficiary, 294–295
  communication about, 130, 133–134
  cost-conscious, 232
  satisfaction, 137, 209, 294–295
Patient-focused care, 169–170, 197, 232
Pay scale, *8*
Pediatrics, 84, 141, 150
Peer review, 28, 31, 88–89, 91, 208
Performance Based Development System
  (PBDS), 27–28, 86–87, 89
Physician, *149*
  DRGs and, 255
  Integrated Clinical Pathways and, 163,
    164
  practice pattern, *43*, *44*
  relationships with, 9, 153, 297, 311
  satisfaction, 137, *155–156*, *174–175*,
    297
  subspecialization, 3, 5, 9, *156*
Porter-O'Grady, Tim, 76, 136, 214–215,
  221
Portfolio, 28, 88–*90*
  See also Job description standards

Postanesthesia care, *199*
Postpartum/normal newborn nursery, 141, *151*, 295, 301–*302*
Power, 12, 24
  celebration of, 310
  change and, 310
  choice and, 70, 76, 80–81
  decisions and, 31, 46–47
  knowledge and, 204, 314
  peace and, 310
  structure, 46–47, 48
Powerlessness, 70–*71*
Preceptor, 28, 32, 44, 87–88, *90*, *107*, 192
  incentive plan, 87–88, *111–113*
Primary nurse, 30
  as consultant, 134, 189, *199*
  job description, 84, *97–99*
  as patient advocate, 189, 295
  role, *43–44*, 85, 86, 132–134, 142–143, 172, 294
  screening, *43*, *143*, 155
  selection, 86–87
  standards, *119–123*
Primm, Peggy, 4, 14, 86, 221, 314
Privileges, 88–*89*, *91*
Process watcher, 59
Profession, characteristics of, *215*
Psyche, 74–77
Pulmonary/Renal, *199*
Pygmalion, 53

Q

Quality of care, 29
Questionnaire
  patient, 137
  physician, 137, *174–175*

R

Ratio, of roles, 44, *49*, 142
Recorder, 58
Referrals, *98*, *100*, 143, 150
  consultation, 172, 203, 209
  discharge, 172, 301–*302*
Refreezing, 225, *226*, 229–230

Registered nurse. *See* Primary nurse, Associate nurse, and Clinical care coordinator
Rehabilitation, *216*
Research, 2, 24, 41, 42, 82
  See also Job descriptions and Job description standards
  Harvard, 15
  Healing Web, The, 15
  interface agreement and, *252*
  used for making decisions, 10, 54
Residency, nursing, 28, 85, 88, 299
Resources, 135, *140*, 194
  See also Job descriptions and Job description standards
Responsibility, 30, 48, *56*, 83, 207–208
  See also Job descriptions and Job description standards
  of group members, 59, 60
  for outcomes, 255–256
Retention, 39
Rewards, 39, 87
Risk taking, 25, 37–38, 64, 82–83
Role
  ambiguity, 206–209
  blurring, 131–132
  designing, 39, 132
  differentiating, 9, 12, 132–133, 190–*191*
  employee, *95–96*, *98–99*, *101–102*, 298
  expectations, 53, 132–133, 144, 208, 296
  preference, 32, 308
  ratio for each, 44, *49*, 142
  socialization, 207
  supervisor, 5, 84, 134, 157, 300
  unit individualization of, 33, 297
Role Choice Tool, 44, 86, *108–110*
Role Introduction Tool, 44, 45

S

Salient factors, 202
Sam, *146–149*
Satisfaction
  customer, *155–156*, 239, *240*, 300

nurse, 138, 299
patient, 137, 209, 300
physician, 137, 155, 300
School of Nursing, 218
Screening, *43–44, 143*, 155
Seize the day, 71–73
Selection process, 86–87
Self-esteem, 34, 138, 197, 207
Self-examination, 72
Self-scheduling, *56–57*, 85–86, *194*, 231
Shared governance, 10, 13, 24, *26*
    See also Councils
    choice and, 70, 79
    costs, 300
    decision making and, 30
    defined, 214
    models, 214–215
    organizational, 234
Sioux Falls, South Dakota, 4
Skills
    See also Communication, Job descrip-
        tions and Job description standards
    critical thinking, 12, 13, 15, 25, *26, 27*
    interpersonal, 12, 15, *27*
    technical, 15, *27*, 142–143
South Dakota Statewide Project for
    Nursing and Nursing Education, 48, *49,
    50, 57*, 137, 138
    celebration of, 308–309, 311, 312–313
    description, 4–5, 83, 86, 141, 300
    pin, *312*
    rationale for participation in, 82
    units, 5, 141–142, 143, 153–154, 307–
        308
Space, 12–13, 76
Standards
    of care, *106*, 158–159, 164
    continuous fiscal improvement, *283–
        284*
    job description, *114–128*
    of practice, 158
State board, 15, 159, *194*
Steiner, Frank, 238, 241, 248, 316
Strengths, weaknesses, opportunities,
    threats (SWOT), 34, 138, 238, 240, 241,
    255, 305

Structure
    linear, 243–*245*
    nursing department organizational, *6, 7,
        9*
    power within organization, 48
    role and, 190–*191*
Summer E, *111, 194*
Supervisor role, 5, 84, 134, 157, 300
Surgical, *216*
Symbols, 23–24, 202
    See also Mythology
    burial, 256, 311
    circles, *27*–28, 243–*244*, 247
    pin, *312*
Synergy, 10, 18, 201
System
    closed, 218, 246
    hierarchical, 48, 79, 218, *219*, 246
    linear, 247
    open, 218, 246, 247
    value, 77
Systems theory, *217*–224, *226*
    compensation and, 291–293

T

Task force
    Integrated Clinical Pathway, *52*, 162
    multidisciplinary, 129, 131
Teaching, 32, *95, 98, 100*, 143, *146*, 165
Team
    See also Consultation
    building, 32, 38
    interdisciplinary, 197, 201, 210
    management, *195–196*
    nursing, *144–145, 146, 150*
    types of members, 12, 32–33, 222
Teamwork, *26*, 32, 44, 138
Technical, 15, *27*, 142–143
Theory
    change, 224–230
    locus of control, 307
    of self-fulfilling prophecy, 307
    systems, *217*–224, *226*
Three-day week, 6–7, *83*
Throughput, *217*–218, *220*, 291–*292*